# Acute Nephrology for the Critical Care Physician

Heleen M. Oudemans-van Straaten
Lui G. Forni • A.B. Johan Groeneveld
Sean M. Bagshaw • Michael Joannidis
Editors

# Acute Nephrology for the Critical Care Physician

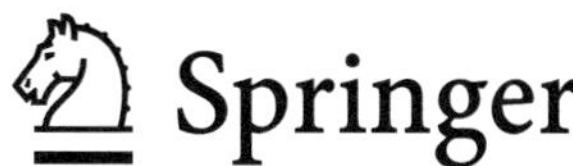 Springer

*Editors*
Heleen M. Oudemans-van Straaten
Department of Intensive Care
VU University Hospital
Amsterdam
The Netherlands

Lui G. Forni
Department of Intensive Care Medicine
Royal Surrey County Hospital NHS
Foundation Trust, Surrey Perioperative
Anaesthesia Critical Care Collaborative
Research Group (SPACeR) and Faculty of
Health Care Sciences
University of Surrey
Guildford
UK

A.B. Johan Groeneveld
Department of Intensive Care
Erasmus Medical Center
Rotterdam
The Netherlands

Sean M. Bagshaw
Department of Critical Care Medicine
Faculty of Medicine and Dentistry
University of Alberta
Edmonton
Alberta
Canada

Michael Joannidis
Division of Intensive Care
and Emergency Medicine
Department of General Internal Medicine
Medical University Innsbruck
Anichstrasse
Innsbruck
Austria

ISBN 978-3-319-17388-7      ISBN 978-3-319-17389-4    (eBook)
DOI 10.1007/978-3-319-17389-4

Library of Congress Control Number: 2015942522

Springer Cham Heidelberg New York Dordrecht London


Springer International Publishing AG Switzerland is part of Springer Science+Business Media
(www.springer.com)

# Preface

This book offers a comprehensive overview of acute nephrology-related problems as encountered by the critical care physician and provides practical commonsense guidance for the management of these challenging cases. In the intensive care unit, acute kidney injury generally occurs as part of multiple organ failure due to septic or cardiogenic shock, systemic inflammation, or following a major surgery. Once the damage is done, acute kidney injury increases the risk of long-term morbidity and mortality. Awareness of its development is therefore crucial. Intensivists have a central role in the field of critical care nephrology since they provide the bridge to consultation with the nephrologist. The critical care physician is primarily responsible for the prevention of AKI, for optimal protection of the kidneys during critical illness, and for its management. Therefore, early recognition and discrimination of the contributing factors are crucial skills, as is decision making regarding the prescription and delivery of high-quality renal replacement therapy. Although the latter is often performed in close collaboration with the nephrologist, the intensivist has the integrated knowledge of and the global responsibility for the patient and therefore can not delegate this role to the nephrologist. The critical care physician navigates the interaction of acute kidney impairment and its management with other failing organs and vice versa – the consequences of other organ failure on the development, treatment, and prognosis of the acute kidney injury. This book represents a comprehensive state-of-the-art overview of critical care nephrology and supplies the knowledge needed to manage the complexity of daily acute nephrology care.

The book has been written by a worldwide panel of experts in the field of acute nephrology from Europe, Canada, the United States, and Australia. It has four parts. The first part deals with acute kidney injury, its epidemiology and outcome, pathophysiology, associated acid-base disturbances, and the complex interaction between the kidney and other organs. Special consideration is given to the rare but devastating condition of acute kidney injury in pregnancy. The second part of the book is assigned to the diagnostic work-up in a patient with acute kidney injury, including the classical work-up, the potential use of biomarkers, and special imaging techniques. The third part discusses measures to be taken to prevent acute kidney injury, including optimization of renal perfusion and the protection of the kidney against endogenous or exogenous toxins. The fourth part offers an overview of the prescription and delivery of acute renal replacement therapy. Considerations on when to start and which dose to prescribe are given, and the pros and cons of hemodialysis, hemofiltration, and continuous and intermittent treatments are discussed. Furthermore, maintaining filter patency and managing the risk of clotting and bleeding in the critically ill patients can be a struggle. The choice of anticoagulation and its consequences are highlighted which is of practical clinical relevance. Renal replacement therapy offers a primitive replacement of the kidneys' excretory function. The metabolic sequelae of renal replacement therapy on acid-base and electrolyte balance are discussed, as are considerations on nutrition and micronutrients. Correct drug dosing during renal replacement therapy is a challenge, but is crucial and may be lifesaving. The altered pharmacokinetics and pharmacodynamics during acute kidney injury and critical illness are explained. Special emphasis has been given to the role of continuous hemofiltration in sepsis, its use as blood purification for intoxications, along with the principles of provision of pediatric CRRT. The final chapter discusses the operational and nursing aspects of continuous renal replacement therapy.

We are grateful to all contributors for the free and enthusiastic sharing of their knowledge and clinical experience with our readers and thank the editorial team of Springer for their professional editing. We especially hope that this book will increase the understanding and know-how of critical care physicians regarding the diagnosis, treatment, and consequences of acute kidney injury in intensive care and hope that it will arouse their interest in the kidney during critical illness. Finally we hope that this will be translated into better outcomes for all our patients.

Amsterdam, The Netherlands                     Heleen M. Oudemans-van Straaten
Edmonton, AB, Canada                                          Sean M. Bagshaw
Leuven, Belgium                                                     Lui G. Forni
Rotterdam, The Netherlands                           A.B. Johan Groeneveld
Innsbruck, Austria                                             Michael Joannidis

# Contents

**Part III  Prevention and Protection**



**Part IV  Renal Replacement Therapy**

# Part I

# Acute Kidney Injury

# AKI: Definitions and Clinical Context

1

Zaccaria Ricci and Claudio Ronco

## 1.1 Acute Kidney Injury

Acute kidney injury (AKI) is a clinical syndrome representing a sudden decline of renal function leading to the decrease of glomerular filtration rate (GFR) [1]. This "conceptual" definition has been utilized for many years in place of a more precise and universally accepted classification: Currently, objective parameters such as urine output and creatinine levels have been included into the so-called KDIGO (Kidney Disease: Improving Global Outcomes) definition [2, 3]. This recent innovation into clinical practice of AKI is improving uncertainties in epidemiology and clinical management. However, still the literature reports that AKI incidence and mortality varies widely (incidence ranges 1–31 % and mortality ranges 28–82 %) [4]. All this depends on the fact that often patients with different characteristics and severity of renal dysfunction are included in the analyses. Furthermore, it has been reported that AKI aetiology and patient clinical condition strongly affect outcome, moving mortality rate from 20 % of the cases with isolated AKI with minimal or absent comorbidities to 80 % in case of AKI associated with severe sepsis or septic shock [5]. Hence, in the description and evaluation of AKI in the clinical context, it becomes very important to diagnose this pathology with a consensus definition, to exactly identify the aetiology and to define the presence of comorbidities often characterizing the susceptibility of the patient to develop the syndrome.

Z. Ricci, MD (✉)
Department of Pediatric Cardiac Intensive Care Unit,
Bambino Gesù Children's Hospital, IRCCS, Piazza S. Onofrio 4, Rome 00165, Italy
e-mail: z.ricci@libero.it

C. Ronco, MD
Department of Nephrology, Dialysis and Transplantation, S. Bortolo Hospital,
Viale Rodolfi, Vicenza 36100, Italy

International Renal Research Institute, Vicenza, Italy
e-mail: cronco@goldnet.it

© Springer International Publishing 2015
H.M. Oudemans-van Straaten et al. (eds.), *Acute Nephrology for the Critical Care Physician*, DOI 10.1007/978-3-319-17389-4_1

### 1.1.1   AKI Definitions

As previously described, a series of definitions have been used in the literature to describe AKI. It might be useful to critically reappraise some of them and to abandon others.

*Acute Tubular Necrosis (ATN):*
This term was used for many years as a surrogate for severe anuric renal dysfunction, based on histopathological findings in animal models of ischaemia-reperfusion. However, in humans, this anatomic-pathological picture rarely occurs [6].

*Acute Renal Failure (ARF):*
Originally referred to describe the effects of the crush syndrome on the victims of London bombing during World War II, the term ARF describes a syndrome characterized by sudden oliguria and rapid decrease of glomerular filtration leading to hyperkalemia and uremic intoxication. A precise biochemical definition was never proposed and the term was generally utilized to describe a syndrome with different causes and disparate levels of severity. Today, this term should be abandoned in favour of AKI [7].

*Acute Kidney Injury (AKI):*
This term was implemented and started to be widely used approximately 12 years ago after the second ADQI conference held in Vicenza, Italy, in 2002 [8]. This is the most recent term indicating an abrupt and persistent reduction of kidney function and accepting the paradigm that causes of injury may be disparate and the level of damage may be variable from negligible to severe. During that conference, the term ARF was substituted with AKI and the new RIFLE criteria (RIFLE stays for Risk, Injury, Failure, Loss and End stage kidney disease) were created, using a biochemical syntax to grade severity based on fall in GFR or urine output [8]. Subsequently, this was modified by AKIN (Acute Kidney Injury Network) that introduced three stages as a measure of severity based on creatinine and urine output values [9]. Those criteria were finally resumed into the KDIGO classification [2, 3] that recently reconciled RIFLE and AKIN into a unique final common definition (Table 1.1).

**Table 1.1**  KDIGO classification

| Stage | Serum creatinine | Urine output |
|---|---|---|
| 1 | 1.5–1.9 times baseline<br>OR<br>$\geq$0.3 mg/dl ($\geq$26.5 mmol/l) increase | <0.5 ml/kg/h for 6–12 h |
| 2 | 2.0–2.9 times baseline | <0.5 ml/kg/h for $\geq$12 h |
| 3 | 3.0 times baseline<br>OR<br>Increase in serum creatinine to $\geq$4.0 mg/dl ($\geq$353.6 mmol/l)<br>OR<br>Initiation of renal replacement therapy<br>OR<br>In patients <18 years, decrease in eGFR to <35 ml/min per 1.73 m$^2$ | <0.3 ml/kg/h for $\geq$24 h<br>OR<br>Anuria for $\geq$12 h |

Modified from [10]

*Kidney attack*:

This term was coined in order to highlight the analogy of the characteristics of the acute injury occurring to the kidney with that of acute coronary syndrome [11]: An insult to these organs (regardless of its nature) causes outcomes that are directly dependent on the intensity of damage and on the time spent before therapy is started. Different from heart attack, where chest pain and EKG abnormalities are fundamental symptoms for early diagnosis, the kidney is a silent organ and clinical evidence for this disorder is scanty, nevertheless a kidney attack may be of enormous importance both for short-term clinical outcomes, and for long-term kidney function. Accurate monitoring for diagnostic criteria for AKI coupled with utilization of novel early biomarkers may frame the syndrome of AKI similar to that of heart attack (see below).

*Subclinical AKI and Renal Angina*:

Emerging evidence suggests that 15–20 % of patients who do not fulfil current serum-creatinine-based or urine output consensus criteria for AKI are nevertheless likely to have acute tubular damage, which is associated with adverse outcomes [12, 13]. In other words, subclinical AKI is diagnosed when renal damage and dysfunction does not reach a threshold sufficient to make serum creatinine rise above 0.3 mg/dl in 48 h or when oliguria is rapidly reversed before the 6 h timeframe. However, such level of renal damage/dysfunction becomes evident only after the structure and function of nephrons that are part of the so-called renal functional reserve are affected. Patients may have up to 50 % of the renal mass compromised before creatinine rises. Thus, other criteria should be included in the diagnosis of AKI such as biomarkers or minimal increases of serum creatinine. In the last case, we may identify a condition defined "renal angina" (RA). Since, different from chest angina, there is no kidney pain, we need to use a composite framework of symptoms, signs and biomarkers to identify this population at risk (Table 1.2). Using patient demographic factors and early signs of injury, RA aims to delineate patients at risk for subsequent severe AKI (AKI beyond the period of functional injury) versus those at low risk. While the concept of RA is an intriguing and logical proposal, it has been validated with the interesting RA index in only one paediatric study [15]. It has been recently demonstrated that in these patients the prognosis is poor [12, 13] and the level of complications such as evolution towards severe AKI, need of dialysis and death is somehow similar to those who have AKI according to KDIGO criteria. This conceptual framework allows defining AKI as a family of syndromes where dysfunction and damage may coexist or represent separate independent entities.

*CRIAKI and NCRIAKI*:

The question may arise if subclinical AKI is an actual clinical condition or it represents a risk condition for developing creatinine positive AKI. Continuing the cardiorenal parallelism, creatinine can be used as the cardiologists use electrocardiogram (EKG) to diagnose myocardial infarction (MI). The typical distinction of "STEMI" (S-T elevation MI) and "NSTEMI" (Non S-T elevation MI) based on EKG could be paralleled by a distinction based on serum creatinine between "CRIAKI" (creatinine increase AKI) and "NCRIAKI" (Non creatinine increase AKI) [16]. As for NSTEMI biomarkers such as troponin are used to rule out MI in case of chest pain, in case of NCRIAKI (or subclinical AKI) biomarkers of tubular damage can be used to rule out

**Table 1.2** The renal angina index (RAI) score is composed by the hazard (or risk) component times renal clinical signs

| Hazard Trance | | | Renal injury | | |
| --- | --- | --- | --- | --- | --- |
| Level | Evaluation | Score | Clinical risk on creatinine | Clinical risk on urine output | Score |
| Very high | Inotropes + mechanical ventilation or septic shock | 5 | No change | No change | 1 |
| High | After cardiac surgery: Thakar score >5; after general surgery: Michigan classes III through V; general ICU: High-risk patients according to Ref [14] | 3 | Increase 0.1 mg/dl over baseline | One hour of oliguria in a appropriately resuscitated subject | 2 |
| Moderate | After cardiac surgery: Thakar score >3; after general surgery: Michigan class II; general ICU: low-risk patients according to Ref [14] | 1 | Increase 0.3 mg/dl over baseline | Three hours of oliguria in a appropriately resuscitated subject | 4 |
| – | – | – | Increase 0.4 mg/dl over baseline | Five hours of oliguria in a appropriately resuscitated subject | 8 |

Modified from Basu et al. [15]
Risk strata are essentially the epidemiologic risk of critically ill adult population: 5 (very high risk), 3 (high risk) and 1 (moderate risk). Clinical signs of injury are based on changes in creatinine and urine output. The composite range of the RAI is therefore: 1, 2, 3, 4, 5, 6, 8, 10, 12, 20, 24 and 40

renal parenchymal damage following an exposure or other risk conditions. The bottom line is that every insult that damages even a limited number of nephrons represents in an episode of kidney attack and it is ultimately an AKI episode. Since the characterization of clinical or subclinical AKI is only dependent on the level of damage and the remnant renal functional reserve, we can no longer dismiss an episode of subclinical AKI as marginal or negligible. Subsequent kidney attacks may reduce the renal functional reserve leading to a point in which every insult will become clinically evident and full recovery cannot be guaranteed [17]. This represents a condition in which fibrosis and sclerosis may become self-sustaining leading to chronic kidney disease (CKD) progression and ultimately end stage kidney failure.

## 1.2 Comorbidities and the Risk of AKI

Apart from AKI definitions and its different grades of severity and clinical hues, it is clear that the syndrome of acute renal dysfunction must be seen in the broader context of the complex clinical picture of the critically ill patient. Critical illness *per se* puts patients at risk of renal damage. The entire clinical history of AKI is based on the combination of two main factors: susceptibility to damage and exposures to specific insults.

## 1.2.1 Susceptibility

The chances of developing AKI after exposure to one or more insults depend on a number of susceptibility factors that vary widely from individual to individual: Recent KDIGO guidelines clearly described the importance of interaction between exposures and susceptibility in the final development of the AKI syndrome [2, 3, 10]. Dehydration or volume depletion, advanced age, female gender, black race, presence of chronic diseases (kidney, heart, lung, liver), diabetes mellitus, cancer, anaemia and poly-transfusion, obesity or cachexia all represent conditions identified as general susceptibility to AKI [10].

Besides these general susceptibility conditions, the presence of a pre-existing kidney disease represents an important factor significantly increasing the risk of developing AKI after an insult. As already remarked before, baseline GFR does not necessarily tell the full story about the anatomical and functional conditions of the kidney because a normal baseline GFR or serum creatinine level can be present despite significant reduction of the functional renal mass [17]. This is due to a remarkable renal functional reserve present in intact kidneys. A patient with intact renal functional reserve may tolerate repeated kidney attacks simply loosing part of the reserve and without clinical evidence of the significant damage. An individual with normal baseline GFR could potentially be at increased risk of AKI due to a loss of reserve. Furthermore, when an episode of AKI is resolved and renal function recovery appears complete by measurement of GFR, this does not necessarily mean that a full restoration of renal mass and reserve has also occurred. Interestingly, the lower the remnant kidney mass, the higher will be the susceptibility to further insults and the higher will be the stress imposed to residual nephrons, resulting in hyperfiltration, sclerosis and progressive kidney disease.

Susceptibility factors are not currently clearly defined and their identification depends on many observational studies on different clinical settings [18]. As a matter of fact, however, such factors represent an insult that may be tolerated by some patients whereas may result in mild to severe AKI in others. For this reason, a careful medical history collection and evaluation should be an indispensable part of the process of risk assessment and AKI diagnosis.

KDIGO recommends to keep monitoring high-risk patients until the risk has subsided [10]. Exact intervals for checking serum creatinine and for which individuals' urine output should be monitored remain matters of clinical judgment; however, as a general rule, high-risk in patients should have serum creatinine measured at least daily and more frequently after an exposure. The same should be true for tight urine output monitoring.

## 1.2.2 Exposures

AKI is a multifactorial syndrome and in most cases one or more exposures can be accounted in its pathogenesis. Haemorrhage, circulatory shock, sepsis, critical illness with one or more organ acutely involved, burns, trauma, cardiac surgery (especially with cardiopulmonary bypass circulation), major non-cardiac surgery, nephrotoxic drugs, radiocontrast agents, poisonous plants and animals all represent possible exposures leading to AKI [10]. The clinical evaluation of exposures in the pathogenesis of AKI includes a careful history and thorough physical examination. Among the most important and preventable exposures, we must consider iatrogenic disorders [19, 20]. In several clinical conditions, drugs required to treat diabetes, oncological diseases, infections, heart failure or fluid overload may affect the delicate balance of a susceptible kidney leading to an acute worsening of organ function. Metformin, normally eliminated by the liver and the kidney, may accumulate if CKD pre-exists, inducing lactic acidosis and AKI. Chemotherapic agents used in solid tumour treatments may induce a tumour lysis syndrome with a sudden increase in circulating uric acid levels potentially toxic for the tubule-interstitial component of the renal parenchyma. Antibiotics may certainly result toxic to the kidney causing interstitial nephritis and tubular dysfunction and contribute to progressive renal insufficiency. The same effect can be induced by contrast media, especially if hyperosmolar dye is utilized for imaging techniques. In all these conditions, a cell cycle arrest may be induced with important tubular-glomerular feedback and a negative impact on glomerular hemodynamics [21]. Patients may already be undergoing treatment with aldosterone blockers or ACE inhibitors or angiotensin receptor blockers (ARB). In such circumstances, the original compensatory mechanism in the kidney is blunted or altered. The maintenance of aldosterone blockers when GFR is reduced below 60 ml/min may lead to secondary hyperkalemia and severe disturbances of the cardiac rhythm. Suspension of ACE inhibitors or ARB may produce an apparent improvement of kidney function due to a blockage of the efferent arteriolar vasodilatation [22]. On the contrary, the use of non-steroidal anti-inflammatory drugs in these conditions may exactly induce the opposite effect [23]. Loop diuretics are another family of medications frequently called into question as far as kidney damage is concerned. Diuretics are a double-sided treatment since they may resolve congestion on one side, but they may worsen renal perfusion and arterial underfilling on the other [24]. Furthermore, it is possible that chronic administration of high-dose loop diuretics may induce drug resistance secondary to substantial histological modifications of Henle loop and decrease of renal function [25].

### 1.2.3 AKI Risk Assessment

In the management of critically ill patients, it is becoming clearer and clearer that the assessment of whether a patient has already suffered a loss of glomerular excretory function would be a precious information for diagnostic, therapeutic and prognostic purposes. Most (if not all) patients at risk of an imminent acute loss of filtration function are asymptomatic, and various biochemical and imaging (i.e. ultrasound) tests are often of limited use early in the course of renal injury. The quality of decision-making also depends on the clinical experience of the physician;

experienced individuals will perform better at interpreting contradictory lines of evidence. Nonetheless, despite the general recognition that AKI is a prognosis-determining disease of epidemic prevalence, all attempts to prevent and treat it in clinical practice have so far failed. Reasons for this failure could include an incomplete understanding of the pathophysiology of AKI, but also the fact that diagnosis of AKI has relied upon detecting impairment of kidney function. Currently available therapeutic measures are only initiated once glomerular function has already declined, when irreversible organ damage might already be present. So far, a practicable alternative parameter for assessing renal function in real time in an unselected population of patients is not currently available. Several scoring systems (such as the Thakar score [26] or the SHARF [27]) have been suggested to quantify the severity of AKI or predict the need for renal replacement therapy (RRT); however, these scores are poorly calibrated, not reproducible in other centres, and tend to underestimate the actual need for RRT.

A body of evidence from experimental and clinical studies has now established a plausible biological role for biomarkers of tubular damage, and presented proof of the concept that such markers might be able to predict AKI [28]. In our view, these novel biomarkers will be crucial in enabling the presence of AKI to be detected even in the absence of other signs and symptoms. In addition to facilitating early diagnosis of AKI, these biomarkers could also describe the severity of this illness [29]. A number of biomarkers of functional change and cellular damage are under evaluation for early diagnosis of AKI, risk assessment for AKI, and prognosis of AKI. Recent work suggests in particular that the prognostic utility of newer plasma and urinary biomarkers, including neutrophil gelatinase-associated lipocalin, kidney injury molecule-1 and IL-18 is significantly higher over clinical assessment alone [10].

In these circumstances, some structural biomarkers may be identified: Such molecules contribute to making an earlier diagnosis of established and evolving AKI and potentially resulting in preventive strategies and/or earlier changes in management such as stopping harmful interventions or mitigating/avoiding current or planned exposures and insults [30]. Structural biomarkers are the mirror of a process occurring in the kidney tissue, and thus they can help to make an accurate differential diagnosis of AKI directing appropriate therapy of AKI (pre-renal vs renal). More accurate risk assessment and prediction of severity provided by these biomarkers could help prognostic stratification of AKI (serial staging of AKI and evolution of the syndrome) with possible directions for management and therapeutic strategies. In a recent paper by Kashani and colleagues [31], the urine concentration of two novel markers – insulin-like growth factor-binding protein 7 [IGFBP7] and tissue inhibitor of metalloproteinases-2 [TIMP-2] was found to be increased in a large cohort of critically ill patients developing AKI. The authors also compared them with known markers of AKI such as NGAL and KIM1. Not only the combined use of these two markers performed better than other known markers, but also their performance allowed prediction of AKI within 12 h with an area under the curve of about 0.8. [TIMP-2] [IGFBP7] significantly improved AKI risk prediction when added into a complex nine-parameter clinical model, including both susceptibilities and exposures of AKI (Age, Serum Creatinine, APACHE III Score, Hypertension, Nephrotoxic drugs, Liver Disease, Sepsis, Diabetes, Chronic Kidney Disease). An intriguing implication of this study is that they are considered to be markers of cell cycle arrest: It is believed that this prevents cells from dividing when the DNA may be damaged and arrests the process of cell division until the damage can be repaired. Interestingly, IGFBP7 is superior to TIMP-2 in surgical patients while TIMP-2 is best in sepsis-induced AKI: A combined marker like this may result (and eventually be further developed in the next years) as a sort of panel of markers identifying various aetiologies of AKI. These two biomarkers, for example, probably predict AKI so effectively because they are involved in slightly different renal damage pathways.

Detecting this alarm at specific time points (i.e. ICU admission) will permit appropriate triage of patients, more intensive monitoring, and perhaps early involvement from specialists in nephrology and critical care. Finally, as new therapies for AKI are being evaluated in the next few years, the use of biomarkers to help select which patients should be enrolled in trials will be an enormous advantage over current study design and planning.

## Conclusion

Although AKI is extremely common with an incidence of about 2,100 per million people, the condition remains difficult to identify and several forms of AKI can be currently described. Indeed, early mortality associated with AKI is still unacceptable, particularly when patients undergo available supportive therapy such as dialysis or hemofiltration. A number of susceptibilities and exposures for AKI have been clearly identified but there is no reliable way for a clinician to use this information to establish a clear risk profile. The concept of renal angina and subclinical AKI have been proposed; both likely describe kidney damage and small changes in renal function occurring in patients already deemed to be at high risk. For all these reasons, the KDIGO guidelines for AKI diagnosis introduced the concept of evaluating critically ill patients at risk for renal dysfunction and only including those with frank disease. In the future, the concept of subclinical AKI will probably be incorporated to better define the spectrum of this syndrome.

If patients could only tell us that their kidneys hurt, then front-line clinicians could stratify AKI "at risk" patients at a time when interventions (such as stopping nephrotoxins) are feasible and most likely to be effective. The promise of the next years will be essentially relying on novel early biomarkers of renal function change and, interestingly, of renal structural change that reliably predict the risk of future overt AKI. These novel early biomarkers, with the integration of clinical risk profiles of patients, will hopefully provide an effective tool for the prevention and eventual modification of AKI in "at risk" patients.

**Key Messages**

- Acute kidney injury (AKI) is currently the most commonly used term to define sudden worsening of kidney function in hospitalized patients.
- AKI implies the concept that renal damage is a continuum with a broad range from mild to severe forms.
- AKI is a clinical syndrome with several different aetiologies, pathophysiologic mechanisms and prognostic features: It is likely, even if currently not described, that different AKIs will require different treatments.
- Definition and (early) diagnosis of AKI is currently the focus of most intense research.
- As a matter of fact, the AKI syndrome as we know is a consequence of multiple (cumulative) insults in susceptible patients as well as single hits of highly nephrotoxic entity: We are currently aware that the amount of time over these insults occurs is unknown and that their clinical expression is almost silent.
- The identification of the risk of AKI is probably more important than the definition and diagnosis of AKI itself.
- The hope of the next decade relies on novel biomarkers and the possibility of being informed on silent hits occurring to the kidneys allowing the operators to act before frank AKI developed.

# References


1. Bellomo R, Kellum JA, Ronco C. Acute kidney injury. Lancet. 2012;380:756–66.
2. Kellum JA, Lameire N; for the KDIGO AKI Guideline Work Group. Diagnosis, evaluation, and management of acute kidney injury: a KDIGO summary (Part 1). Crit Care. 2013; 17:204.
3. Lameire N, Kellum JA; for the KDIGO AKI Guideline Work Group. Contrast-induced acute kidney injury and renal support for acute kidney injury: a KDIGO summary (Part 2). Crit Care. 2013;17:205.
4. Ali T, Khan I, Simpson W, et al. Incidence and outcomes in acute kidney injury: a comprehensive population-based study. J Am Soc Nephrol. 2007;18:1292–8.
5. McCullough PA, Shaw AD, Haase M, Bouchard J, Waikar SS, Siew ED, Murray PT, Mehta RL, Ronco C. Diagnosis of acute kidney injury using functional and injury bio- markers: workgroup statements from the tenth Acute Dialysis Quality Initiative Consensus Conference. Contrib Nephrol. 2013;182:13–29. Basel, Karger.
6. Prowle J, Bagshaw SM, Bellomo R. Renal blood flow, fractional excretion of sodium and acute kidney injury: time for a new paradigm? Curr Opin Crit Care. 2012;18(6):585–92.
7. Thadhani R, Pascual M, Bonventre JV. Acute renal failure. N Engl J Med. 1996;334(22):1448–60.
8. Bellomo R, Ronco C, Kellum JA, Mehta RL, Palevsky P, Acute Dialysis Quality Initiative workgroup. Acute renal failure – definition, outcome measures, animal models, fluid therapy and information technology needs: the Second International Consensus Conference of the Acute Dialysis Quality Initiative (ADQI) Group. Crit Care. 2004;8(4):R204–12.

9. Mehta RL, Kellum JA, Shah SV, Molitoris BA, Ronco C, Warnock DG, Levin A, Acute Kidney Injury Network. Acute Kidney Injury Network: report of an initiative to improve outcomes in acute kidney injury. Crit Care. 2007;11:R31.

10. Kidney disease: improving global outcomes (KDIGO) acute kidney injury work group. KDIGO clinical practice guideline for acute kidney injury. Kidney Int Suppl. 2012;2:1–138.

11. Kellum JA, Bellomo R, Ronco C. Kidney attack. JAMA. 2012;307:2265–6.

12. Uchino S, Bellomo R, Bagshaw SM, Goldsmith D. Transient azotaemia is associated with a high risk of death in hospitalized patients. Nephrol Dial Transplant. 2010;25(6):1833–9.

13. Haase M, Kellum JA, Ronco C. Subclinical AKI–an emerging syndrome with important consequences. Nat Rev Nephrol. 2012;8(12):735–9.

14. Malhotra R, Macedo E, Bouchard J, Wynn S, Mehta RL. Prediction of acute kidney injury (AKI) by risk factors classification [Abstract]. J Am Soc Nephrol. 2009;20:979A.

15. Basu RK, Zappitelli M, Brunner L, Wang Y, Wong HR, Chawla LS, Wheeler DS, Goldstein SL. Derivation and validation of the renal angina index to improve the prediction of acute kidney injury in critically ill children. Kidney Int. 2014;85:659–67.

16. Ronco C, McCullough PA, Chawla LS. Kidney attack versus heart attack: evolution of classification and diagnostic criteria. Lancet. 2013;382(9896):939–40.

17. Ronco C. Kidney attack: overdiagnosis of acute kidney injury or comprehensive definition of acute kidney syndromes? Blood Purif. 2013;36:65–8.

18. Rewa O, Bagshaw SM. Acute kidney injury-epidemiology, outcomes and economics. Nat Rev Nephrol. 2014;10(4):193–207.

19. Goldstein SL, Kirkendall E, Nguyen H, Schaffzin JK, Bucuvalas J, Bracke T, Seid M, Ashby M, Foertmeyer N, Brunner L, Lesko A, Barclay C, Lannon C, Muething S. Electronic health record identification of nephrotoxin exposure and associated acute kidney injury. Pediatrics. 2013;132:e756–67.

20. Ricci Z, Ronco C. New insights in acute kidney failure in the critically ill. Swiss Med Wkly. 2012;142:w13662.

21. Legrand M, Dupuis C, Simon C, Gayat E, Mateo J, Lukaszewicz AC, Payen D. Association between systemic hemodynamics and septic acute kidney injury in critically ill patients: a retrospective observational study. Crit Care. 2013;17:R278.

22. Coca SG, Garg AX, Swaminathan M, Garwood S, Hong K, Thiessen-Philbrook H, Passik C, Koyner JL, Parikh CR, TRIBE-AKI Consortium. Preoperative angiotensin-converting enzyme inhibitors and angiotensin receptor blocker use and acute kidney injury in patients undergoing cardiac surgery. Nephrol Dial Transplant. 2013;28:2787–99.

23. Lafrance JP, Miller DR. Selective and non-selective non-steroidal anti-inflammatory drugs and the risk of acute kidney injury. Pharmacoepidemiol Drug Saf. 2009;18:923–31.

24. Felker GM, Lee KL, Bull DA, Redfield MM, Stevenson LW, Goldsmith SR, LeWinter MM, Deswal A, Rouleau JL, Ofili EO, Anstrom KJ, Hernandez AF, McNulty SE, Velazquez EJ, Kfoury AG, Chen HH, Givertz MM, Semigran MJ, Bart BA, Mascette AM, Braunwald E, O'Connor CM, NHLBI Heart Failure Clinical Research Network. Diuretic strategies in patients with acute decompensated heart failure. N Engl J Med. 2011;364:797–805.

25. Neuberg GW, Miller AB, O'Connor CM, et al.; PRAISE Investigators. Diuretic resistance predicts mortality in patients with advanced heart failure. Am Heart J. 2002;144:31–8.

26. Thakar CV, Arrigain S, Worley S, Yared JP, Paganini EP. A clinical score to predict acute renal failure after cardiac surgery. J Am Soc Nephrol. 2005;16:162–8.

27. Lins RL, Elseviers MM, Daelemans R, Arnouts P, Billiouw JM, Couttenye M, Gheuens E, Rogiers P, Rutsaert R, Van der Niepen P, De Broe ME. Re-evaluation and modification of the Stuivenberg Hospital Acute Renal Failure (SHARF) scoring system for the prognosis of acute renal failure: an independent multicentre, prospective study. Nephrol Dial Transplant. 2004;19:2282–8.

28. Parikh CR, Coca SG, Thiessen-Philbrook H, Shlipak MG, Koyner JL, Wang Z, Edelstein CL, Devarajan P, Patel UD, Zappitelli M, Krawczeski CD, Passik CS, Swaminathan M, Garg AX, TRIBE-AKI Consortium. Postoperative biomarkers predict acute kidney injury and poor outcomes after adult cardiac surgery. J Am Soc Nephrol. 2011;22:1748–57.

29. Koyner JL, Garg AX, Coca SG, Sint K, Thiessen-Philbrook H, Patel UD, Shlipak MG, Parikh CR, TRIBE-AKI Consortium. Biomarkers predict progression of acute kidney injury after cardiac surgery. J Am Soc Nephrol. 2012;23:905–14.
30. Ronco C, Ricci Z. The concept of risk and the value of novel markers of acute kidney injury. Crit Care. 2013;17:117.
31. Kashani K, Al-Khafaji A, Ardiles T, Artigas A, Bagshaw SM, Bell M, Bihorac A, Birkhahn R, Cely CM, Chawla LS, Davison DL, Feldkamp T, Forni LG, Gong MN, Gunnerson KJ, Haase M, Hackett J, Honore PM, Hoste EA, Joannes-Boyau O, Joannidis M, Kim P, Koyner JL, Laskowitz DT, Lissauer ME, Marx G, McCullough PA, Mullaney S, Ostermann M, Rimmelé T, Shapiro NI, Shaw AD, Shi J, Sprague AM, Vincent JL, Vinsonneau C, Wagner L, Walker MG, Wilkerson RG, Zacharowski K, Kellum JA. Discovery and validation of cell cycle arrest biomarkers in human acute kidney injury. Crit Care. 2013;17:R25.

# Epidemiology of AKI

**Ville Pettilä, Sara Nisula, and Sean M. Bagshaw**

## 2.1 Incidence of AKI

### 2.1.1 Population-Based Incidence

The reported incidence rates of AKI are strongly influenced both by the definition of AKI used and the studied population (all citizens/all hospitalized patients/all ICU-treated patients/only those with renal replacement therapy). So far only two studies [1, 2] (both using RIFLE criteria) have used any of the recent definitions (RIFLE, AKIN, KDIGO – See Chap. 1) to evaluate the population-based incidence. The first retrospective study from Scotland representing a population of 523,390 reported the population-based incidence of hospital-treated AKI as 214/100,000/year [1]. Another retrospective study from one USA county area comprising a population of 124,277 reported a population-based incidence of 290/100,000/year for ICU-treated AKI [2]. Previously, the community-based incidence of non-RRT-requiring and RRT-requiring AKI in Northern California was estimated to be 384.1 and 24.4 per 100,000/year, respectively [3]. Most recently, in the FINNAKI study, the population-based incidence of ICU-treated AKI was 74.6/100,000 adults/year using both KDIGO creatinine and urine output criteria [4].


V. Pettilä, MD, PhD (✉) • S. Nisula, MD, PhD
Division of Intensive Care, Department of Anesthesiology, Intensive and Pain Medicine, Helsinki University Hospital, Haartmaninkatu 4, Helsinki 00029 HUS, Finland
e-mail: ville.pettila@hus.fi

S.M. Bagshaw, MD, MSc
Division of Critical Care Medicine, Faculty of Medicine and Dentistry, University of Alberta, 2-124E Clinical Sciences Building, 8440-112 ST NW, Edmonton, AB T6R 2K5, Canada
e-mail: bagshaw@ualberta.ca



© Springer International Publishing 2015

15

H.M. Oudemans-van Straaten et al. (eds.), *Acute Nephrology for the Critical Care Physician*, DOI 10.1007/978-3-319-17389-4_2

## 2.1.2   Proportion of AKI Patients

Recently, a systematic review comprising 49 million patients (312 cohort studies) from mostly high-income countries indicated that AKI occurs in 1 in 5 adults and 1 in 3 children in association with an acute care hospitalization [5]. Since the first unified criteria (RIFLE) for AKI were published, several studies [4, 6–18] have evaluated the proportion of AKI patients among all ICU patients. The proportion of AKI patients according to different stages are presented in Fig. 2.1. The incidence of AKI in these studies varies significantly from 10.8 % [8] to 67.2 % [6].

Plausible explanations for differences in reported incidences between studies are differences in study designs (retrospective vs. prospective), study populations/case mix, inclusion of urine output criteria, sample sizes and variety in observation periods. Large, multicentre retrospective registry studies comprising more than 10,000 patients have reported incidences from 22 % [13] to 57.0 % [14]. Only few prospective studies [4, 8, 15, 16, 19] have been published, the largest of them including 2,901 patients [4].

Importantly, in only half of the abovementioned studies, both Cr and urine output criteria were included in the definition [4, 6, 8, 10, 11, 15, 16, 19]. The observation period for development of AKI varied from 24 h [10] to the entire hospital stay [6].

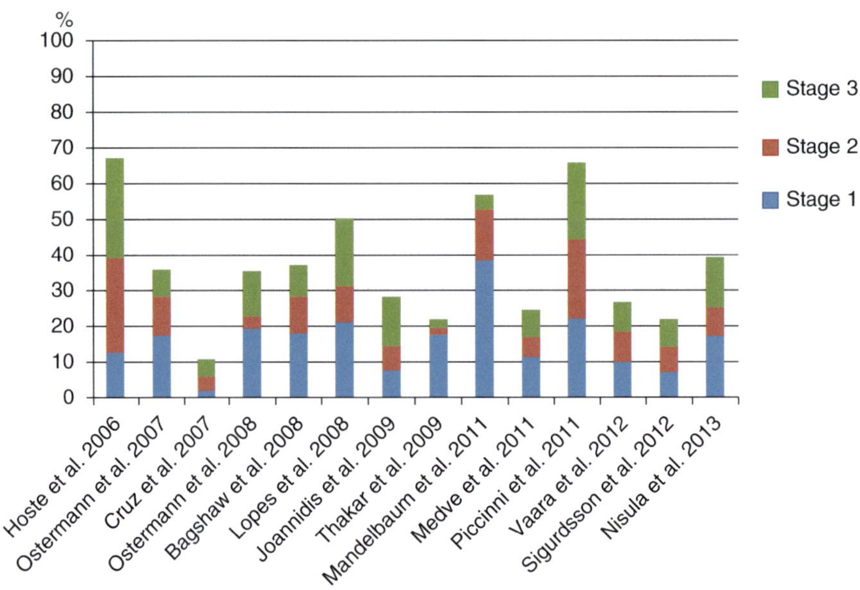


**Fig. 2.1**  Proportion of patients (%) with different acute kidney injury (AKI) stages, according to the recent new classifications (RIFLE/AKI/KDIGO)

## 2.2    Risk Factors Associated with AKI

Several different predisposing factors and transient insults may affect the kidneys and lead to AKI. The risk for each patient to develop AKI is dependent first on chronic conditions and patient-related factors and second on type and intensity of acute exposures and insults [20]. The most relevant risk factors associated with AKI are summarized in Table 2.1. Estimating an individual absolute risk for AKI is challenging, and attempts to develop risk-prediction scores exist, but are mostly limited to patients with contrast media administration [21] or those after cardiac surgery [22].

**Table 2.1**  Risk factors associated with AKI

| |
| --- |
| *Predisposing factors/chronic diseases* |
| Advanced age |
| Gender |
| Black race |
| Chronic kidney disease |
| Diabetes mellitus |
| Heart failure |
| Pulmonary disease |
| Chronic liver disease and/or complications of portal hypertension |
| Proteinuria |
| Hypertension |
| Coronary artery disease |
| Peripheral vascular disease |
| Malignancy |
| Genetic factors |
| *Acute diseases/drugs* |
| Severe sepsis |
| Trauma |
| Any critical illness |
| Hypovolemia |
| Hypotension |
| Anaemia |
| Any major surgery, e.g. cardiac surgery |
| Radiocontrast media |
| Fluid overload |
| Synthetic colloids |
| Chloride-rich solutions (i.e. 0.9 % saline) |
| Drug toxicity, drug interaction or nephrotoxic medication: |
| ACE inhibitors, acyclovir, aminoglycosides, amphotericin, NSAIDs, diuretics, aspirin, metformin, methotrexate, statins |

## 2.2.1 Predisposing Factors/Chronic Diseases

The incidence of AKI is increasing with advanced age [11, 13, 15, 16, 21, 23] – up to 45 % in ICU patients over 80 years [4]. Conflicting data relate gender to AKI – in some studies female gender [24, 25], but in some studies male gender [26, 27] has been overrepresented [16].Chronic kidney disease (CKD) is by far the most relevant predisposing susceptibility for increased risk for development of AKI [4, 6, 11, 23, 26–28], even with a minimal elevation in creatinine values. Proteinuria per se (with an eGFR >60 mL/min/1.73 m$^2$) carries an adjusted relative risk of 4.4 for AKI [5]. Among the most common diseases at the population level which predispose to AKI are diabetes mellitus [15, 21, 23, 25, 27], heart failure [23, 26, 27], hypertension [27], pulmonary disease [23, 25] and liver disease [13, 23, 27]. Patients with malignant conditions have a higher risk of AKI in the ICU [24, 25] which may be related to either direct invasion to the kidneys, or via modifiable additional factors, such as severe sepsis or nephrotoxic chemotherapeutic agents.

## 2.2.2 Acute Diseases/Drugs

Sepsis is the most important factor associated with AKI. Up to 50 % of AKI cases are related to sepsis [29–31]. In addition to sepsis, other forms of critical illness, such as major trauma [26] may lead to severe hypovolemia [32] or sustained hypotension [33, 34] predisposing to AKI. Colloids are disadvantageous for the kidneys. Several studies have confirmed that the use of hydroxyethyl starch in critically ill patients, in particular in septic states, increase the risk for AKI and the risk for RRT. The clinical evidence to date, linking gelatin or albumin to increased risk for AKI is inconclusive. Excessive fluid overload has been acknowledged as an independent risk factor for AKI and adverse outcome [35].

Any emergency [23, 27] or major surgery [27], especially cardiac surgery with cardiopulmonary bypass exposure predisposes to AKI due to potential changes in hemodynamics, intravascular volume, delivery of oxygen and the systemic inflammation reaction (systemic inflammatory response syndrome, SIRS) caused by the surgery.

Radiocontrast media and multiple drugs are known to be nephrotoxic. Up to one-fourth of severe AKI cases are estimated to be related to drug toxicity [30]. CKD, sepsis, liver failure, heart failure and malignancies as comorbidities increase the risk for drug-induced kidney injury [36].

Due to the multifactorial etiology of AKI, most patients who develop AKI have several factors predisposing to AKI simultaneously or temporally over time (Fig. 2.2). In the FINNAKI study, a large prospective observational study, only pre-ICU hypovolemia (odds ratio, OR 2.2), pre-ICU use of diuretics (OR 1.7), colloid use (OR 1.4) and chronic kidney disease (OR 2.6, 95 % CI 1.9–3.7) were independently associated with the development of AKI [4].

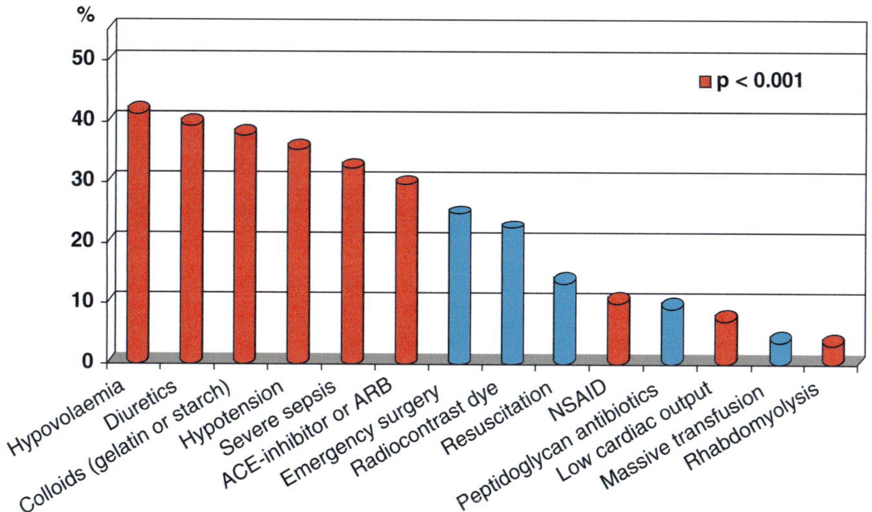



**Fig. 2.2** Proportion of AKI patients (%) with different predisposing factors preceding ICU admission. Factors more common in AKI patients compared to patients without AKI ($p < 0.001$) with *red* colour [4]

## 2.3 Outcomes of AKI Patients

### 2.3.1 Hospital Mortality

Regrettably most of the AKI studies have focused on short-term mortality. ICU mortality is generally accepted as unreliable due to differences in discharge and end-of-life policies. Hospital mortality may also be biased, and thus variable, due to differences in discharging patients to rehabilitation centres or other hospitals. The reported hospital mortality of AKI patients has varied between 13.3 % [6] and 49.1 % [15] in ten studies [4, 6, 7, 9–12, 15, 18, 19] (Table 2.2). Differences in study designs and patient populations/case mix explain some of the variation. Studies do not consistently report severity scores, but on the basis of the given SAPS II points there was a large variation in disease severity among ICU patients.

### 2.3.2 Long-Term Fixed-Time Mortality (90 Days, 6 Months)

The only study with a fixed long-term mortality reported the 90-day mortality rate for AKI patients as 33.7 % [4]. Two prospective studies have reported the 6-month mortality rates of 46.5 % [37] and 35.3 % [38], and two retrospective studies as 58.5 %

**Table 2.2** Hospital and 90-day mortality in patients with acute kidney injury classified according to the new definitions (RIFLE, AKIN, KDIGO)

| Author, year | Design | Criteria | Number of patients | AKI<br>Hospital mortality (%) | Stage 3/ RIFLE F<br>Hospital mortality (%) | AKI<br>90-day mortality (%) |
|---|---|---|---|---|---|---|
| Åhlström, 2006 [19] | Prospective, single centre | RIFLE Cr + UO | 658 | 16.7 | 23.0 | – |
| Hoste, 2006 [6] | Retrospective, single centre | RIFLE Cr + UO | 5,383 | 13.3 | 26.3 | – |
| Ostermann, 2007 [7] | Retrospective, multicentre | RIFLE Cr | 41,972 | 36.1 | 56.8 | – |
| Ostermann, 2008 [9] | Retrospective, multicentre | AKIN Cr | 22,303 | 40.4 | 57.9 | – |
| Bagshaw, 2008 [10] | Retrospective, multicentre | RIFLE Cr | 120,123 | 24.5 | 32.6 | – |
| Lopes, 2008 [11] | Retrospective, single centre | RIFLE Cr + UO | 662 | 41.3 | 55.0 | – |
| Joannidis, 2009 [12] | Retrospective, multicentre | AKIN Cr | 14,356 | 36.4 | 41.2 | – |
| Medve, 2011 [15] | Prospective, multicentre | AKIN Cr + UO | 459 | 49.1 | 73.5 | – |
| Sigurdsson, 2012 [18] | Retrospective, single centre | RIFLE Cr | 1,012 | 37.6 | 51.0 | – |
| Nisula, 2013 [4] | Prospective, multicentre | KDIGO Cr + UO | 2,901 | 25.6 | 32.2 | 33.7 |

*Cr* creatinine, *UO* urine output

[39] and 38.0 % [40]. The survival curves of AKI patients [38, 41] suggest that most of deaths among AKI patients occur within 60 days, and so the follow up of 60–90 days would be adequate for a reliable analysis of mortality rate. The mortality rates from different studies for RRT-treated AKI-patients are presented in Fig. 2.3.

## 2.3.3 Trends in Mortality

A systematic review indicated that mortality of AKI patients has remained high throughout years [42]. However, two studies suggested that mortality both among AKI [43] patients and among RRT-treated patients [44] has decreased.

## 2.3.4 Factors Associated with Mortality

Pre-existing co-morbidities, such as diabetes [45] and CKD [7, 10], and advanced age [46] increase the mortality rate. Fluid overload [47, 48] and hydroxyethyl starch use [49] are associated with excess mortality. Additionally, delay in ICU admission

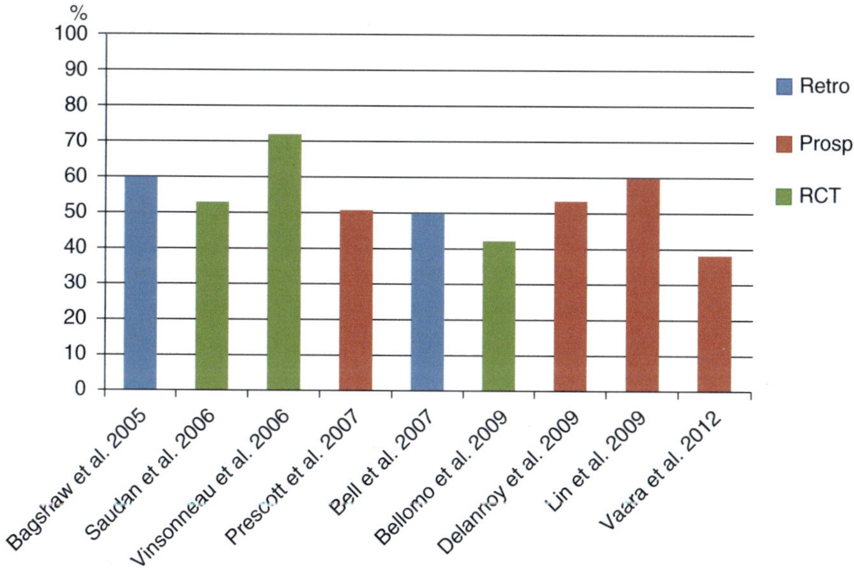

**Fig. 2.3** 90-day mortality (%) in patients with severe AKI who received renal replacement therapy (RRT)

[30, 46], use of mechanical ventilation [30], sepsis [45] and severity of illness and number of organ failures [45] have been associated with increased mortality in AKI patients. Variations in the severity of illness plausibly have an effect on not only the incidence of AKI, but also mortality. RIFLE or AKIN stages, representing worsening severity of AKI, have been independently associated with mortality in most studies [6–12, 15, 18, 19]. Furthermore, even mild stages of AKI have been associated with increased mortality [6]. Most recently, there was a linear increase in 90-day mortality according to the advancing KDIGO stages: from 16.6 % without AKI to 29.3 % in stage 1, 34.1 % for stage 2 and 39.0 % for stage 3 AKI [4].

Recently, a sequentially propensity-matched analysis calculated that the absolute excess mortality attributable to AKI at 90 days was 8.6 % and that statistically 19.6 % of deaths (population attributable risk, 90-day mortality) among ICU patients could be avoided if there was no AKI [50].

## 2.3.5 Health-Related Quality of Life (HRQoL) of AKI Survivors

The HRQoL of patients with AKI has been evaluated in at least three studies [37, 38, 40]. The HRQoL by Short Form-36 questionnaire at 6 months was lower in physical domains among patients with postoperative AKI. However, the patients graded their HRQoL better than before ICU admission [40].

Another study found no difference in HRQoL (by SF-36) at 6 months between patients with and without AKI [37]. More recently, a prospective multi-centre study reported that the HRQoL (assessed by the EuroQoL-5D) of AKI patients remained unchanged during critical illness and was not different from that of patients without AKI 6 months after ICU admission [38]. Despite their lower HRQoL scores, patients with AKI perceive their health comparable to the general population [38].

Studies comprising only AKI patients treated with RRT (stage 3) have reported impaired physical health component in comparison with controls [51–53]. Notably, surviving AKI-RRT patients perceived their health as excellent [51] and would decide to undergo the same treatment again [52]. More recently, the HRQoL of critically ill patients who survived with or without RRT was not different and comparable to the general population [17]. These HRQoL findings support the active treatment of AKI patients with RRT despite high long-term mortality and remarkable societal costs and low cost efficiency especially in patients with more advanced age and co-morbidities [54].

## 2.4  Summary

Multiple chronic diseases, such as diabetes and chronic kidney disease, and acute illness, most commonly sepsis (half of the cases) predispose to AKI. The modifiable factors, such as hypotension, fluid overload, nephrotoxic drugs and starch should be monitored for and avoided. In summary, one of five hospitalized adult patients and two of five critically ill adult patients develop AKI. AKI portends an increased risk of death with higher risk with increasing severity of AKI – approximately one in four AKI patients die in the hospital, and one in three during 90 days. If RRT has been administered due to more severe AKI (stage 3), one in two patients will die in 90 days. Although impaired relative to matched population norms, the HRQoL among AKI survivors is comparable to the HRQoL of the critically ill survivors without AKI. Of note, despite lower measured HRQoL among AKI survivors, these patients perceive their HRQoL to be comparable to that of an age- and sex-matched critically ill control population. Large observational and interventional studies are further needed to better understand the development and long-term outcomes of AKI and to ameliorate the recovering process after AKI.

**Key Points**
1. Several non-modifiable chronic diseases along with numerous potentially avoidable factors contribute to the risk of developing AKI in critical illness.
2. One of 5 hospitalized adult patients and 2 of 5 critically ill adult patients develop AKI.
3. Increasing severity of AKI is associated with an incremental risk of death – up to half of the RRT-treated AKI patients die within 3 months.
4. AKI survivors describe their quality of life to be comparable to that of other survivors without AKI after critical illness.
5. At present the long-term kidney recovery and associated outcomes among AKI survivors are incompletely understood and represent important gaps in knowledge and evidence-based care.

# References


1. Ali T, Khan I, Simpson W, et al. Incidence and outcomes in acute kidney injury: a comprehensive population-based study. J Am Soc Nephrol. 2007;18(4):1292–8.
2. Cartin-Ceba R, Kojicic M, Li G, et al. Epidemiology of critical care syndromes, organ failures, and life-support interventions in a suburban US community. Chest. 2011;140(6):1447–55.
3. Hsu CY, McCulloch CE, Fan D, Ordonez JD, Chertow GM, Go AS. Community-based incidence of acute renal failure. Kidney Int. 2007;72(2):208–12.
4. Nisula S, Kaukonen KM, Vaara ST, et al. Incidence, risk factors and 90-day mortality of patients with acute kidney injury in Finnish intensive care units: the FINNAKI study. Intensive Care Med. 2013;39(3):420–8.
5. Susantitaphong P, Cruz DN, Cerda J, et al. World incidence of AKI: a meta-analysis. Clin J Am Soc Nephrol. 2013;8(9):1482–93.
6. Hoste EA, Clermont G, Kersten A, et al. RIFLE criteria for acute kidney injury are associated with hospital mortality in critically ill patients: a cohort analysis. Crit Care. 2006;10(3):R73.
7. Ostermann M, Chang RW. Acute kidney injury in the intensive care unit according to RIFLE. Crit Care Med. 2007;35(8):1837–43; quiz 52.
8. Cruz DN, Bolgan I, Perazella MA, et al. North East Italian Prospective Hospital Renal Outcome Survey on Acute Kidney Injury (NEiPHROS-AKI): targeting the problem with the RIFLE Criteria. Clin J Am Soc Nephrol. 2007;2(3):418–25.
9. Ostermann M, Chang R, Riyadh ICUPUG. Correlation between the AKI classification and outcome. Crit Care. 2008;12(6):R144.
10. Bagshaw SM, George C, Dinu I, Bellomo R. A multi-centre evaluation of the RIFLE criteria for early acute kidney injury in critically ill patients. Nephrol Dial Transplant Off Publ Eur Dial Transplant Assoc Eur Ren Assoc. 2008;23(4):1203–10.
11. Lopes JA, Fernandes P, Jorge S, et al. Acute kidney injury in intensive care unit patients: a comparison between the RIFLE and the Acute Kidney Injury Network classifications. Crit Care. 2008;12(4):R110.
12. Joannidis M, Metnitz B, Bauer P, et al. Acute kidney injury in critically ill patients classified by AKIN versus RIFLE using the SAPS 3 database. Intensive Care Med. 2009;35(10):1692–702.
13. Thakar CV, Christianson A, Freyberg R, Almenoff P, Render ML. Incidence and outcomes of acute kidney injury in intensive care units: a Veterans Administration study. Crit Care Med. 2009;37(9):2552–8.
14. Mandelbaum T, Scott DJ, Lee J, et al. Outcome of critically ill patients with acute kidney injury using the Acute Kidney Injury Network criteria. Crit Care Med. 2011;39(12):2659–64.
15. Medve L, Antek C, Paloczi B, et al. Epidemiology of acute kidney injury in Hungarian intensive care units: a multicenter, prospective, observational study. BMC Nephrol. 2011;12:43.
16. Piccinni P, Cruz DN, Gramaticopolo S, et al. Prospective multicenter study on epidemiology of acute kidney injury in the ICU: a critical care nephrology Italian collaborative effort (NEFROINT). Minerva Anestesiol. 2011;77(11):1072–83.
17. Vaara ST, Pettila V, Reinikainen M, Kaukonen KM, Finnish Intensive Care Consortium. Population-based incidence, mortality and quality of life in critically ill patients treated with renal replacement therapy: a nationwide retrospective cohort study in Finnish intensive care units. Crit Care. 2012;16(1):R13.
18. Sigurdsson MI, Vesteinsdottir IO, Sigvaldason K, Helgadottir S, Indridason OS, Sigurdsson GH. Acute kidney injury in intensive care units according to RIFLE classification: a population-based study. Acta Anaesthesiol Scand. 2012;56(10):1291–7.
19. Ahlstrom A, Kuitunen A, Peltonen S, et al. Comparison of 2 acute renal failure severity scores to general scoring systems in the critically ill. Am J Kidney Dis Off J Natl Kidney Found. 2006;48(2):262–8.
20. Kidney Disease: Improving Global Outcomes (KDIGO) Acute Kidney Injury Work Group. KDIGO Clinical Practice Guideline for Acute Kidney Injury. Kidney Int. 2012;2(Suppl):1–138.

21. Mehran R, Aymong ED, Nikolsky E, et al. A simple risk score for prediction of contrast-induced nephropathy after percutaneous coronary intervention: development and initial validation. J Am Coll Cardiol. 2004;44(7):1393–9.
22. Candela-Toha A, Elias-Martin E, Abraira V, et al. Predicting acute renal failure after cardiac surgery: external validation of two new clinical scores. Clin J Am Soc Nephrol. 2008;3(5):1260–5.
23. Selby NM, Crowley L, Fluck RJ, et al. Use of electronic results reporting to diagnose and monitor AKI in hospitalized patients. Clin J Am Soc Nephrol. 2012;7(4):533–40.
24. Thakar CV, Liangos O, Yared JP, et al. ARF after open-heart surgery: influence of gender and race. Am J Kidney Dis Off J Natl Kidney Found. 2003;41(4):742–51.
25. Thakar CV, Arrigain S, Worley S, Yared JP, Paganini EP. A clinical score to predict acute renal failure after cardiac surgery. J Am Soc Nephrol. 2005;16(1):162–8.
26. Xue JL, Daniels F, Star RA, et al. Incidence and mortality of acute renal failure in Medicare beneficiaries, 1992 to 2001. J Am Soc Nephrol. 2006;17(4):1135–42.
27. Colpaert K, Hoste EA, Steurbaut K, et al. Impact of real-time electronic alerting of acute kidney injury on therapeutic intervention and progression of RIFLE class. Crit Care Med. 2012;40(4):1164–70.
28. Coca SG, Peixoto AJ, Garg AX, Krumholz HM, Parikh CR. The prognostic importance of a small acute decrement in kidney function in hospitalized patients: a systematic review and meta-analysis. Am J Kidney Dis Off J Natl Kidney Found. 2007;50(5):712–20.
29. Bagshaw SM, Uchino S, Bellomo R, et al. Septic acute kidney injury in critically ill patients: clinical characteristics and outcomes. Clin J Am Soc Nephrol. 2007;2(3):431–9.
30. Uchino S, Kellum JA, Bellomo R, et al. Acute renal failure in critically ill patients: a multinational, multicenter study. JAMA. 2005;294(7):813–8.
31. Poukkanen M, Vaara ST, Pettila V, et al. Acute kidney injury in patients with severe sepsis in Finnish Intensive Care Units. Acta Anaesthesiol Scand. 2013;57(7):863–72.
32. Finlay S, Bray B, Lewington AJ, et al. Identification of risk factors associated with acute kidney injury in patients admitted to acute medical units. Clin Med. 2013;13(3):233–8.
33. Brienza N, Giglio MT, Marucci M, Fiore T. Does perioperative hemodynamic optimization protect renal function in surgical patients? A meta-analytic study. Crit Care Med. 2009;37(6):2079–90.
34. Poukkanen M, Wilkman E, Vaara ST, et al. Hemodynamic variables and progression of acute kidney injury in critically ill patients with severe sepsis: data from the prospective observational FINNAKI study. Crit Care. 2013;17(6):R295.
35. Prowle JR, Kirwan CJ, Bellomo R. Fluid management for the prevention and attenuation of acute kidney injury. Nat Rev Nephrol. 2014;10(1):37–47.
36. Perazella MA. Drug use and nephrotoxicity in the intensive care unit. Kidney Int. 2012;81(12):1172–8.
37. Hofhuis JG, van Stel HF, Schrijvers AJ, Rommes JH, Spronk PE. The effect of acute kidney injury on long-term health-related quality of life: a prospective follow-up study. Crit Care. 2013;17(1):R17.
38. Nisula S, Vaara ST, Kaukonen KM, et al. Six-month survival and quality of life of intensive care patients with acute kidney injury. Crit Care. 2013;17(5):R250.
39. Abosaif NY, Tolba YA, Heap M, Russell J, El Nahas AM. The outcome of acute renal failure in the intensive care unit according to RIFLE: model application, sensitivity, and predictability. Am J Kidney Dis Off J Natl Kidney Found. 2005;46(6):1038–48.
40. Abelha FJ, Botelho M, Fernandes V, Barros H. Outcome and quality of life of patients with acute kidney injury after major surgery. Nefrologia Publ Off Soc Esp Nefrol. 2009;29(5):404–14.
41. Bell M, Liljestam E, Granath F, Fryckstedt J, Ekbom A, Martling CR. Optimal follow-up time after continuous renal replacement therapy in actual renal failure patients stratified with the RIFLE criteria. Nephrol Dial Transplant Off Publ Eur Dial Transplant Assoc Eur Ren Assoc. 2005;20(2):354–60.

42. Ympa YP, Sakr Y, Reinhart K, Vincent JL. Has mortality from acute renal failure decreased? A systematic review of the literature. Am J Med. 2005;118(8):827–32.
43. Bagshaw SM, George C, Bellomo R, Committee ADM. Changes in the incidence and outcome for early acute kidney injury in a cohort of Australian intensive care units. Crit Care. 2007;11(3):R68.
44. Waikar SS, Curhan GC, Wald R, McCarthy EP, Chertow GM. Declining mortality in patients with acute renal failure, 1988 to 2002. J Am Soc Nephrol. 2006;17(4):1143–50.
45. Zhou J, Yang L, Zhang K, Liu Y, Fu P. Risk factors for the prognosis of acute kidney injury under the Acute Kidney Injury Network definition: a retrospective, multicenter study in critically ill patients. Nephrology (Carlton). 2012;17(4):330–7.
46. Brivet FG, Kleinknecht DJ, Loirat P, Landais PJ. Acute renal failure in intensive care units–causes, outcome, and prognostic factors of hospital mortality; a prospective, multicenter study. French Study Group on Acute Renal Failure. Crit Care Med. 1996;24(2):192–8.
47. Grams ME, Estrella MM, Coresh J, et al. Fluid balance, diuretic use, and mortality in acute kidney injury. Clin J Am Soc Nephrol. 2011;6(5):966–73.
48. Vaara ST, Korhonen AM, Kaukonen KM, et al. Fluid overload is associated with an increased risk for 90-day mortality in critically ill patients with renal replacement therapy: data from the prospective FINNAKI study. Crit Care. 2012;16(5):R197.
49. Perner A, Haase N, Guttormsen AB, et al. Hydroxyethyl starch 130/0.42 versus Ringer's acetate in severe sepsis. N Engl J Med. 2012;367(2):124–34.
50. Vaara ST, Pettila V, Kaukonen KM, et al. The attributable mortality of acute kidney injury: a sequentially matched analysis*. Crit Care Med. 2014;42(4):878–85.
51. Morgera S, Kraft AK, Siebert G, Luft FC, Neumayer HH. Long-term outcomes in acute renal failure patients treated with continuous renal replacement therapies. Am J Kidney Dis Off J Natl Kidney Found. 2002;40(2):275–9.
52. Delannoy B, Floccard B, Thiolliere F, et al. Six-month outcome in acute kidney injury requiring renal replacement therapy in the ICU: a multicentre prospective study. Intensive Care Med. 2009;35(11):1907–15.
53. Johansen KL, Smith MW, Unruh ML, et al. Predictors of health utility among 60-day survivors of acute kidney injury in the Veterans Affairs/National Institutes of Health Acute Renal Failure Trial Network Study. Clin J Am Soc Nephrol. 2010;5(8):1366–72.
54. Laukkanen A, Emaus L, Pettila V, Kaukonen KM. Five-year cost-utility analysis of acute renal replacement therapy: a societal perspective. Intensive Care Med. 2013;39(3):406–13.

# Renal Outcomes After Acute Kidney Injury

**3**


John R. Prowle, Christopher J. Kirwan, and Rinaldo Bellomo


## 3.1 Introduction

During critical illness the occurrence of Acute Kidney Injury (AKI) is strongly associated with increased risk of death. However, in those who survive, it has traditionally been assumed that the majority will recover pre-morbid renal function with just a few patients being left dependent of renal replacement therapy (RRT) as a result of distinct pathological processes such as cortical necrosis and renal infarction. In fact, as long ago as the 1950s it had been established that when accurate determinations of glomerular filtration rate (GFR) are made, persistent reduction in renal function could be demonstrated months and years after an episode of AKI [1, 2]. More recently, following standardization in the diagnosis and staging of AKI, the longer-term consequences of AKI on renal function in survivors have become better recognised [3] and episodes of AKI have been established as a major risk factor for the development of chronic kidney disease (CKD).

Chronic Kidney Disease is a major health care challenge for the twenty-first century. It has been estimated that in 8.5 % of adults in the United Kingdom have CKD with its prevalence increasing [4]. The clinical and economic impact of CKD is very significant, even mild CKD has been associated with increased long-term


J.R. Prowle • C.J. Kirwan
Adult Critical Care Unit, The Royal London Hospital, Barts Health NHS Trust, London, UK

Department of Renal medicine and Transplantation, Barts Health NHS Trust, London, UK

R. Bellomo (✉)
Australian and New Zealand Intensive Care Research Centre, Carlton, VIC, Australia

Department of Epidemiology and Preventive Medicine, Monash University, Melbourne, VIC, Australia

Department of Intensive Care, Austin Health, 145 Studley Road, Heidelberg, VIC 3084, Australia
e-mail: rinaldo.bellomo@austin.org.au



© Springer International Publishing 2015

27

H.M. Oudemans-van Straaten et al. (eds.), *Acute Nephrology for the Critical Care Physician*, DOI 10.1007/978-3-319-17389-4_3

morbidity and mortality, in particular cardiovascular disease and death [5]. The annual cost of CKD to the National Health Service in England and Wales has been estimated at £1.45 billion, more than the annual cost of breast, lung, colon and skin cancer combined [6]. Evidence-based guidelines exist for the prevention, recognition, treatment and follow-up of CKD [7], however, CKD often arises insidiously, goes undiagnosed and is left untreated. It is therefore crucial that survivors of critical illness be appropriately screened and managed in a similar fashion to other patient groups at high risk of CKD.

In this chapter, we review the epidemiological evidence for an association between AKI and the development or worsening of CKD, and the underlying pathophysiology of this process. We discuss difficulties in accurately diagnosing renal dysfunction in survivors of critical illness from ICU and, finally we suggest a structure for renal follow-up in this population.

## 3.2 AKI and the Development of CKD

### 3.2.1 Epidemiology of CKD After AKI

Considerable epidemiological evidence now exists to implicate AKI as a major risk factor for CKD [8–11]. For instance in a study involving a cohort of almost 250,000 US Medicare patients [9], elderly individuals who experienced AKI were at significantly increased risk of developing of end-stage renal disease (ESRD) compared to individuals with no history of AKI. The highest risk was in individuals developing AKI on a background of pre-existing CKD. In all, one quarter of patients developing ESRD had a prior clinical episode of AKI. Similarly, in over 5,000 patients admitted to US Veterans Health Administration Hospitals without a prior diagnosis of CKD, a diagnostic coding for *Acute Tubular Necrosis* was associated with a significantly increase in the risk of later developing CKD stage 4 and 5 or death compared to controls without an AKI diagnosis [10]. Episodes of AKI requiring renal replacement therapy (RRT) may confer the highest risk of CKD. For example, a retrospective analysis of over 500,000 patients without advanced CKD (estimated-GFR >45 ml/ml/1.73 $m^2$) requiring RRT for AKI within a managed health care consortium in California, found a 28-fold increase in risk of developing stage 4 or 5 CKD and more than a twofold increased risk of death [11]. The severity of AKI has been linked with the risk of subsequent CKD in another analysis of US Veterans Health Administration patients [12], with greater odds of CKD associated with the a more severe AKI category in the RIFLE classification, and with the greatest odds for those patients requiring RRT. Finally, recurrent AKI may confer particular risk of CKD. For example, in a cohort of 3,679 patients with diabetes followed for 10 years, hospitalization complicated by AKI of any severity was associated with an independent 3.6-fold increase in rate of developing CKD stage 4, with a doubling of risk for each further AKI episode [13].

The above studies highlight a strong epidemiological association between AKI and the development of CKD, however, this may not be apparent soon after recovery from major illness. This is significant because without evidence of CKD, patients are unlikely to receive specific renal follow-up, but may still be likely to have increased risk of later renal dysfunction. In a cohort of 1,610 patients who had AKI and recovered to normal serum creatinine, half developed CKD after 36 months. In addition, these patients had a 1.5-fold higher risk of death during follow-up compared to matched controls without AKI [14]. In another large study of patients hospitalized within an integrated health care system in the United States, 719 patients who had AKI during admission and recovered to baseline creatinine level were identified. These individuals had an almost fourfold increased risk of developing incident stage 3 CKD compared to controls without AKI in propensity-stratified analyses [15]. Similarly, in a study of 126 children whose creatinine returned to baseline after AKI [16], 10 % had developed CKD and half were identified as having increased risk of developing CKD within 3 years. Importantly, the most common renal abnormality at follow-up was micro-albuminuria, which is strongly associated with progression of adult CKD and which may long-precede any alteration in GFR. Collectively, these studies suggest that the decision on renal specialist follow-up for patients surviving AKI cannot be easily based on serum creatinine at hospital discharge. Difficultly in recognising risk of CKD after AKI may account for very low reported rates of referral for nephrology follow-up [17], even in survivors of severe AKI, short of immediately needing ongoing RRT.

## 3.2.2  Pathophysiology of CKD After AKI

While there are many potential causes of CKD, once substantial chronic renal damage has occurred, progression of CKD involves common pathophysiological processes involving the development of proteinuria, systemic hypertension, and glomerulosclerosis and tubulo-interstitial fibrosis leading to a progressive decline in GFR. Chronic inflammation is thought to play an important role in the development of tubulo-interstial fibrosis and this can occur as a sequela of acute inflammation during AKI [18]. In AKI there is an early neutrophil cellular infiltration followed by a later monocytic-lymphocytic infiltrate during the recovery phase. A severe early neutrophilic response may cause irreversible nephron loss, however, the nature of the delayed mononuclear cell infiltrate (chronic phase) correlates better with the nature and extent of recovery after AKI. Depending on the local inflammatory microenvironment, monocytes and lymphocytes may direct repair, regeneration, and tissue remodeling, or promote fibroblastic metaplasia, proliferation and fibrosis. Once fibrosis is triggered, interactions between inflammatory cells, fibroblasts, endothelial and epithelial cells perpetuate its development, which, in conjunction with the development of peri-tubular capillary rarefaction and hypoxia, mediates progressive renal injury. Once irreversible loss of nephron units has occurred, renal blood flow auto-regulation to neighboring nephron units is impaired, allowing systemic blood pressure to be directly transmitted to glomerular arterioles. In combination with hypertensive systemic neuro-endocrine responses to diminished GFR, this causes intra-glomerular hypertension and hyperfiltration, for a time preserving GFR at the expense progressive arteriosclerosis, glomerulosclerosis and further tubular atrophy. In CKD of all forms these processes are accelerated by secondary risk factors, unrelated to the aetiology of CKD, such as genetic background, gender, episodes of recurrent AKI, degree of proteinuria, essential hypertension, sodium intake, obesity, smoking, systemic inflammation and hyperlipidaemia (Fig. 3.1) [19].

Evidence for the above mechanisms can be found in the outcomes of animal models of AKI. In rats after renal ischaemia/reperfusion (I/R) injury, creatinine levels return to the normal range after 4 weeks, despite a persistent GFR reduction of ~50 % [20]. Furthermore, a high salt diet causes hypertension and proteinuria in animals exposed to renal I/R, but not in sham operated controls [20]. Similarly a high salt diet reduces renal clearances and increases interstitial inflammation specifically in kidneys subjected to I/R [21]. The pathophysiology of chronic renal injury in these models may involve oxidative stress, alteration in gene expression, loss of peri-tubular capillaries [22], and the haemodynamic and fibrotic effects of angiotensin II [23].

Thus, after AKI, initial chronic damage may be subtle and not be associated with obvious abnormality in serum biochemistry, but still of great prognostic significance. Importantly, management of risk factors may attenuate these pathophysiological processes and slow the progression of CKD.

## 3.3    Diagnosis of CKD in AKI Survivors

Diagnosis of persistent renal dysfunction as an outcome of AKI can be confounded by many factors hampering our ability to define its nature, extent and significance (Table 3.1). The reciprocal relationship between creatinine and GFR implies that, quite large declines in renal function from a normal baseline can occur with only small rises in steady state creatinine, so that GFR can fall by almost half before creatinine becomes clearly abnormal. This is particularly important when assessing renal outcomes because even if the reduction in total nephron mass is relatively small, this can still trigger slow, progressive decline in renal function. Furthermore, in critical illness, acute falls in creatinine generation rate are observed both in clinical settings [24] and animal models [25]. Such reduced creatinine generation, in turn, decreases both the rate of rise and the absolute creatinine increment after a fall in GFR [26]. Importantly, the largest falls in creatinine generation are associated with greatest illness severity [24]. The decreased ability of serum creatinine to reflect the magnitude of decrease in GFR suggests that some patients may develop 'sub-clinical' AKI and then CKD. Neutrophil gelatinase–associated lipocalin (NGAL) a biomarker of renal tubular injury is associated with risk of death and other adverse outcomes even in the absence AKI diagnosis based on serum creatinine [27], suggesting that sub-clinical AKI could be common and clinically relevant. It is uncertain whether sub-clinical AKI is a risk factor for CKD. However, as subtle chronic kidney damage can predispose to progressive renal dysfunction, it is possible that some survivors of major illness could be at increased risk of CKD even in the absence of a formal AKI diagnosis during their illness.

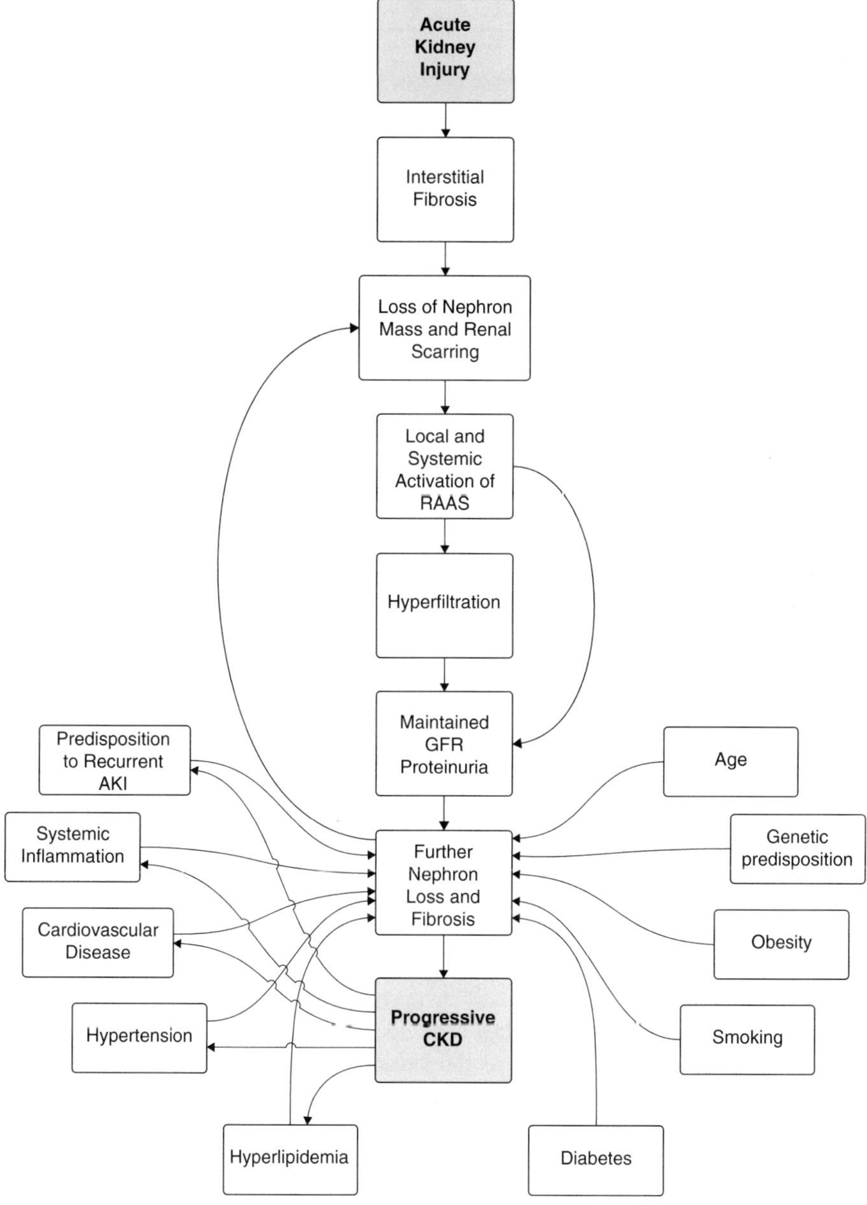



**Fig. 3.1** Common pathogenesis of CKD after AKI. Initial loss of nephrons and interstitial scarring leads to hyperfiltration and proteinuria. Hyperfiltration may maintain total GFR, but at the expense of progressive renal injury, which in turn accelerates these processes. Many risk factors may accelerate the progression of CKD, in many cases with positive feedback as CKD in turn is a significantly associated with development of cardiovascular disease, hypertension, systemic inflammation and risk of recurrent AKI. *AKI* acute kidney injury, *CKD* chronic kidney disease, *RAAS* renal/angiotensin aldosterone system

**Table 3.1** Impediments to recognition and staging of CKD after AKI

| |
| --- |
| Sub-clinical AKI may go unrecognised during acute critical illness |
| Milder interstitial injury after AKI may not be associated with reduction in GFR initially, but still be a risk factor for progressive CKD |
| Hyperfiltration and loss of renal reserve may mask reduction in resting GFR, despite being a potential risk factor for CKD progression |
| Significant reduction in GFR from a previously normal baseline may not cause creatinine to rise above the normal range, despite underlying nephron loss |
| Loss of muscle mass after critical illness and in chronic disease may confound ability of serum creatinine to accurately reflect the severity of reduction in GFR |

Even when the AKI is diagnosed, assessing renal function during recovery can be confounded by pre-existing or acquired alteration in muscle mass, liver function [28] and diet. Steady-state serum creatinine is determined by the equilibrium between creatinine production and creatinine excretion. Many critically ill patients have pre-morbid chronic disease and are likely to have reduced creatinine generation at baseline. The use of creatinine-based eGFR in the general population has recently been the subject of a meta-analysis [29]. The prevalence of CKD rose significantly when cystatin-c, a renal filtration marker less dependent on muscle mass, was used for eGFR estimation, with better prediction of all-cause mortality and cardiovascular death. These results suggest that variations in creatinine generation might confound CKD diagnosis in the general population and that these missed diagnoses are clinically significant. Critical illness is then associated with further profound and progressive loss of skeletal muscle protein [30–32] and muscle thickness [32–34], with a strong inverse correlation between muscle thickness and duration of critical illness [33, 34]. Thus, estimates of renal function after critical illness based on ICU or hospital discharge creatinine can fail to detect significant loss of GFR, and will not be directly comparable to a baseline creatinine.

Even when GFR is accurately assessed, measurements may not represent the extent of chronic kidney damage after AKI. Many patients who have developed chronic renal scarring can have relatively normal GFR for an extended period until overt CKD eventually occurs. It has been speculated that loss of *renal functional reserve* [35] occurs in early CKD as the kidney lacks capacity to augment GFR in response to demand despite preserved baseline GFR [36]. This may occur when the nephron number is reduced, but total GFR is persevered by glomerular hyperfiltration [37]. Such patients have no capacity to increase GFR as their renal reserve is maximally recruited at baseline. Hyperfiltration may be triggered by neuroendocrine responses to renal damage, including local and systemic generation of angiotensin II, and is associated with glomerulosclerosis and eventual deterioration in renal function. These processes are strongly associated with the development of proteinuria. Irrespective of GFR, microalbuminuria (urinary albumin: creatinine ratio >3.5 mg/mmol) is associated with increased all cause mortality, cardiovascular mortality, progressive CKD, end stage renal disease and risk of new AKI, with increasing risk with more severe levels of proteinuria [38, 39]. Thus, proteinuria is a key prognostic indicator for progression of CKD after AKI at all levels of GFR including apparently normal renal function.

There has been considerable recent research into the development of novel renal biomarkers to accelerate and refine the diagnosis of AKI. However, less is known on how these markers relate to chronic renal outcomes after AKI. Plasma NGAL concentrations at AKI diagnosis do correlate with degree of renal recovery [40] and prediction of renal recovery may be refined by combining markers and clinical risk factors [41]. This suggests that those measures that correlate with renal tubular injury may provide an early prognosis for renal recovery after critical illness. However, existing studies have examined renal recovery as freedom from renal replacement therapy and further research is needed to refine the use novel diagnostics to discriminate severity of CKD in patients who come off, or never need, renal replacement therapy. In addition specific markers of renal recovery or fibrosis may be developed to improve prediction of long-term renal outcomes [41]. Finally, serial measurement of AKI biomarkers may be useful to screen for new AKI during recovery from critical illness allowing measures to minimise subsequent recurrent renal injury, which may have a strong impact on recovery of renal function.

## 3.4 Primary Prevention of CKD After AKI

In the treatment of AKI, avoidance of recurrent renal injury is crucial to achieving maximal renal recovery, thus the treatment of AKI merges into the prevention of CKD. Use of intermittent haemodialysis for RRT in AKI has been associated with poorer renal recovery than continuous modalities of RRT [42], possibly related to intra-dialytic falls in cardiac output with rapid ultrafiltration, causing renal hypoperfusion and recurrent ischaemic injury [43]. This concern has led to recommendations for the preferred use of CRRT in the treatment of haemodynamically unstable patients with AKI [44]. More controversially, it has been recently suggested that the kidney might be best protected in AKI by pharmacological intervention (ACE-inhibition or Angiotensin II blockade) to reduce glomerular filtration and decreasing renal vascular resistance, thus reducing oxygen demand while increasing renal oxygen delivery, even if this were at the expense of acute need for renal support [45]. While this strategy cannot currently be recommended for clinical use it is a provocative suggestion that warrants experimental investigation.

## 3.5 Managing CKD After AKI

Given the diagnostic difficulties outlined above, it seems appropriate to consider all survivors of critical illness at risk of CKD. In particular, in patients who had clinically overt AKI, follow-up for development of CKD should be considered, irrespective of apparent degree of renal recovery. CKD in general has well-developed clinical guidelines [7] for monitoring and treatment and in the absence of evidence to the contrary, we should apply these principles to the management of AKI survivors with or at risk of CKD. Follow-up will involve measurement of serum creatinine, blood pressure, urinalysis and cardiovascular risk factors; in some patients formal measurement of GFR may be helpful. AKI survivors should be regarded, as having a long-term risk factor for CKD and continued screening should be considered. Patients with more severe renal dysfunction or other specific risk factors may benefit from specialist follow-up with a nephrologist [46] while others could be followed-up in primary care and be referred back to renal services if required. Treatment of hypertension and modification of cardiovascular risk factors are central to management of patients with or at risk of CKD. In particular, in patients with diabetes or hypertension and proteinuria, ACE inhibitors or A2 receptor blocking agents should be considered, as these may reduce proteinuria and the rate of progression of CKD [47]. Finally, recurrent episodes of AKI are a particular concern resulting in a step-wise loss of renal function, and any follow-up programme should address the prevention and early detection of new episodes of AKI.

### 3.5.1 Proposed Follow-Up Pathway After AKI

Given the above concerns, we would like to propose a framework for the ideal follow-up of adult patients surviving critical illness complicated by significant AKI (Fig. 3.2). Patients with pre-existing CKD and a new episode of AKI they should *at least* have CKD criteria re-assessed in 90 days to check for CKD progression, if earlier follow-up is not indicated. As more-severe AKI is more likely to result in earlier progression to CKD, in the absence of other evidence, we propose that patients with AKI-KDIGO stage 2 during critical illness should be considered for a specific follow-up pathway. However, many other survivors of critical illness could be at increased risk of CKD, and specific risk factors for CKD (diabetes, hypertension, cardiovascular disease) may indicate monitoring for new CKD within follow-up of that chronic condition. Thus, all patients with AKI stage 2 or greater should receive follow-up of renal function with early review in those with more severe renal dysfunction at discharge (Fig. 3.2). Other patients should have their CKD criteria re-assessed after 90 days with measurement of serum creatinine, calculation of estimated GFR, measurement of urinary albumin-creatinine ratio, urinalysis for micro-haematuria, blood pressure measurement and renal ultrasound (if not recently performed). At this stage patients may require specialist referral, or be deemed appropriate for primary care follow-up at a frequency commensurate with their level of renal dysfunction [48]. Even in the absence of evidence of CKD at 90 days, survivors of significant AKI should have at least one further check for CKD criteria at 1 year to check for late progression, or indefinite follow-up, depending on the presence of other CKD risk factors.

Systems are required to identify and flag AKI survivors for follow-up. This can be problematic as hospital discharge may be many weeks or months from an episode of AKI and the discharging service may not be the one that actively managed the patient during their critical illness. In the UK, only a fraction of patients who required renal replacement therapy in the ICU and recover renal function receive

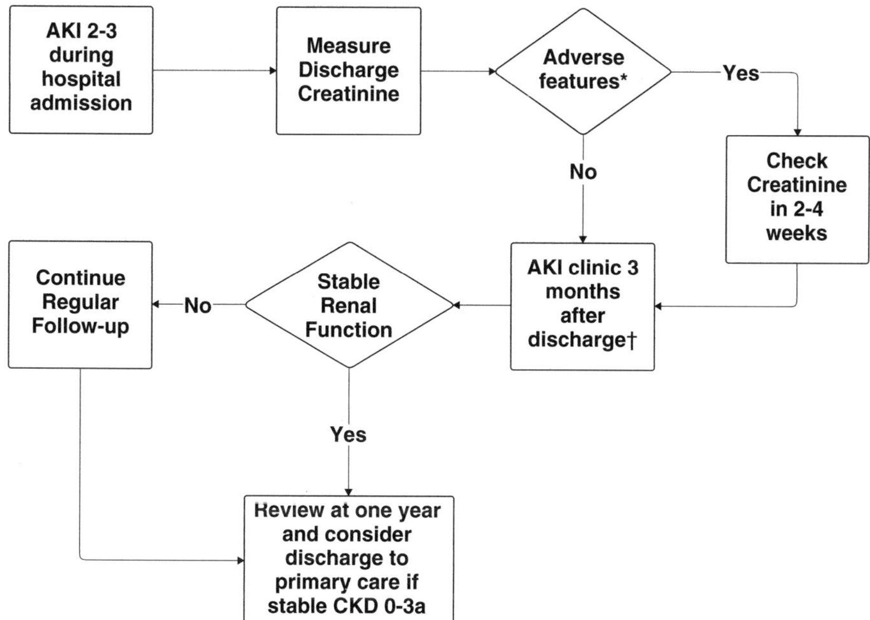


**Fig. 3.2** Outline of a pathway for follow-up of patients who survive and episode of AKI 2 or 3 whilst in hospital. * Adverse features suggesting need for early follow-up include a significant increase in serum creatinine from pre-morbid baseline to discharge (new overt CKD or unrecovered AKI) or the presence of significant renal impairment (suggested as a serum creatinine of >175 μmol/L (2 mg/dl) or eGFR <30 ml/min/1.73 m$^2$). Consider formal measurement of GFR or Creatinine Clearance in patients with prolonged critical illness or significant loss of muscle mass. † Patients with specific features including persistent hematuria or proteinuria (Urine Protein: Creatinine Ratio >100), proven or suspected glomerulonephritis, refractory hypertension, familial renal disease, recurrent or extensive nephrolithiasis, or likely progression to ESRD within 1 year should be referred directly to the appropriate specialist nephrology clinic

nephrology follow-up. In addition, AKI is frequently omitted from hospital discharge summaries and clinical coding, as AKI occurs as a complication of major illness rather than as a presenting complaint. Thus, even when seen in other (non-nephrology) specialist clinics, renal function is often not assessed. These experiences are not isolated: in an analysis of 3,929 survivors of AKI with CKD at discharge carried out in the United States, 1 year mortality was 22 %, however, only 8.5 % received nephrology referral before death, need for chronic dialysis, or experiencing an improvement in kidney function [17]. Unless we adequately identify and monitor patients who have had AKI, we will be unable to improve their outcomes. In many cases appropriate long-term follow-up can be accomplished in primary care, but this is only possible if patients are identified and appropriate clinical guidelines are provided by specialists. There is thus a clear impetus for establishing mechanisms to adequately identify and follow-up patients with AKI in particular after critical illness.

**Conclusion**

As well as being strongly associated with increased morbidity and mortality in the ICU, acute kidney injury is a significant risk factor for the development of chronic kidney disease, and, as a result, adverse long-term outcomes. However, the acute and chronic effects of critical illness can complicate the recognition and staging of CKD after AKI. Thus, this important condition is often neglected, despite the fact that appropriate management can modify risk factors, slow CKD progression, and enable a planned transition to chronic dialysis if required. Robust pathways for monitoring and treating these patients need to be developed and tested.

## References


1. Lowe KG. The late prognosis in acute tubular necrosis; an interim follow-up report on 14 patients. Lancet. 1952;1(6718):1086–8.
2. Finkenstaedt JT, Merrill JP. Renal function after recovery from acute renal failure. N Engl J Med. 1956;254(22):1023–6.
3. Chawla LS, Kimmel PL. Acute kidney injury and chronic kidney disease: an integrated clinical syndrome. Kidney Int. 2012;82(5):516–24.
4. Stevens PE, O'Donoghue DJ, de Lusignan S, et al. Chronic kidney disease management in the United Kingdom: NEOERICA project results. Kidney Int. 2007;72(1):92–9.
5. Go AS, Chertow GM, Fan D, McCulloch CE, Hsu CY. Chronic kidney disease and the risks of death, cardiovascular events, and hospitalization. N Engl J Med. 2004;351(13):1296–305.
6. Kerr M, Bray B, Medcalf J, O'Donoghue DJ, Matthews B. Estimating the financial cost of chronic kidney disease to the NHS in England. Nephrol Dial Transplant. 2012;27 Suppl 3: iii73–80.
7. The National Collaborating Centre for Chronic Conditions (UK). Chronic kidney disease: national clinical guideline for early identification and management in adults in primary and secondary care. London: Royal College of Physicians (UK); 2008; Available from: http://www.nice.org.uk/nicemedia/live/12069/42119/42119.pdf.
8. Mehta RL, Pascual MT, Soroko S, Chertow GM. Diuretics, mortality, and nonrecovery of renal function in acute renal failure. JAMA. 2002;288(20):2547–53.
9. Ishani A, Xue JL, Himmelfarb J, et al. Acute kidney injury increases risk of ESRD among elderly. J Am Soc Nephrol. 2009;20(1):223–8.
10. Amdur RL, Chawla LS, Amodeo S, Kimmel PL, Palant CE. Outcomes following diagnosis of acute renal failure in U.S. veterans: focus on acute tubular necrosis. Kidney Int. 2009;76(10): 1089–97.
11. Lo LJ, Go AS, Chertow GM, et al. Dialysis-requiring acute renal failure increases the risk of progressive chronic kidney disease. Kidney Int. 2009;76(8):893–9.
12. Chawla LS, Amdur RL, Amodeo S, Kimmel PL, Palant CE. The severity of acute kidney injury predicts progression to chronic kidney disease. Kidney Int. 2011;79(12):1361–9.
13. Thakar CV, Christianson A, Himmelfarb J, Leonard AC. Acute kidney injury episodes and chronic kidney disease risk in diabetes mellitus. Clin J Am Soc Nephrol. 2011;6(11): 2567–72.
14. Bucaloiu ID, Kirchner HL, Norfolk ER, Hartle 2nd JE, Perkins RM. Increased risk of death and de novo chronic kidney disease following reversible acute kidney injury. Kidney Int. 2012;81(5):477–85.
15. Jones J, Holmen J, De Graauw J, Jovanovich A, Thornton S, Chonchol M. Association of complete recovery from acute kidney injury with incident CKD stage 3 and all-cause mortality. Am J Kidney Dis. 2012;60(3):402–8.

16. Mammen C, Al Abbas A, Skippen P, et al. Long-term risk of CKD in children surviving episodes of acute kidney injury in the intensive care unit: a prospective cohort study. Am J Kidney Dis. 2012;59(4):523–30.
17. Siew ED, Peterson JF, Eden SK, et al. Outpatient nephrology referral rates after acute kidney injury. J Am Soc Nephrol. 2012;23(2):305–12.
18. Venkatachalam MA, Griffin KA, Lan R, Geng H, Saikumar P, Bidani AK. Acute kidney injury: a springboard for progression in chronic kidney disease. Am J Physiol Renal Physiol. 2010;298(5):F1078–94.
19. Metcalfe W. How does early chronic kidney disease progress? A background paper prepared for the UK Consensus Conference on early chronic kidney disease. Nephrol Dial Transplant. 2007;22 Suppl 9:ix26–30.
20. Pechman KR, De Miguel C, Lund H, Leonard EC, Basile DP, Mattson DL. Recovery from renal ischemia-reperfusion injury is associated with altered renal hemodynamics, blunted pressure natriuresis, and sodium-sensitive hypertension. Am J Physiol Regul Integr Comp Physiol. 2009;297(5):R1358–63.
21. Basile DP, Leonard EC, Tonade D, Friedrich JL, Goenka S. Distinct effects on long-term function of injured and contralateral kidneys following unilateral renal ischemia-reperfusion. Am J Physiol Renal Physiol. 2012;302(5):F625–35.
22. Basile DP, Donohoe D, Roethe K, Osborn JL. Renal ischemic injury results in permanent damage to peritubular capillaries and influences long-term function. Am J Physiol Renal Physiol. 2001;281(5):F887–99.
23. Basile DP, Leonard EC, Beal AG, Schleuter D, Friedrich J. Persistent oxidative stress following renal ischemia-reperfusion injury increases ANG II hemodynamic and fibrotic activity. Am J Physiol Renal Physiol. 2012;302(11):F1494–502.
24. Wilson FP, Sheehan JM, Mariani LH, Berns JS. Creatinine generation is reduced in patients requiring continuous venovenous hemodialysis and independently predicts mortality. Nephrol Dial Transplant. 2012;27(11):4088–94.
25. Doi K, Yuen PS, Eisner C, et al. Reduced production of creatinine limits its use as marker of kidney injury in sepsis. J Am Soc Nephrol. 2009;20(6):1217–21.
26. Endre ZH, Pickering JW, Walker RJ. Clearance and beyond: the complementary roles of GFR measurement and injury biomarkers in acute kidney injury (AKI). Am J Physiol Renal Physiol. 2011;301(4):F697–707.
27. Haase M, Devarajan P, Haase-Fielitz A, et al. The outcome of neutrophil gelatinase-associated lipocalin-positive subclinical acute kidney injury: a multicenter pooled analysis of prospective studies. J Am Coll Cardiol. 2011;57(17):1752–61.
28. Sherman DS, Fish DN, Teitelbaum I. Assessing renal function in cirrhotic patients: problems and pitfalls. Am J Kidney Dis. 2003;41(2):269–78.
29. Shlipak MG, Matsushita K, Ärnlöv J, et al. Cystatin C versus creatinine in determining risk based on kidney function. N Engl J Med. 2013;369(10):932–43.
30. Hill AA, Plank LD, Finn PJ, et al. Massive nitrogen loss in critical surgical illness: effect on cardiac mass and function. Ann Surg. 1997;226(2):191–7.
31. Monk DN, Plank LD, Franch-Arcas G, Finn PJ, Streat SJ, Hill GL. Sequential changes in the metabolic response in critically injured patients during the first 25 days after blunt trauma. Ann Surg. 1996;223(4):395–405.
32. Puthucheary ZA, Rawal J, McPhail M, et al. Acute skeletal muscle wasting in critical illness. JAMA. 2013;310(15):1591–600.
33. Gruther W, Benesch T, Zorn C, et al. Muscle wasting in intensive care patients: ultrasound observation of the M. quadriceps femoris muscle layer. J Rehabil Med Off J Eur Board Phys Rehabil Med. 2008;40(3):185–9.
34. Reid CL, Campbell IT, Little RA. Muscle wasting and energy balance in critical illness. Clin Nutr. 2004;23(2):273–80.
35. Bosch JP, Saccaggi A, Lauer A, Ronco C, Belledonne M, Glabman S. Renal functional reserve in humans. Effect of protein intake on glomerular filtration rate. Am J Med. 1983;75(6):943–50.

36. Ronco C, Rosner MH. Acute kidney injury and residual renal function. Crit Care. 2012;
    16(4):144.
37. Brenner BM, Lawler EV, Mackenzie HS. The hyperfiltration theory: a paradigm shift in
    nephrology. Kidney Int. 1996;49(6):1774–7.
38. Chronic Kidney Disease Prognosis Consortium, Matsushita K, van der Velde M, et al.
    Association of estimated glomerular filtration rate and albuminuria with all-cause and cardio-
    vascular mortality in general population cohorts: a collaborative meta-analysis. Lancet.
    2010;375(9731):2073–81.
39. Levey AS, de Jong PE, Coresh J, et al. The definition, classification, and prognosis of chronic
    kidney disease: a KDIGO Controversies Conference report. Kidney Int. 2011;80(1):17–28.
40. Srisawat N, Murugan R, Lee M, et al. Plasma neutrophil gelatinase-associated lipocalin pre-
    dicts recovery from acute kidney injury following community-acquired pneumonia. Kidney
    Int. 2011;80(5):545–52.
41. Srisawat N, Wen X, Lee M, et al. Urinary biomarkers and renal recovery in critically ill patients
    with renal support. Clin J Am Soc Nephrol. 2011;6(8):1815–23.
42. Schneider AG, Bellomo R, Bagshaw SM, et al. Choice of renal replacement therapy modality
    and dialysis dependence after acute kidney injury: a systematic review and meta-analysis.
    Intensive Care Med. 2013;39(6):987–97.
43. Manns M, Sigler MH, Teehan BP. Intradialytic renal haemodynamics–potential consequences
    for the management of the patient with acute renal failure. Nephrol Dial Transplant.
    1997;12(5):870–2.
44. Glassford NJ, Bellomo R. Acute kidney injury: how can we facilitate recovery? Curr Opin Crit
    Care. 2011;17(6):562–8.
45. Chawla LS, Kellum JA, Ronco C. Permissive hypofiltration. Crit Care. 2012;16(4):317.
46. Harel Z, Wald R, Bargman JM, et al. Nephrologist follow-up improves all-cause mortality of
    severe acute kidney injury survivors. Kidney Int. 2013;83(5):901–8.
47. Jafar TH, Stark PC, Schmid CH, et al. Proteinuria as a modifiable risk factor for the progres-
    sion of non-diabetic renal disease. Kidney Int. 2001;60(3):1131–40.
48. Kidney Disease: Improving Global Outcomes (KDIGO) CKD Work Group. KDIGO 2012
    clinical practice guideline for the evaluation and management of chronic kidney disease.
    Kidney Int Suppl. 2013;3:1–150.

# Etiology and Pathophysiology of Acute Kidney Injury

4


Anne-Cornélie J.M. de Pont, John R. Prowle,
Mathieu Legrand, and A.B. Johan Groeneveld


## 4.1 Introduction

Acute kidney injury (AKI) is estimated to complicate around 5 % of critical care admissions [1]. AKI frequently occurs in the context of multiple organ failure and entails mortality rates in excess of 40 % despite appropriate therapy [1]. Etiologies for AKI are varied and multiple factors often coexist in critically ill patients. While sepsis and nephrotoxin exposure are major risk factors for AKI in the ICU, direct ischemia/reperfusion (I/R) injury may also play a role, especially in hypovolemic and cardiogenic shock. It seems likely that most patients develop AKI as a result of multiple risk factors [2]. Despite these diverse causes, the ultimate presentation of established AKI is relatively uniform, with renal tubular injury mediating a decline in glomerular filtration rate and in the most severe cases oliguric renal failure. This chapter focuses on the causes and pathophysiology of AKI in critical illness. For


A.C.J.M. de Pont (✉)
Department of Intensive Care, Academic Medical Center, University of Amsterdam,
Amsterdam, The Netherlands
e-mail: a.c.depont@amc.uva.nl

J.R. Prowle
Adult Critical Care Unit, The Royal London Hospital, Bart's and the London NHS Trust,
London, UK
e-mail: john.prowle@bartshealth.nhs.uk

M. Legrand
Department of Anesthesiology and Critical Care,
Hôpital Européen Georges Pompidou Assistance Publique-Hopitaux de Paris,
Sorbonne Paris Cité, Paris, France
e-mail: mathieu.legrand@gmail.com

A.B.J. Groeneveld
Department of Intensive Care Medicine, Erasmus Medical Centre,
Doctor Molewaterplein 50-60, Rotterdam, The Netherlands
e-mail: a.b.j.groeneveld@erasmusmc.nl



© Springer International Publishing 2015
H.M. Oudemans-van Straaten et al. (eds.), *Acute Nephrology for the Critical
Care Physician*, DOI 10.1007/978-3-319-17389-4_4

clarity we separately discuss AKI etiologies, although it should be reemphasized that in the real world these mechanisms often coexist [3–5].

## 4.2 Sepsis

Nearly 50 % of the cases of AKI in the intensive care unit occur in the context of sepsis [1]. We will briefly summarize mechanisms of sepsis-induced AKI.

### 4.2.1 Renal Hemodynamics in Sepsis

While a fall in renal blood flow has been considered an important factor in septic AKI, there is growing evidence that blood flow to the kidneys may not be severely compromised in septic shock and that an inflammatory component is largely responsible for a decline in renal function [6].

Renal blood flow has been estimated by a wide variety of techniques including renal vein thermodilution and Doppler ultrasound [7–10]. The most easily applied ultrasound technique, Doppler renal resistive index, provides the pulsatility or resistance index in renal arteries and measures renal vascular resistance rather than absolute blood flow [11]. Phase contrast-enhanced magnetic resonance imaging is another method [12], but cannot be applied at the bedside. Measurements of effective renal blood flow by plasma clearance of para-aminohippuric acid (*PAH*) or other substances normally excreted by the tubules may be inaccurate, since in sepsis-induced AKI the extraction of these substances by the renal tubules may decline to less than 50 %. In experimental studies, renal blood flow has also been assessed with the help of microspheres and flow probes around the renal artery, while the renal microcirculation has been studied using visualizing techniques [13, 14].

Most studies in sepsis indicate a fall in renal perfusion during AKI, but other studies suggest a normal to elevated renal blood flow [7, 12]. In a recent review, renal blood flow during sepsis was either preserved or increased in one-third of the studies included and cardiac output seemed a direct determinant of renal blood flow [15]. While the kidney may initially participate in the general vasodilated state of sepsis, development of AKI may be accompanied by selective renal vasoconstriction causing a relative reduction in renal blood flow and glomerular filtration rate. During sepsis and shock, renal blood flow and glomerular filtration may become more dependent on perfusion pressure than normal; therefore, low cardiac output and arterial hypotension are considered major risk factors for AKI during sepsis. However, even in the case of a normal or elevated cardiac output and in the absence of a severe fall in blood pressure, reduction in glomerular filtration may occur as a result of renal vasoconstriction or inflammatory responses [6]. Indeed, targeting a higher mean arterial pressure in patients with sepsis did neither result in improvement of renal function, nor in a lower incidence of AKI [16, 17].

For filtration, glomeruli need an adequate plasma flow and capillary pressure. Both renal blood flow and glomerular pressure are defended by autoregulation.

However, during progressive reduction in cardiac output, prostaglandin-induced renal vasodilation is overwhelmed by intrarenal vasoconstrictive responses to maintain systemic and intra-glomerular pressure, causing an abrupt fall in glomerular filtration.

During a fall in renal perfusion, glomerular filtration is normally better autoregulated than renal blood flow, due to a rise in tone of the efferent over the afferent glomerular arterioles, resulting in a rise in filtration fraction (i.e., filtration divided by renal plasma flow). However, regardless of absolute blood flow, filtration fraction in sepsis is usually low, probably due to a fall in efferent over afferent arteriolar tone [18]. Increased tubuloglomerular feedback may finally contribute to a sustained fall in glomerular perfusion and filtration in established AKI independent of systemic hemodynamics [19].

The unique microvascular architecture of the kidney shows a network with high capillary density within the cortex to ensure filtration function and poor capillary density in the medulla organized serially to facilitate osmotic gradient generation for urine concentration [13]. A consequence of this architecture is that an oxygen gradient exists between the cortex and the inner medulla from around 70 mmHg in the cortex to <20 mmHg in the inner medulla. The low oxygen tension in the medulla results from physiological oxygen shunting within the kidney, low regional medullary blood flow and high oxygen consumption within the medulla for tubular function [20]. The combination of low oxygen delivery and high oxygen demand puts the medulla and thus the proximal tubule at high risk of ischemia.

## 4.2.2 Regulation of Renal Hemodynamics in Sepsis

Figure 4.1 gives an overview of the systems affecting renal blood flow and metabolism in sepsis. The sympathetic nervous system directly controls renal vascular tone and is activated early during sepsis. This may contribute to renal vasoconstriction, stimulation of renin release, and redistribution of renal blood flow from the cortex to the medulla.

The renin–angiotensin–aldosterone system (RAAS) is activated during sepsis and hypotension. Renin release is stimulated by the fall in renal perfusion and is also influenced by prostaglandins, the sympathetic nervous system, and the kallikrein system. Angiotensin II may potentiate norepinephrine release, but also stimulates production of vasodilating prostaglandins, kallikrein, and nitric oxide (NO). Angiotensin II constricts efferent arterioles, thereby reducing renal blood flow but increasing filtration fraction. Besides its vascular effects, angiotensin II may also contract mesangial cells, reducing the surface area available for filtration.

The production of renal prostaglandins depends on the availability of arachidonic acid and phospholipase ($PLA_2$). Activation of $PLA_2$ and increased production of arachidonic acid metabolites can be triggered by several factors such as endotoxin, cytokines, platelet activating factor (PAF), tissue hypoxia, reactive oxygen species (ROS), and angiotensin II. Prostaglandins interact in a complex fashion with other regulatory systems, since they may mediate renin secretion, reduce

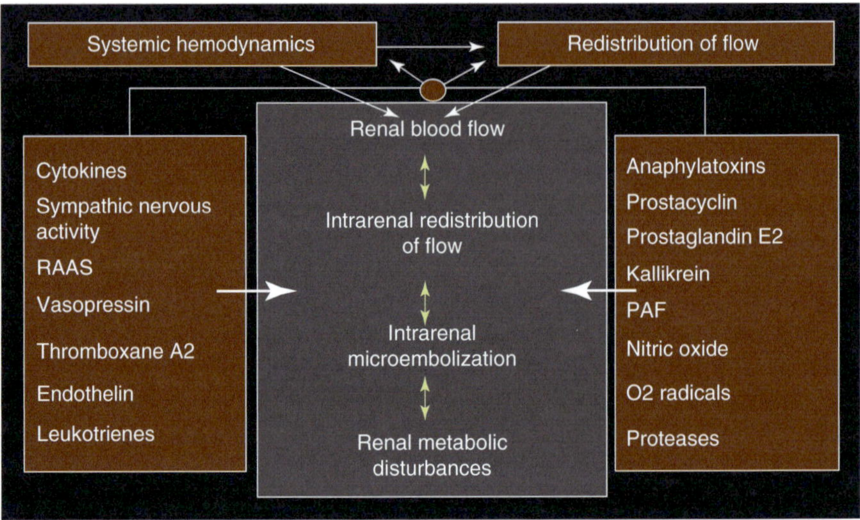


**Fig. 4.1** An overview of the systems affecting renal blood flow and metabolism in sepsis

catecholamine actions, and contribute to the release of vasopressin. Normal renal hemodynamics does not depend on the vasoactive prostaglandins. During a fall in cardiac output, however, vasodilating prostaglandin $E_2$ and prostacyclin $PGI_2$ are released. Conversely, activation of the lipoxygenase pathway during sepsis yields leukotrienes having vasoconstrictive properties, which adversely interfere with the filtration coefficient. Their blockade may be beneficial for renal perfusion and function. Inhibition of the cyclooxygenase-derived compounds by non-steroidal anti-inflammatory drugs (NSAIDs) reduces renal blood flow during experimental sepsis, suggesting a predominantly vasodilating effect of prostaglandins generated via cyclooxygenase in the kidney.

The balance between endothelin and NO may play a critical role in renal perfusion during sepsis. Endothelin is a potent renal vasoconstrictor and expression of endothelin receptors is increased during sepsis. The kidney produces endothelin upon stimuli including endotoxin and tumor necrosis factor (TNF)-α. Endothelin may constrict afferent more than efferent vessels, which decreases renal blood flow and glomerular filtration.

During sepsis, morphological and functional alterations of the renal microcirculation have been observed, involving vasoconstriction and capillary clotting [21, 22]. Oxidative stress and the NO-system have been described as major contributors to these phenomena. ROS can injure the endothelium, damage the glycocalyx, and impair the endothelium-dependent vasoreactivity [18, 23, 24]. NO is formed by enzymatic cleavage from L-arginine by NO-synthetase. Especially NO derived from endothelial NO-synthetase (eNOS) plays an essential role in maintaining the renal vascular homeostasis. It dilates afferent vessels in response to shear stress and angiotensin II-mediated vasoconstriction, and inhibits tubuloglomerular feedback, increasing renal blood flow. It also inhibits platelet aggregation and leukocyte activation. eNOS-derived NO thus regulates vascular tone, influences the filtration coefficient, mediates the effects of macula densa stimulation, defends medullary oxygen supply, and mediates pressure-induced sodium excretion.

On the other hand, activation of inducible NO-synthase (iNOS) has been shown to promote renal injury. Endotoxin induces the activation of iNOS, leading to the formation of intracellular ROS and reactive nitrogen species (RNS) [25, 26]. Intracellular ROS and RNS are able to damage mitochondria, leading to apoptosis. In addition, iNOS-derived NO enables shedding of tubular epithelial cells by cytokines [27]. In an attempt to mitigate renal injury caused by iNOS, septic patients were treated with an NO-synthetase inhibitor. Although this treatment increased the percentage of shock reversal, it did not change the incidence of AKI [28].

Adenosine also plays a role in the pathophysiology of sepsis-associated AKI. During stress caused by inflammation and hypoxia, adenosine triphosphate (ATP) can be released from the cell, stimulating inflammation by attracting phagocytes and activating inflammasomes [29]. The enzyme alkaline phosphatase can convert ATP to adenosine, which has anti-inflammatory and tissue protective effects [30]. A small randomized controlled trial of alkaline phosphatase in patients with sepsis showed significant improvement of a composite endpoint consisting of creatinine clearance and requirement of renal replacement therapy [31].

## 4.2.3 Cell Signaling and Inflammation

During sepsis, multiple cell lines, cytokines, vasoactive substances as well as the coagulation and the complement cascade participate in the inflammatory response to infection [32]. Essential for host defense is the recognition of molecular patterns by so-called toll-like receptors (TLRs) localized on the membrane of different cell types. TLRs recognize molecules derived from bacteria, viruses, fungi, and parasites known as pathogen-associated molecular patterns (PAMPs). TLRs are also able to recognize molecules released during tissue injury, known as damage-associated molecular patterns (DAMPs). In the kidney, TLR-2 and TLR-4 are expressed both in endothelial, glomerular, and epithelial cells of Bowman's capsule and the proximal and distal tubules [33]. Activation of TLRs triggers a series of events leading to the expression of pro-inflammatory genes [34]. Moreover, TLRs can be upregulated in the presence of interferon-γ and TNF.

Several studies in animal models of sepsis have demonstrated the role of TNF in the development of acute kidney injury: mice lacking a TNF receptor are resistant to endotoxin-induced acute kidney injury and TNF-receptor negative kidneys are resistant to endotoxin-induced damage when transplanted into TNF-positive mice [32]. In human sepsis, elevated serum levels of two soluble TNF-receptors are strongly associated with the development of acute kidney injury [35]. TNF is believed to induce apoptotic cell death through intracellular signaling. Renal tubular cells express cell surface 'death receptors' of the TNF superfamily, including TNF-receptor 1, Fas and FN14 receptor. TNF, TNF-like weak inducer of apoptosis (TWEAK) and Fas ligand can all activate caspases (cysteine-dependent aspartate directed proteases), enzymes with the ability to initiate apoptosis [36].

In a cascade-like manner, caspases activate other target caspases by cleaving away prodomains, ultimately activating effector caspases such as caspase-3, which cleaves multiple structural molecules, resulting in the morphologic changes that define apoptosis [37]. Treatment with a caspase-3 inhibitor was demonstrated to have a renoprotective effect in mice [38]. Caspase-1 has the ability to activate interleukin-1β and interleukin-18, cytokines playing an important role in the inflammatory process occurring during septic acute kidney injury. Blocking the activation of these cytokines also had a renoprotective effect in mice [39]. Moreover, in a murine sepsis model, combined inhibition of IL-1 and IL-18 protected animals against a lethal challenge with endotoxin [40].

Inflammation is an important component of both the initiation and extension of injury in AKI [41]. Endothelial injury stimulates the recruitment of leukocytes to the renal tissue and promotes leukocyte adhesion and migration. Leukocyte adhesion is mediated by adhesion molecules known as selectins, of which intercellular adhesion molecule-1 (ICAM-1) appears to be essential to the transendothelial migration of leukocytes [42]. The low microcirculatory blood flow observed during sepsis further facilitates the interaction between inflammatory cells and the endothelium through prolonged exposure to leukocytes and inflammatory mediators, which amplify the local inflammatory response and renal injury.

Coagulation plays an important role in the pathogenesis of sepsis. Inflammatory mediators such as endotoxin and cytokines may activate the coagulation cascade, which results in thrombin formation. Thrombin itself is a proinflammatory agent with the ability to activate inflammatory cells, which in turn produce cytokines, thus promoting an amplifying loop. The literature on the role of the coagulation cascade in the pathogenesis of acute kidney injury is scarce. Recently, the contribution of microparticles to various pathophysiologic processes has gained interest. Microparticles are small lipid bilayer vesicular bodies originating from activated or apoptotic cells. They often carry phosphatidylserine in their outer layer, which may act as a surface for activated clot formation. In addition, microparticle bound coagulation factors such as tissue factor may initiate coagulation during sepsis. A recent study among patients with severe sepsis showed that patients with renal injury had significantly increased numbers of circulating microparticles [43]. This finding suggests that activation of the coagulation pathway also plays a role in the pathogenesis of septic acute kidney injury.

### 4.2.4   Tissue Injury and Apoptosis

Historically, renal tubular epithelial cell necrosis was regarded as the characteristic lesion in septic AKI. However, analysis of kidney biopsies from patients who died of septic shock showed limited evidence for acute tubular necrosis, but did show tubular and glomerular cell apoptosis and infiltration of monocytes [44]. During experimental sepsis, glomeruli and interstitium are also infiltrated by activated neutrophils [32, 45]. Tubular apoptosis rather than necrosis may thus prevail in vulnerable proximal tubules. However, the relevance of apoptosis to organ dysfunction has been debated [44].

## 4.3    Ischemia and Reperfusion (I/R)

The I/R injury of the kidney mainly occurs in clinical conditions such as cardiovascular surgery, shock, trauma, resuscitation, and other situations associated with hypotension, low cardiac output or both [46]. The time interval of complete blood flow interruption that leads to renal injury in animals is 30–45 min, but in humans the period can be longer, as observed during vascular and renal surgery [47]. Reperfusion during shock resuscitation stimulates inflammatory factors, therefore, I/R injury shares many pathways with the pathogenesis of AKI in inflammatory states.

### 4.3.1    Hemodynamics

Severe renal hypoperfusion leads to ischemia, which may only be partially reversed during reperfusion [13]. However, in the absence of other risk factors, near 100 % occlusion of the renal circulation is required to cause significant ischemic renal injury [48]. Doppler and contrast-enhanced ultrasonography yield an index of renal vascular resistance and regional perfusion at the bedside and show marked increases in resistance in patients at risk for developing AKI [9, 10, 13, 14, 49].

When injured tubules reabsorb less sodium and water, this results in a negative feedback to the RAAS system at the macula densa and activation of the tubuloglomerular feedback, causing afferent vasoconstriction contributing to a sustained fall in perfusion and filtration. In particular the blood flow to the cortico-medullary junction, an area with baseline supply dependence for oxygenation, can remain compromised during reperfusion. The microvasculature in this region becomes congested due to interstitial edema, red blood cell trapping, leukocyte adherence, and extravasation upon reperfusion [50]. A fall in renal blood flow due to microvascular injury and tubuloglomerular feedback, a rise in the pre- to post-glomerular capillary resistance ratio and increased tubular luminal pressure opposing filtration across the tubular epithelium can all contribute to the low glomerular filtration following I/R [51].

### 4.3.2    Endothelial and Vascular Smooth Muscle Injury

Endothelial and vascular smooth muscle cells are damaged by ischemia, which contributes to vascular dysfunction [52, 53]. This includes diminished capability to autoregulate vascular tone following endothelial dysfunction. The endothelium-dependent relaxation to acetylcholine may be less effective in defending against constriction of the renal artery after I/R, and this may be associated with increased endothelin and impaired NO production by eNOS, in part downregulated by iNOS [54, 55].

### 4.3.3    Tubular Injury

Renal tubular cells are polarized, the apical and basolateral side having different composition and function. The tight junction separates the apical and basolateral membrane and provides a barrier to parallel transport of water and solutes. The adherens junction is located directly basal to the tight junction and contributes to cell polarity [56]. ATP depletion disrupts both the tight and adherens junction, leading to loss of cell polarity, increase in permeability and back-leak of glomerular filtrate. Prolonged ATP depletion leads to disruption of the actin cytoskeleton, collapse and detachment of tubular cells with shedding in the tubular lumen and excretion into the urine [56].

### 4.3.4 Cell Signaling and Inflammation

Factors which may trigger inflammatory injury after renal I/R include activation of the complement system, adherence of the membrane attack complex, microvascular thrombosis, generation of ROS, and stimulation of tubular NFκB [34]. In addition, histones derived from dying cells trigger TLRs, thereby contributing to the perpetuation of AKI [57]. These processes lead to the generation of multiple cytokines and pro-inflammatory molecules that mediate inflammatory injury after I/R [58–61]. In response to endothelial activation, inflammatory mediators, cytokines, and chemokines induce rolling, sticking, and infiltration of activated neutrophils to the interstitium, which contributes to interstitial edema and may limit the recovery of renal blood flow [50, 60]. Cytoskeletal alterations may be involved in the transmigration of neutrophils via loosened intercellular junctions. After mild I/R of the kidneys, endotoxin exposure and neutrophil priming can further contribute to AKI, and as a consequence, retention of activated neutrophils and further release of proteases and ROS. Following neutrophil infiltration, a monocyte/macrophage infiltrate may become apparent up to 24 h after renal I/R, which may be involved in tissue repair [62] or conversely in development of fibrosis and chronic renal injury [53, 63].

### 4.3.5 Tissue Apoptosis, Necrosis, and Repair

Apoptotic and necrotic forms of cell death coexist in I/R kidneys [36, 64, 65; Fig. 4.2]. The relative contribution of the two types of cell death depends on the severity of the injury. The degree of cellular ATP and GTP depletion may play a crucial role in determining the mode of cell death [64, 66]. Survival mechanisms may allow the cells to produce growth factors such as hepatocyte growth factor (HGF) that may regenerate proximal and distal tubules [65, 67–71]. Collectively, a range of factors may promote inflammation, apoptosis, and ultimately fibrosis after renal injury, as opposed to tubular regeneration, redifferentiation, and full restoration of renal function [71].

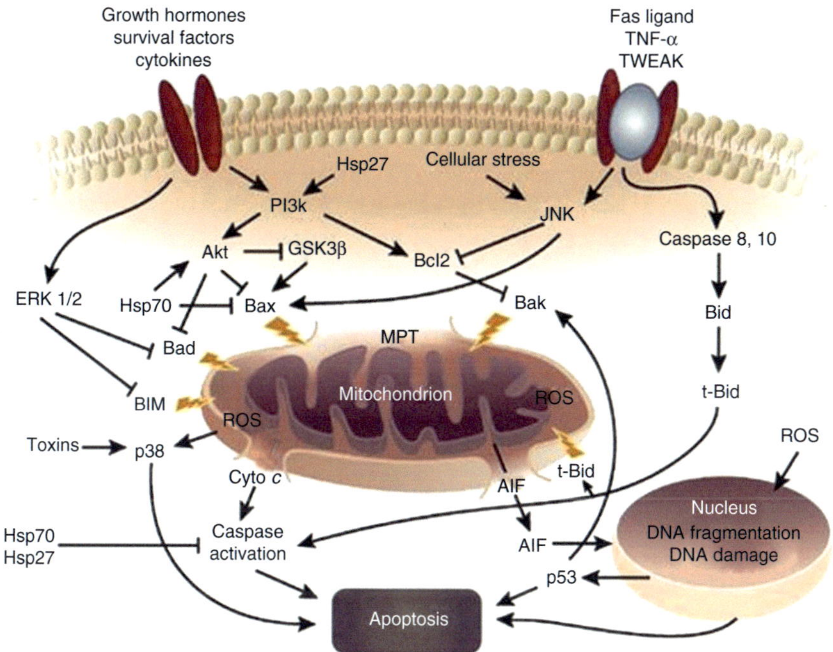


**Fig. 4.2** Interaction between inflammation and apoptosis (Reproduced with permission from Nature publishing Group [36]). *Abbreviations*: *AIF* apoptosis-inducing factor, *Akt* protein kinase B, *Bax*, *Bad*, *Bak*, and truncated or *t-Bid* are proapoptotic BCL2 proteins, *Bcl2* antiapoptotic BCL2 protein, *Cyto c* cytochrome c, *ERK1/2* extracellular regulated kinase 1/2, *GSK3b* glycogen synthase kinase 3-b, *Hsp* heat stress protein, *JNK* Jun-N-terminal kinase, *MPT* outer mitochondrial membrane pore transition, *p38* mitogen-activated protein kinase, *p53* a tumor-suppressor protein, *PI3k* phosphatidylinositol 3-kinase, *ROS*, reactive oxygen species generated by mitochondria or other sources, *TNF-α* tumor necrosis factor-α, *TWEAK* TNF-related weak inducer of apoptosis. *ERK1/2 and JNK* are stress-regulated kinases, *Hsp70* is heat stress protein 70 kDa an antiapoptotic protein, *Hsp27* is heat stress protein 27 kDa is a TNF family member, *BID* stands for BH3 interacting-domain death agonist. It is a pro-apoptotic member of the Bcl-2 protein family

## 4.4  Nephrotoxicity

Nephrotoxin exposure accounts for up to 25 % of the cases of AKI in the intensive care unit [72]. Nephrotoxicity may be promoted by factors relating to the patient, the kidney and the ingested toxic substance [73]. Critically ill patients are vulnerable to nephrotoxicity due to compromised renal perfusion. The kidney itself is prone for toxicity because it takes up toxins and concentrates them in interstitium and medulla. Renal tubular cells have a high metabolic rate requiring a substantial amount of energy and their environment is relatively hypoxic, increasing the risk of hypoxic injury to the tubular cells. Toxins may potentiate renal injury induced by other causes. Moreover, hypoalbuminemia often occurs in critically ill patients, leading to a higher plasma free fraction of potentially toxic agents [74].

The most important nephrotoxins are drugs frequently used in the ICU, such as antibiotics, analgesics, and radiocontrast [72–78]. However, outpatient exposure to nephrotoxins such as heavy metals and certain herbs may also cause nephrotoxicity [79, 80] (Table 4.1). All compartments of the kidney can be injured by toxic substances: renal vessels, glomeruli, tubular system, collecting ducts, and interstitium (Table 4.2). The pathophysiologic mechanisms of the injury to the different compartments of the kidney are briefly described.

### 4.4.1 Agents Altering Hemodynamics

Substances causing vasoconstriction of the renal vasculature, such as norepinephrine, vasopressin, radiocontrast, calcineurin inhibitors, and amphotericin B decrease renal perfusion and glomerular capillary hydrostatic pressure, thereby decreasing the glomerular filtration rate [73, 75]. When renal perfusion is decreased, it becomes prostaglandin dependent. In this situation, NSAIDs may further compromise glomerular perfusion by increasing the vascular tone of the afferent arteriole. Lowering the vascular tone of the efferent arteriole with angiotensin converting enzyme inhibitors or angiotensin receptor blockers may further decrease glomerular filtration pressure and thus glomerular filtration rate.

### 4.4.2 Agents Causing Injury to Small Vessels

Several drugs can induce renal vascular disease. Thrombotic microangiopathy can be induced by platelet aggregation inhibitors, calcineurin inhibitors, chemotherapeutics, interferon, quinine, and cocaine [76, 81]. Renal vasculitis may be induced by penicillamine, allopurinol, and phenytoin and hyaline arteriolopathy can be induced by calcineurin inhibitors. Finally, anticoagulants and fibrinolytics may cause cholesterol emboli [81].

### 4.4.3 Agents Causing Glomerular Injury

Several drugs can induce glomerulopathies: NSAIDs, penicillins and quinolones may cause minimal change nephropathy, whereas pamidronate, lithium, and interferon may cause focal and segmental glomerulosclerosis. In addition, NSAIDs, penicillamine and captopril can cause membranous glomerulonephritis [81].

**Table 4.1**  Groups of nephrotoxic agents

| Antimicrobial agents | Lead |
|---|---|
| Aminoglycosides | Mercury |
| Antiviral agents | Uranium |
| Amphotericin B | Herbal agents |
| Quinolones | Taxus |
| Sulfonamides | Euphorbia |
| Sulfadiazine | Immunosuppressives |
| Analgesics | Calcineurin inhibitors |
| NSAIDs | Tacrolimus |
| Selective COX-2 inhibitors | Osmotic agents |
| Chemotherapeutics | Dextrans |
| Ifosfamide | Immunoglobulins |
| Methotrexate | Mannitol |
| Platins | Starches |
| Contrast agents | Vasodilators |
| Radiocontrast | Angiotensin converting enzyme inhibitors |
| Gadolinium | Angiotensin receptor blockers |
| Heavy metals | Vasopressors |
| Bismuth | Norepinephrine |
| Cadmium | Vasopressin |
| Copper | Lead |

**Table 4.2**  Pathophysiologic mechanisms of nephrotoxicity

| Impact on hemodynamics | Cisplatin |
|---|---|
| Norepinephrine | Ifosfamide |
| Vasopressine | Adefovir |
| NSAIDs | Cidofovir |
| Angiotensin converting enzyme inhibitors | Foscarnet |
| Angiotensin receptor blockers | Cocaine |
| Radiocontrast | Osmotic agents |
| Amphotericin B | Mannitol |
| Small vessel injury | Immunoglobulins |
| Thrombotic microangiopathy | Dextrans |
| Calcineurin inhibitors | Starches |
| Chemotherapeutics | Urinary obstruction |
| Platelet aggregation inhibitors | Crystal precipitation |
| Interferon | Sulfonamides |
| Quinine | Quinolones |
| Cocaine | Nitrofurantoin |
| Vasculitis | Acyclovir |
| Allopurinol | Indinavir |
| Penicillamine | Methotrexate |

(continued)

**Table 4.2** (continued)

| | |
|---|---|
| Phenytoine | Triamterene |
| Hyaline arteriolopathy | Myoglobin precipitation |
| Calcineurin inhibitors | Antibiotics |
| Cholesterol emboli | Neuroleptics |
| Thrombolytic agents | Illicit drugs |
| Heparin | Statins |
| Warfarin | Retroperitoneal fibrosis |
| Glomerular injury | Dopamine agonists |
| Minimal change nephropathy | Ergot alkaloids |
| Lithium | Interstitial nephritis |
| NSAIDs | Antibiotics |
| Interferon | Beta-lactams |
| Penicillin | Quinolones |
| Quinolones | Macrolides |
| Focal and segmental glomerulosclerosis | Rifampin |
| Pamidronate | Sulfonamides |
| Lithium | Tetracyclines |
| Heroine | Antivirals |
| Interferon | Acyclovir |
| Membranous glomerulonephritis | Indinavir |
| NSAIDs | Cocaine |
| Penicillamine | NSAIDs |
| Captopril | Diuretics |
| Tubular injury | Thiazide diuretics |
| Direct toxicity | Loop diuretics |
| Aminoglycosides | H2 receptor blockers |
| Amphotericin B | Anticonvulsants |
| Radiocontrast | |

## 4.4.4 Agents Causing Tubular Injury

The role of the proximal tubule in concentrating and reabsorbing glomerular filtrate renders it vulnerable to toxicity. Therefore, tubular toxicity most often occurs in the proximal tubule. Tubular damage can occur through direct toxicity, causing cell membrane damage, formation of ROS, mitochondrial dysfunction, apoptosis, and cell cast formation. Agents most frequently implied in tubular toxicity are radiocontrast, antimicrobials such as aminoglycosides and amphotericin B; chemotherapeutics such as cisplatin and ifosfamide; and antiviral agents such as adefovir, cidofovir, and foscarnet [72, 73, 82]. Cocaine and heavy metals may also cause tubular damage by means of direct toxicity. The mechanism by which osmotic agents induce tubular injury is different: uptake of hyperosmolar molecules in the tubular cell causes an oncotic gradient entailing cell swelling and tubular obstruction. This type of tubular injury is described for mannitol, immunoglobulins, dextrans, and starches [76].

## 4.4.5 Agents Causing Injury by Urinary Obstruction

Some substances can cause precipitation of crystals in the distal tubular lumen, entailing urinary obstruction. This mechanism is generally pH-dependent and is described for antibiotics such as sulfonamides and triamterene and for antiviral agents such as acyclovir and indinavir [76]. Chemotherapeutic agents causing tumor lysis syndrome may cause precipitation of uric acid and calcium phosphate crystals. Rhabdomyolysis can be elicited by a great number of drugs and may induce tubular obstruction by causing intratubular myoglobin precipitation [83]. Urinary obstruction can also be caused by substances inducing retroperitoneal fibrosis, such as dopamine agonists and derivatives of ergot alkaloids such as ergotamine [84].

## 4.4.6 Agents Causing Injury to the Interstitium

The interstitium can be damaged by acute or chronic tubulointerstitial nephritis (TIN). Acute interstitial nephritis is most commonly induced by a non-dose-dependent allergic response to a drug or toxic substance: the substance elicits the production of antibodies against components of the tubular basement membrane, either by acting as a haptene or by mimicking an antigen normally present in the basement membrane. The immune complexes formed may be deposited in the interstitium [85, 86]. Substances most often implied in TIN are NSAIDs, thiazide and loop diuretics, antibiotics such as beta-lactams, quinolones, macrolides, sulfonamides, tetracyclines and rifampin, $H_2$-blockers, proton pump inhibitors, anticonvulsants, and antivirals. Cocaine-induced TIN has also been described [87].

> **Conclusions**
>
> AKI in critical illness reflects a combination of baseline risk and diverse etiological factors, in particular inflammatory responses and reduction in renal perfusion. Most severe renal injury occurs in patients with a baseline hazard such as chronic kidney disease or diabetes mellitus in combination with inflammatory or ischemic injury and nephrotoxin exposure. There is increasing evidence that long-term risk for chronic kidney disease is increased in patients with AKI. Prevention is therefore of paramount importance, and insight into the pathogenesis is essential to the development of appropriate interventions. Unfortunately, despite a wealth of experimental evidence in animal models, there are so far no specific therapeutic interventions in humans, beyond avoidance of hemodynamic instability, minimization of nephrotoxin exposure, and best supportive care. Applying our understanding of the pathophysiology of AKI to its treatment is the challenge for the future.

**Key Notes**

- Etiologic factors for the development of acute kidney injury are ischemia and reperfusion, inflammation, and toxic injury.
- In the intensive care unit, acute kidney injury occurs most often in the context of sepsis.
- During sepsis, renal blood flow may either be decreased or increased.
- The combination of low oxygen delivery and high oxygen demand puts the proximal tubule at high risk of ischemia.
- During sepsis, renal vasoconstriction is mediated by the sympathetic nervous system, the renin–angiotensin–aldosterin system, leukotrienes and endothelin, and loss of endothelial nitric oxide (NO), while vasodilatation is mediated by prostaglandins and endothelium derived NO-synthase.
- During sepsis, the inflammatory response in the kidney is mediated by activated leukocytes, reactive oxygen species, toll-like receptors 2 and 4 recognizing pathogen associated molecular patterns, cytokines (in particular tumor necrosis factor) and caspases, which can induce apoptosis. Inducible NO-synthase, extracellular adenosine triphosphate, and the coagulation system can also have a proinflammatory effect.
- Kidney biopsies of patients who died in septic shock showed not only tubular necrosis, but also monocyte infiltration and apoptosis.
- Since reperfusion after ischemia stimulates the inflammatory response, ischemic renal injury shares many pathways with septic renal injury.
- Energy depletion disrupts both the tight and adherens junctions between tubular cells, leading to increase in permeability and back-leak of glomerular filtrate.
- Prolonged energy depletion leads to collapse of tubular cells with shedding in the tubular lumen and excretion into the urine.
- The inflammatory response after ischemia and reperfusion is mediated by activated leukocytes, the complement system, cytokines, chemokines, reactive oxygen species, histones, and microvascular thrombosis.
- Nephrotoxin exposure accounts for up to 25 % of the cases of acute kidney injury in the intensive care unit and may be promoted by factors relating to the patient, the kidney and the ingested toxic substance.
- The most important nephrotoxins are drugs frequently used in the ICU, such as antibiotics, analgesics, and radiocontrast.
- All compartments of the kidney can be injured by toxic substances: renal vessels, glomeruli, tubular system, collecting ducts, and interstitium.

## References


1. Uchino S, Kellum JA, Bellomo R, et al. Acute renal failure in critically ill patients: a multinational, multicenter study. JAMA. 2005;294:813–8.
2. Bellomo R, Auriemma S, Fabbri A, et al. The pathophysiology of cardiac surgery-associated acute kidney injury (CSA-AKI). Int J Artif Organs. 2008;31:166–78.
3. Versteilen AM, DiMaggio F, Leemreis JR, et al. Molecular mechanisms of acute renal failure following ischemia/reperfusion. Int J Artif Organs. 2004;27:1019–29.
4. Lameire N, Van Biesen W, Vanholder R. Acute renal failure. Lancet. 2005;365:417–30.
5. Kinsey GR, Okusa MD. Pathogenesis of acute kidney injury: foundation for clinical practice. Am J Kidney Dis. 2011;58:291–301.
6. Langenberg C, Wan L, Egi M, et al. Renal blood flow and function during recovery from experimental septic acute kidney injury. Intensive Care Med. 2007;33:1614–8.
7. Prowle JR, Ishikawa K, May CN, et al. Renal blood flow during acute renal failure in man. Blood Purif. 2009;28:216–25.
8. Dewitte A, Coquin J, Meyssignac B, et al. Doppler resistive index to reflect regulation of renal vascular tone during sepsis and acute kidney injury. Crit Care. 2012;16:R165.
9. Schnell D, Darmon M. Renal Doppler to assess renal perfusion in the critically ill: a reappraisal. Intensive Care Med. 2012;38:1751–60.
10. Schnell D, Deruddre S, Harrois A, et al. Renal resistive index better predicts the occurrence of acute kidney injury than cystatin C. Shock. 2012;38:592–7.
11. Darmon M, Schortgen F, Vargas F, et al. Diagnostic accuracy of Doppler renal resistive index for reversibility of acute kidney injury in critically ill patients. Intensive Care Med. 2011; 37:68–76.
12. Prowle JR, Molan MP, Hornsey E, et al. Measurement of renal blood flow by phase-contrast magnetic resonance imaging during septic acute kidney injury: a pilot investigation. Crit Care Med. 2012;40:1768–76.
13. Legrand M, Mik EG, Johannes T, et al. Renal hypoxia and dysoxia after reperfusion of the ischemic kidney. Mol Med. 2008;14:502–16.
14. Schneider A, Johnson L, Goodwin M, et al. Bench-to-bedside review: contrast enhanced ultrasonography – a promising technique to assess renal perfusion in the ICU. Crit Care. 2011;15:157.
15. Langenberg C, Bellomo R, May C, et al. Renal blood flow in sepsis. Crit Care. 2005;9: R363–74.
16. Asfar P, Meziani F, Hamel JF, et al. High versus low blood pressure target in patients with septic shock. N Engl J Med. 2014;370:1583–93.
17. Bourgoin A, Leone M, Delmas A, et al. Increasing mean arterial pressure in patients with septic shock: effects on oxygen variables and renal function. Crit Care Med. 2005;33:780–6.
18. Morrell ED, Kellum JA, Hallows KR, et al. Epithelial transport during septic acute kidney injury. Nephrol Dial Transplant. 2014;29:1312–9.
19. Le Dorze M, Legrand M, Payen D, et al. The role of the microcirculation in acute kidney injury. Curr Opin Crit Care. 2009;15:503–8.
20. Abdelkader A, Ho J, Ow CP, et al. Renal oxygenation in acute renal ischemia-reperfusion injury. Am J Physiol Renal Physiol. 2014;306:F1026–38.
21. Tiwari MM, Brock RW, Megyesi JK, et al. Disruption of renal peritubular blood flow in lipopolysaccharide-induced renal failure: role of nitric oxide and caspases. Am J Physiol Renal Physiol. 2005;289:F1324–32.

22. Legrand M, Bezemer R, Kandil A, et al. The role of renal hypoperfusion in development of renal microcirculatory dysfunction in endotoxemic rats. Intensive Care Med. 2011;37: 1534–42.
23. Legrand M, Almac E, Mik EG, et al. L-NIL prevents renal microvascular hypoxia and increase of renal oxygen consumption after ischemia-reperfusion in rats. Am J Physiol Renal Physiol. 2009;296:F1109–17.
24. Legrand M, Kandil A, Payen D, et al. Effects of sepiapterin infusion on renal oxygenation and early acute renal injury after suprarenal aortic clamping in rats. J Cardiovasc Pharmacol. 2011;58:192–8.
25. Heemskerk S, Pickkers P, Bouw MP, et al. Upregulation of renal inducible nitric oxide synthase during human endotoxemia and sepsis is associated with proximal tubule injury. Clin J Am Soc Nephrol. 2006;1:853–62.
26. Quoilin C, Mouithys-Mickalad A, Lécart S, et al. Evidence of oxidative stress and mitochondrial respiratory chain dysfunction in an *in vitro* model of sepsis-induced kidney injury. Biochim Biophys Acta. 1837;2014:1790–800.
27. Glynne PA, Picot J, Evans TJ. Coexpressed nitric oxide synthase and apical $\beta 1$ integrins influence tubule cell adhesion after cytokine-induced injury. J Am Soc Nephrol. 2001;12: 2370–83.
28. Bakker J, Grover R, McLuckie A, et al. Administration of the nitric oxide synthetase inhibitor $N^{G}$-methyl-L-arginine hydrochloride (546C88) by intravenous infusion for up to 72 hours can promote the resolution of shock in patients with severe sepsis: results of a randomized, double-blind, placebo-controlled multicenter study (study no. 144–002). Crit Care Med. 2004; 32:1–12.
29. Peters E, Heemskerk S, Masereeuw R, et al. Alkaline phosphatase: a possible treatment for sepsis-associated acute kidney injury in critically ill patients. Am J Kidney Dis. 2014;63: 1038–48.
30. Peters E, van Elsas A, Heemskerk S, et al. Alkaline phosphatase as a treatment of sepsis-associated acute kidney injury. J Pharmacol Exp Ther. 2013;344:2–7.
31. Pickkers P, Heemskerk S, Schouten J, et al. Alkaline phosphatase for treatment of sepsis-induced acute kidney injury: a prospective randomized double-blind placebo-controlled trial. Crit Care. 2012;16:R14.
32. Wan L, Bagshaw SM, Langenberg C, et al. Pathophysiology of septic acute kidney injury: what do we really know? Crit Care Med. 2008;36(4Suppl):S198–203.
33. Gonçalves GM, Zamboni DS, Câmara NO. The role of innate immunity in septic acute kidney injuries. Shock. 2010;34 Suppl 1:22–6.
34. Sanz AB, Sanchez-Nin MD, Ramos AM, et al. NF-κB in renal inflammation. J Am Soc Nephrol. 2010;21:1254–62.
35. Iglesias J, Marik PE, Levine JS, et al. Elevated serum levels of the type I and type II receptors for tumor necrosis factor-alpha as predictive factors for ARF in patients with septic shock. Am J Kidney Dis. 2003;41:62–75.
36. Havasi A, Borkan SC. Apoptosis and acute kidney injury. Kidney Int. 2011;80:29–40.
37. Guo R, Wang Y, Minto AW, et al. Acute renal failure in endotoxemia is dependent on caspase activation. J Am Soc Nephrol. 2004;15:3093–102.
38. Lee SY, Lee YS, Choi HM, et al. Distinct pathophysiologic mechanismas of septic acute kidney injury: role of immune suppression and renal tubular cell apoptosis in murine model of septic acute kidney injury. Crit Care Med. 2012;40:2997–3006.
39. Liu HF, Liang D, Wang LM, et al. Effects of specific interleukin-1β converting enzyme inhibitor on ischemic acute renal failure in murine models. Acta Pharmacol Sin. 2005;26:1345–51.
40. Van den Berghe T, Demon D, Bogaert P, et al. Simultaneous targeting of IL-1 and IL-18 is required for protection against inflammatory and septic shock. Am J Respir Crit Care Med. 2014;189:282–91.
41. Gomez H, Ince C, De Backer D, et al. A unified theory of sepsis-induced acute kidney injury: inflammation, microcirculatory dysfunction, bioenergetics, and the tubular cell adaptation to injury. Shock. 2014;41:3–11.

42. Wu X, Guo R, Wang Y, et al. The role of ICAM-1 in endotoxin-induced acute renal failure. Am J Physiol Renal Physiol. 2007;293:F1262–71.

43. Tőkés-Füzesi M, Woth G, Emyey B, et al. Microparticles and acute renal dysfunction in septic patients. J Crit Care. 2013;28:141–7.

44. Lerolle N, Nochy D, Guérot E, et al. Histopathology of septic shock induced acute kidney injury: apoptosis and leukocytic infiltration. Intensive Care Med. 2010;36:471–8.

45. Langenberg C, Bagshaw SM, May CN, et al. The histopathology of septic acute kidney injury: a systematic review. Crit Care. 2008;12:R38.

46. Sear JW. Kidney dysfunction in the postoperative period. Br J Anaesth. 2005;95:20–32.

47. Parekh DJ, Weinberg JM, Ercole B, et al. Tolerance of the human kidney to isolated controlled ischemia. J Am Soc Nephrol. 2013;24:506–17.

48. Saotome T, Ishikawa K, May CN, et al. The impact of experimental hypoperfusion on subsequent kidney function. Intensive Care Med. 2010;36:533–40.

49. Bossard G, Bourgoin P, Corbeau JJ, et al. Early detection of postoperative acute kidney injury by Doppler renal resistive index in cardiac surgery with cardiopulmonary bypass. Br J Anaesth. 2011;107:891–8.

50. Versteilen AM, Blaauw N, Di Maggio F, et al. ρ-Kinase inhibition reduces early microvascular leukocyte accumulation in the rat kidney following ischemia-reperfusion injury: roles of nitric oxide and blood flow. Nephron Exp Nephrol. 2011;118:e79–86.

51. Ramaswamy D, Corrigan G, Polhemus C, et al. Maintenance and recovery stages of postischemic acute renal failure in humans. Am J Physiol Renal Physiol. 2002;282:F271–80.

52. Kwon O, Hong S-M, Sutton TA, et al. Preservation of peritubular capillary endothelial integrity and increasing pericytes may be critical to recovery from postischemia acute kidney injury. Am J Physiol Renal Physiol. 2008;295:F351–9.

53. Bonventre JV, Yang L. Cellular pathophysiology of ischemic acute kidney injury. J Clin Invest. 2011;121:4210–21.

54. Kakoki M, Hirata Y, Hayakawa H, et al. Effects of tetrahydrobiopterin on endothelial dysfunction in rats with ischemic acute renal failure. J Am Soc Nephrol. 2000;11:301–9.

55. Arfian N, Emoto N, Vigon-Zellweger N, et al. ET-1 deletion from endothelial cells protects the kidney during the extension phase of ischemia/reperfusion injury. Biochem Biophys Res Commun. 2012;425:443–9.

56. Sheridan AM, Bonventre JV. Cell biology and molecular mechanisms of injury in ischemic acute renal failure. Curr Opin Nephrol Hypertens. 2000;9:427–34.

57. Allam R, Scherbaum CR, Darisipudi MN, et al. Histones form dying renal cells aggravate kidney injury via TLR2 and TLR4. J Am Soc Nephrol. 2012;23:1375–88.

58. Arumugam TV, Shiels IA, Strachan AJ, et al. A small molecule C5a receptor antagonist protects kidneys from ischemia/reperfusion injury in rats. Kidney Int. 2003;63:134–42.

59. Melnikov VY, Faubel S, Siegmund B, et al. Neutrophil-independent mechanisms of caspase-1-and IL-18-mediated ischemic acute tubular necrosis in mice. J Clin Invest. 2002;110:1083–91.

60. Singbartl K, Ley K. Leukocyte recruitment and acute renal failure. J Mol Med. 2004;82:91–101.

61. He Z, Lu L, Altman C, et al. Interleukin-18 binding protein transgenic mice are protected against ischemic kidney injury. Am J Physiol Renal Physiol. 2008;295:F1414–21.

62. Menke J, Iwata Y, Rabacal WA, et al. CSF-1 signals directly to renal tubular epithelial cells to mediate repair in mice. J Clin Invest. 2009;119:2330–42.

63. Kinsey GR, Sharma R, Okusa MD. Regulatory T cells in AKI. J Am Soc Nephrol. 2013;24:1720–6.

64. Saikumar P, Venkatachalam MA. Role of apoptosis in hypoxia/ischemic damage in the kidney. Semin Nephrol. 2003;23:511–21.

65. Price PM, Safirstein RL, Megyesi J. The cell cycle and acute kidney injury. Kidney Int. 2009;76:604–13.

66. Kelly KJ, Plotkin Z, Dagher PC. Guanosine supplementation reduces apoptosis and protects renal function in the setting of ischemic injury. J Clin Invest. 2001;108:1291–8.

67. Nigam SK, Lieberthal W. Acute renal failure. III. The role of growth factors in the process of renal regeneration and repair. Am J Physiol Renal Physiol. 2000;279:F3–11.
68. Vargas GA, Hoeflich A, Jehle PM. Hepatocyte growth factor in renal failure: promise and reality. Kidney Int. 2000;57:1426–36.
69. Liu KD. Molecular mechanisms of recovery from acute renal failure. Crit Care Med. 2003; 31(Suppl):S572–81.
70. Cuttle L, Zhang X-J, Endre ZH, et al. Bcl-XL translocation in renal tubular epithelial cells in vitro protects distal cells from oxidative stress. Kidney Int. 2001;59:1779–88.
71. Dai C, Yang J, Liu Y. Single injection of naked plasmid encoding hepatocyte growth factor prevents cell death and ameliorates acute renal failure in mice. J Am Soc Nephrol. 2002; 13:411–22.
72. Pannu N, Nadim MK. An overview of drug-induced acute kidney injury. Crit Care Med. 2008;36(Supppl):S216–23.
73. Perazella MA. Renal vulnerability to drug toxicity. Clin J Am Soc Nephrol. 2009;4:1275–83.
74. Perazella MA. Drug use and nephrotoxicity in the intensive care unit. Kidney Int. 2012;81: 1172–8.
75. Sharp LS, Rozycki GS, Feliciano DV. Rhabdomyolysis and secondary renal failure in critically ill surgical patients. Am J Surg. 2004;188:801–6.
76. Schetz M, Dasta J, Goldstein S, et al. Drug-induced acute kidney injury. Curr Opin Crit Care. 2005;11:555–65.
77. McCullough PA. Contrast-induced acute kidney injury. J Am Coll Cardiol. 2008;51: 1419–28.
78. Hoste EJA, Doom S, De Waele J, et al. Epidemiology of contrast-associated acute kidney injury in ICU patients: a retrospective cohort analysis. Intensive Care Med. 2011;37: 1921–31.
79. Isnard Bagnis C, Deray G, Baumelou A, et al. Herbs and the kidney. Am J Kidney Dis. 2004; 44:1–11.
80. Reyes JL, Molina-Jijón E, Rodríguez-Muñoz R, et al. Tight junction proteins and oxidative stress in heavy metals induced nephrotoxicity. Biomed Res Int. 2013;2013:730789.
81. Perazella MA. Drug-induced nephropathy: an update. Expert Opin Drug Saf. 2005;4: 689–706.
82. Oliveira JFP, Silva CA, Barbieri CD, et al. Prevalence and risk factors for aminoglycoside nephrotoxicity in intensive care units. Antimicrob Agents Chemother. 2009;53:2887–9.
83. Zimmerman J, Shen MC. Rhabdomyolysis. Chest. 2013;144:1058–65.
84. Vaglio A, Salvarani C, Buzio C. Retroperitoneal fibrosis. Lancet. 2006;367:241–51.
85. Perazella MA, Markowitz GS. Drug-induced acute interstitial nephritis. Nat Rev Nephrol. 2010;6:461–70.
86. Rossert J. Drug-induced acute interstitial nephritis. Kidney Int. 2001;60:804–17.
87. Alfaro R, Vesavada N, Pauesakon P, et al. Cocaine-induced acute interstitial nephritis: a case report and review of the literature. J Nephropathol. 2013;2:204–9.

# Acid–Base

**5**

Victor A. van Bochove, Heleen M. Oudemans-van Straaten, and Paul W.G. Elbers

## 5.1 Introduction

A thorough understanding of acid–base balance is a prerequisite for practicing medicine and pivotal for those treating the critically ill. Acidity of fluids including that of plasma is determined by their hydrogen concentration or $[H^+]$, often confusingly expressed as its negative logarithm or pH. Plasma $[H^+]$ is tightly regulated around 40 nM (pH 7.4) and influences most physiological processes. Acid–base analysis often yields important diagnostic information, and its physiology represents the crossroads between electrolyte balance and the respiratory system.

The last century gave rise to three commonly used approaches to acid–base problems in clinical medicine. In 1908, Henderson described his equation for carbonic acid equilibrium, which was rewritten in logarithmic form by Hasselbalch in 1917. Ole Siggaard-Andersen introduced Base Excess in 1964. Finally, in 1981, Peter Stewart published his quantitative approach. Recently, the Stewart approach has become increasingly popular, especially in the setting of critical care medicine. This chapter will discuss all of these approaches and use their context to consider renal acid–base handling.


V.A. van Bochove • H.M. Oudemans-van Straaten • P.W.G. Elbers (✉)
Department of Intensive Care Medicine,
VU University Medical Center Amsterdam,
De Boelelaan 1117, Amsterdam 1081 HV, The Netherlands
e-mail: p.elbers@vumc.nl



© Springer International Publishing 2015
H.M. Oudemans-van Straaten et al. (eds.), *Acute Nephrology for the Critical Care Physician*, DOI 10.1007/978-3-319-17389-4_5

## 5.2 The Stewart Approach

Often referred to as the physicochemical or quantitative approach, the basis of Stewart method is that all chemical equilibrium equations in which [H⁺] takes part must be satisfied simultaneously (Table 5.1). Water dissociation plays a pivotal role as a reservoir for H⁺ ions. The key message of the Stewart approach is that [H⁺] is only dependent on three independent variables: the strong ion difference (SID), the total amount of weak acids ($A_{TOT}$) and the partial pressure of carbon dioxide $PCO_2$.

$$\left[ H^+ \right] = f\left( SID, A_{TOT}, PCO_2 \right)$$

These three independent parameters can all be normal, decreased or increased and thus six major acid base disturbances can be distinguished. This also implies that bicarbonate does not play any role in determining [H⁺]. Instead, [$HCO_3^-$] is also determined by the three independent parameters.

### 5.2.1 Strong Ion Difference (SID)

Strong ions are always fully dissociated. Na⁺, K⁺ and Cl⁻ are the most important examples, but others include Mg⁺, Ca²⁺, sulfate and lactate. SID is the sum of strong cations minus the sum of strong anions. Its normal plasma value is about 40 mEq/L.

When SID increases, physicochemistry dictates that [H⁺] must decrease. An example is prolonged vomiting causing plasma [Cl⁻] to decrease and therefore [SID] to increase. When SID decreases, physicochemistry dictates that [H⁺] must increase. Examples include lactic acidosis and ketoacidosis. Ketones and lactate are also strong negative ions that decrease [SID] directly and therefore cause [H⁺] to rise.

### 5.2.2 Total Amount of Weak Acids ($A_{TOT}$)

The total amount of weak acids is expressed as $A_{TOT}$. It mainly consists of albumin and to a lesser extent of phosphate. By definition, weak acids are only partially

**Table 5.1** The Stewart equations

1. Water dissociation equilibrium: $\left[ H^* \right] \times \left[ OH^- \right] = K_w'$

2. Electrical neutrality equation: $\left[ SID \right] + \left[ H^* \right] = \left[ HCO_3^- \right] + \left[ A^- \right] + \left[ CO_3^{2-} \right] + \left[ OH^- \right]$

3. Weak acid dissociation equilibrium: $\left[ K_A \right] \times \left[ HA \right] \leftrightarrow \left[ H^+ \right] \times \left[ A^- \right]$

4. Conservation of mass for "A": $\left[ A_{TOT} \right] \leftrightarrow \left[ A^- \right] + \left[ HA \right]$

5. Bicarbonate ion formation equilibrium: $\left[ PCO_2 \right] \times \left[ K_C \right] = \left[ H^+ \right] \times \left[ HCO_3^- \right]$

6. Carbonate ion formation equilibrium: $\left[ K_3 \right] \times \left[ HCO_3^- \right] = \left[ H^+ \right] \times \left[ CO_3^{2-} \right]$

dissociated. When $A_{TOT}$ increases, physicochemistry dictates that [H⁺] must increase, for example in the case of hyperphosphatemia in renal failure. When $A_{TOT}$ decreases, [H⁺] must also decrease, as is the case in hypoalbuminemia, a common problem in critically ill patients.

## 5.2.3 The Partial Pressure of Carbon Dioxide (PCO₂)

Tissues produce $CO_2$. All approaches to acid–base treat $PCO_2$ similarly. Physicochemistry dictates that if $PCO_2$ rises, for example due to increased dead space ventilation, [H⁺] must rise too. If $PCO_2$ decreases, [H⁺] must also decrease. An example would be psychogenic hyperventilation.

## 5.2.4 Strong Ion Gap (SIG) and Urine SID

Both SIG and Urine SID may be used to further differentiate between causes of acid–base abnormalities (Tables 5.2 and 5.3). Urine SID is defined as urine [Na⁺] + [K⁺] − [Cl⁻]. In metabolic acidosis, a positive urine SID may suggest renal tubular acidosis.

SIG is the difference between the apparent SID ($SID_a$) and the effective SID ($SID_e$). $SID_a$ consists of the sum of the measured strong ions:

$$SID_a = \left[ Na^+ \right] + \left[ K^+ \right] + \left[ Ca^{2+} \right] + \left[ Mg^{2+} \right] - \left[ Cl^- \right]$$

$SID_e$ is an approximation of the true SID, calculating the remaining ion space after accounting for the negative charge on albumin and bicarbonate, and can be calculated from the other independent variables using the following formula, where albumin (Alb) is expressed in g/L and phosphate ($P_i$) in mM:

**Table 5.2** Differential diagnosis of metabolic acidosis

| Adjusted AG >8 12 mEq/L Low SID with SIG >0–2 mEq/L | Normal adjusted AG, Low SID with normal SIG |
| --- | --- |
| Lactate | NaCl 0.9 % infusion |
| Ketones | Diarrhea |
| End-stage renal failure | Early renal insufficiency |
| Salicylate intoxication | Acetazolamide |
| Methanol intoxication | Ureteroenterostomy |
| Ethylene glycol intoxication | Parenteral nutrition |
|  | Anion exchange resins |
|  | Small bowel/pancreatic drainage |
|  | Renal tubular acidosis (Urine SID >0) |
|  | Type I: Urine pH >5.5 |
|  | Type II: Urine pH <5.5/low serum K⁺ |
|  | Type IV: Urine pH <5.5/high serum K⁺ |

**Table 5.3** Differential diagnosis for increased SID metabolic alkalosis

| | |
|---|---|
| Chloride loss <sodium loss (urine [Cl⁻] <10 mmol/L) | Vomiting, gastric drainage, chloride wasting diarrhea, postdiuretic use, posthypercapnea |
| Chloride loss <sodium loss (urine [Cl⁻] >10 mmol/L) | Mineralocorticoid excess (Conn's syndrome, Cushing syndrome, Liddle syndrome, Bartter syndrome, exogenous corticoids, excessive licorice intake), ongoing diuretic use |
| Exogenous sodium load | Massive blood transfusions, parenteral nutrition, plasma volume expanders, sodium lactate, sodium citrate |
| Other | Severe deficiency of $Mg^{2+}$ or $K^+$ |

$$\mathrm{SID_e} = \left[\mathrm{HCO_3^-}\right] + \left(0.123 * \mathrm{pH} - 0.631\right) * \left[\mathrm{Alb}\right] + \left(\mathrm{pH} - 0.469\right) * \left[\mathrm{P_i}\right]$$

Thus SIG represents the sum of any unmeasured strong positive and negative ions. Its normal value is $0 \pm 2$ mEq/L. When positive, unmeasured anions exceed unmeasured cations.

### 5.2.5 Osmol Gap

This is the gap between the measured osmolality and the calculated osmolality.

$$\text{Calculated osmolaity} = 2 \times \left[\mathrm{Na^+}\right] + \left[\text{glucose}\right] + \left[\text{urea}\right]$$

where glucose and urea are expressed in mM. The normal value of the osmol gap is 10–15 mM. A high osmol gap suggests the presence of ethanol, ethylene glycol or methanol.

### 5.2.6 Effect of Resuscitation Fluids

Normal plasma has a SID of approximately 40 mEq/L. Thus, if fluids with a different SID are given, SID will change. Examples include 0.9 or 0.45 % saline with equal amounts of sodium and chloride thus a SID of 0 mM. The same is true for glucose 5 %, which does not contain any strong ions and hence also has a SID of 0 mM.

Balanced salt solutions contain variable amounts of negative ions that are metabolized, such as lactate or acetate. This explains their increased SID, which is about 28 mM for lactated Ringer's for example. Similarly, 8.4 % $NaHCO_3$ is essentially sodium without strong anions, resulting in a high SID of 1,000 mM. In clinical medicine, the effect of resuscitation fluids on SID is counterbalanced by simultaneous dilution of $A_{TOT}$ and renal SID handling.

## 5.3    The Henderson-Hasselbalch Approach

As can be seen from Table 5.1, the Henderson-Hasselbalch equation is actually one of the Stewart equations:

$$\left[H^+\right] \sim PCO_2 / \left[HCO_3^-\right]$$

The ratio of $[HCO_3^-]$ and $PCO_2$ has a fixed relationship to $[H^+]$. All acid–base disturbances are thus explained by changes in either $[HCO_3^-]$ or $PCO_2$. Singling out this equation is attractive as it facilitates dividing acid–base abnormalities in respiratory and non-respiratory or metabolic disorders. However, it should be noted that because $PCO_2$ and $HCO_3^-$ are interdependent, relying solely on this equation might lead to circular reasoning.

Compensatory changes to acid–base disturbances may also be respiratory or metabolic and reflected in same direction changes in $PCO_2$ of $[HCO_3^-]$. Respiratory compensation, either spontaneously or by altering the settings of mechanical ventilation may occur within minutes. Metabolic compensation is slower and may take hours to days, and is mainly regulated by the kidney. To determine whether the compensation is sufficient and to identify mixed acid–base disorders, rules of thumb have been proposed (Table 5.4).

**Table 5.4**  Rules of thumb for compensation

| Primary acid–base disturbance | Compensation rule |
| --- | --- |
| Metabolic acidosis | $\Delta PaCO_2 / \Delta\left[HCO_3^-\right] = 1.2$ mEq/L <br> $\Delta PaCO_2 = \Delta SBE$ |
| Metabolic alkalosis | $\Delta PaCO_2 / \Delta\left[HCO_3^-\right] = 0.7$ mEq/L <br> $\Delta PaCO_2 = 0.6 \times \Delta SBE$ |
| Acute respiratory acidosis | $\Delta\left[HCO_3^-\right] / \Delta PaCO_2 = 0.1$ mEq/L <br> $\Delta SBE = 0$ |
| Chronic respiratory acidosis | $\Delta\left[HCO_3^-\right] / \Delta PaCO_2 = 0.3$ mEq/L <br> $\Delta SBE = 0.4 \times \Delta PaCO_2$ |
| Acute respiratory alkalosis | $\Delta\left[HCO_3^-\right] / \Delta PaCO_2 = 0.2$ mEq/L <br> $\Delta SBE = 0$ |
| Chronic respiratory alkalosis | $\Delta\left[HCO_3^-\right] / \Delta PaCO_2 = 0.4$ mEq/L <br> $\Delta SBE = 0.4 \times \Delta PaCO_2$ |

### 5.3.1 Anion Gap and Urine Anion Gap

The anion gap (AG) should be calculated to differentiate between causes of metabolic acidosis and to assess the presence of mixed acid–base disorders. AG is an estimate of the relative abundance of unmeasured anions and is used to determine if a metabolic acidosis is due to an accumulation of nonvolatile acids or a $HCO_3^-$ loss:

$$AG = \left[ Na^+ \right] - \left[ Cl^- \right] - \left[ HCO_3^- \right]$$

Its normal value is 3–11 mEq/L. This is mainly due to albumin, which is partially ionized. Therefore, the anion gap should be adjusted as follows:

$$\text{Adjusted AG} = \text{observed AG} + 0.25 \times \left( 42 - \left[ Albumin \right] \right)$$

where albumin is given in g/L. Values above 11 m Eq/L for the adjusted anion gap suggest a metabolic acidosis due to nonvolatile acids (Table 5.2). A normal adjusted anion gap metabolic acidosis is sometimes confusingly referred to as hyperchloremic metabolic acidosis. The urine anion gap is the same as the urine strong ion difference and can be used to further differentiate between causes of metabolic acidosis.

### 5.3.2 Delta Ratio

In high anion gap metabolic acidosis the delta ratio may be used to detect the possible coexistence of a normal anion gap acidosis.

$$\text{Delta ratio} = \Delta AG \,/\, \Delta HCO_3^- = \left( \text{measured AG} - 12 \right) / \left( 24 - \text{measured} \, HCO_3^- \right)$$

Interpretation of the delta ratio (Table 5.5) should be done with caution due to possible inaccuracies.

## 5.4 Base Excess and Standard Base Excess

The third approach to acid–base is the base excess (BE) method. The base excess is defined as the concentration of strong acid or base required to return the pH of an in vitro specimen of whole blood with a $PCO_2$ of 40 mmHg and a temperature of

**Table 5.5** Delta gap

| | |
|---|---|
| Delta ratio <0.4 | Hyperchloremic normal anion gap acidosis |
| Delta ratio 0.4–0.8 | Combined high AG and normal AG acidosis |
| Delta ratio 1–2 | Uncomplicated high AG acidosis |
| Delta ratio >2 | Preexisting elevated $HCO_3^-$ (examples: concurrent metabolic alkalosis, preexisting compensated respiratory acidosis) |

37 °C to 7.4. A negative BE is also referred to as base deficit. The BE is based on the Van Slyke equation:

$$BE = \left( \left[ HCO_3^- \right] - 24.4 + \left( 2.3 \times Hb + 7.7 \right) \times \left( pH - 7.4 \right) \right) \times \left( 1 - 0.023 \times Hb \right)$$

with Hb and $HCO_3^-$ in mM. However, this formula proves not to be $PCO_2$ invariant in vivo. This is because in vivo $CO_2$ equilibration occurs throughout the total extracellular compartment, including interstitial fluid. To adjust for this the standard base excess (SBE) was developed, in which Hb is fixed at its approximate mean extracellular concentration of 5 mg/dL:

$$SBE = 0.93 \times \left[ HCO_3^- \right] - 24.4 + 14.8 \times \left( pH - 7.4 \right)$$

SBE is used to assess the metabolic component of an acid–base disturbance and to assess the compensatory regulation (Table 5.4). The primary acid–base disturbance is detected by comparing pH and $PCO_2$. Then, the SBE formulae are used to determine the metabolic component and compensatory response. If the measured response is different, a mixed acid base disturbance may be present.

## 5.5  Stewart at the Bedside: A Unifying Approach

Although its principles may be simple, using the Stewart approach at the bedside may be somewhat intimidating. One possibility is to use the online analysis module on acidbase.org. Alternatively, Story has proposed a unified and simplified approach to acid base. Focusing on the effect of SID, $A_{TOT}$ and unmeasured anions on base excess (BE), this approach only requires three easy to remember formulas (Table 5.6).

1. Determine the problem and its severity by assessing the pH. Remember that acidosis and alkalosis refer to processes that influence [H⁺] or pH. A normal pH does not rule out acid–base pathology.
2. Assess the relative contribution of respiratory versus non-respiratory components using $PCO_2$ and BE. Remember that normal values do not rule out acid–base pathology.

**Table 5.6** Formulas for the simplified Stewart approach

| | |
|---|---|
| SID effect on BE | $\left( \left[ Na^+ \right] - \left[ Cl^- \right] \right) - 40$ |
| $A_{TOT}$ effect on BE | 0.25 * (42- [alb]) |
| Unmeasured ions effect on BE | SBE-SID effect – $A_{TOT}$ effect |

Please note that the normal value for [Na⁺] – [Cl⁻] may differ between laboratories. Albumin (alb) in g/L

3. Use Stewart derived BE partitioning to quantify contribution of various non-respiratory acid–base disorders.
   (a) Calculate the approximate influence of SID on BE.
   (b) Calculate the approximate influence of $A_{TOT}$ on BE.
   (c) If measured BE differs from the sum of 3a and 3b, unmeasured ions must be present.

## 5.6 When and How to Treat Acid–Base Disorders

There is no consensus on treatment of acid–base disorders apart from addressing its cause. As acid–base disturbances influences every aspect of physiology including the cardiovascular, respiratory and immune systems, it is reasonable to start symptomatic treatment in the critically ill with severe deviations of pH from normal. These may arbitrarily be defined as pH <7.1 or pH >7.6. Ventilator settings and sedative infusions may be adjusted to modify $PCO_2$, although trade-offs need to be made clinically because of the adverse effects of overzealous sedation and ventilator induced lung injury at high tidal volumes or plateau pressures. When using a buffer, it should be remembered that administering sodium bicarbonate may transiently decrease intracellular pH, if ventilator settings are not changed simultaneously. In addition, there is no trial that has shown a benefit in terms of mortality when using sodium bicarbonate to attenuate acidosis. In this respect, tromethamine (THAM) may be better suited, as it does not induce intracellular acidosis. However, its clinical benefit is yet to be confirmed.

## 5.7 Renal Acid–Base Handling

In acid–base homeostasis, the kidneys are pivotal. In critical care medicine, their role is often compensatory, by regulating plasma electrolyte concentrations. However, the kidneys may also cause acid–base disturbances, for example in acute kidney injury or various types of renal tubular acidosis.

When discussing renal acid–base handling, it is important to point out that different explanations for observed cellular mechanisms exist depending on which approach to acid–base medicine is adhered to. For example, the Stewart approach may view sodium bicarbonate transporters as SID regulator, whereas the other approaches may relate its effect to bicarbonate transport itself. Interestingly, most of the physiological concepts dealing with renal transporters have been developed before the Stewart approach became popular. Thus, it may prove necessary to revise these concepts. A detailed discussion of controversies in this is beyond the scope of this book.

Renal acid–base handling is mainly dependent on SID and $PCO_2$. In the proximal convoluted tubule hydrogen ions are excreted into the tubular lumen through a $Na^+$-$H^+$ exchanger. There, mediated by carbonic anhydrase, the hydrogen ions react with the filtered bicarbonate to form $H_2CO_3$, which dissociates into $CO_2$ and $H_2O$. These diffuse through the aquaporin channels into the cytosol. There, again mediated by carbonic anhydrase, the reaction is reversed and hydrogen and bicarbonate ions are formed again. Bicarbonate is then absorbed into the circulation together with $Na^+$ by a $Na^+$-$HCO_3^-$ cotransporter. Chloride reabsorption has three main routes: (1) passive due to the electrochemical concentration gradient, (2) active by chloride channels and (3) coupled through various chloride-anion exchangers.

In the distal convoluted tubule, chloride, hydrogen and bicarbonate are handled by $H^+$-ATPase, $H^+$-$K^+$-ATPase and $Cl^-$-$HCO_3^-$ exchangers, situated within the cell membrane of type A-cells and type B-cells respectively. Depending on the acid–base status, the different components are either up regulated or down regulated. For example in acidosis hydrogen is excreted through the $H^+$-ATPase and $H^+$-$K^+$-ATPase and chloride is excreted through pendrin and band 3 protein. In alkalosis, chloride excretion is less due to down regulation of pendrin and band 3 protein.

## 5.7.1  Renal Tubular Acidosis (RTA)

In type 1 renal tubular acidosis (RTA) or distal RTA, there is a defect in the ability to secret hydrogen and chloride ions in the distal tubules due to for example mutations in the anion exchangers. As a reaction type B-cells will change and become type-A cells in order to try to increase the hydrogen secretion. As a reaction bicarbonate reabsorption is decreased. Therefore plasma bicarbonate is low and urine pH is increased.

In type 2 RTA or proximal RTA, a reduced capacity in the reabsorption of bicarbonate exists, due to inherited or acquired causes. In inherited RTA 2 a defect in transporters, such as Na/H exchanger (NHE), kNBC1 or NHE3 can exist. The causes are not fully known yet. Further RTA 2 can occur as part of a syndrome such as Fanconi's. Acquired causes include heavy metal poisoning and drugs related RTA. Since distal bicarbonate reabsorption is still possible, plasma bicarbonate is normally slightly decreased and blood pH low normal.

Type 3 RTA or mixed RTA is based on inhibition of carbonic anhydrase (CA). CA-II and CA-IV both play a role in the reabsorption of bicarbonate in the proximal tubule. CA-II also plays a role in the hydrogen excretion in the distal tubule. Inhibition of CA, due to treatment with acetazolamide, or autoimmune diseases such as Sjögren's disease cause a combination of proximal and distal RTA and is therefore named mixed RTA.

Type 4 RTA is characterized by a decreased renal excretion of ammonium and inhibition of $H^+$/ATPase in type-A cells caused by an aldosterone deficiency or resistance. Ammonium is normally used as a buffer for the excreted hydrogen ions. In the absence of ammonium, less hydrogen can be buffered and thus less hydrogen can be excreted, causing an acidosis. Causes of aldosterone deficiency include Addison's disease, congenital adrenal hyperplasia and drugs inhibiting aldosterone synthesis. Causes of aldosterone resistance include congenital causes, such as pseudohypoaldosteronism type 1 and 2 and acquired causes, such as interstitial nephropathies and drugs. RTA type 4 is commonly associated with a hyperkalemia.

### 5.7.2 Acute Kidney Injury (AKI)

Acute kidney injury (AKI) is a leading contributor of acid–base disturbances in the critically ill patient and often complex due to the coexistence of acidotic and alkalotic factors. Due to lowered chloride excretion by the kidneys, hyperchloremia may develop, leading to a decreased SID and therefore acidosis. In later stages of AKI in the critically ill, other causes of acidosis may develop, some only partially related to AKI. These include unmeasured anions, hyperlactatemia, hypocalcemia (decreasing SID) and hyperphosphatemia (increasing $A_{TOT}$). Two main causes of alkalosis may be present: hypoalbuminemia (lowering $A_{TOT}$) and hyperkalemia (increasing SID). The combination of coexisting acidosis and alkalosis can make the understanding of acid–base balance particularly difficult in the critically ill patient with AKI.

### 5.7.3 Chronic Kidney Disease (CKD)

The acid–base disturbances in chronic kidney disease (CKD) are similar to AKI. These start to develop when the glomerular filtration rate is less than 20–25 % of normal. Again, mechanisms include both impairment of SID handling and accumulation of $A_{TOT}$. The extent and relative contribution of each depends on the underlying cause of CKD, medication and renal replacement therapy.

### 5.7.4 Renal Replacement Therapy (RRT)

The best and fastest way to correct AKI or CKD induced acidosis is renal replacement therapy (RRT). The correction of metabolic acidosis is based on substituting the ultrafiltrate with a SID generator. These include bicarbonate-, lactate- and citrate based substitution fluids. Their effect is based on the metabolisation of the anions and therefore increasing SID and correcting the metabolic acidosis. However, when the metabolisation of the lactate or citrate is impaired, for example in the case of liver failure, the increasing strong anion load can lead to a decreased SID and therefore cause worsening of the metabolic acidosis.

---

**Conclusion**

Stewart's strong ion approach, Siggaard-Andersen's standard base excess approach and the Henderson-Hasselbalch based bicarbonate centered approach are popular frameworks for understanding acid–base disorders in the critically ill. Basic concepts, views of renal acid–base handling and clinical application of these methods were discussed in this chapter. Provided that hypoalbuminemia is corrected for in the latter two, all methods are mathematically compatible and may perform equally well in clinical practice, especially in uncomplicated acid–base disorders.

However, if acid–base disorders become increasingly complex, which is the case in many critically ill patients, Stewart's approach may be superior. Although considered difficult, this method disentangles and quantifies the various factors responsible for complex mixed acid–base disorders, thus arguably providing the best overview. In addition, by explicitly clarifying the relationship between electrolyte disorders and acid–base physiology, the Stewart approach helps to demystify the effects of resuscitation fluids on acid–base balance.

The kidney is pivotal in acid–base physiology, mostly by modifying SID. Our understanding of renal electrolyte handling may need to be revised as a result of the principles of the physiochemical approach. Both in acute and chronic kidney injury, accumulation of weak acids and impaired SID handling may give rise to complex acid base disorders, especially if complicated by hypoalbuminemia.

**Key Messages**

- Three approaches to acid–base disorders are in common use: The bicarbonate centered, base excess and the Stewart approach. All methods are mathematically compatible provided that appropriate corrections are used for the first two. However, the Stewart approach may be superior in terms of versatility and improved understanding of complex acid–base disturbances.
- The Stewart approach states that only three independent parameters determine [H+]. These parameters are the Strong Ion Difference (SID), the total amount of weak acids ($A_{TOT}$) and the partial pressure of carbon dioxide ($PCO_2$).
- SID is the sum strong cations minus the sum of strong anions. Strong ions are always fully dissociated. $Na^+$ and $Cl^-$ are the most important examples. $A_{TOT}$ is mainly represented by albumin and to a lesser extent by phosphate. If SID decreases, or if $PCO_2$ increases or if $A_{TOT}$ increases, physicochemistry dictates that $[H^+]$ must increase and vice versa.
- The kidney is pivotal in regulating non-respiratory acid–base physiology, mainly by modulating SID. Acidosis in kidney failure is complex and also includes accumulation of weak acids such as phosphate. Our understanding of renal electrolyte handling may need to be revised in the context of the Stewart approach.

# Further Reading

Fencl V, Jabor A, Kazda A, Figge J. Diagnosis of metabolic acid–base disturbances in critically ill patients. Am J Respir Crit Care Med. 2000;162(6):2246–51.
Elbers PWG, Gatz R, AcidBase.org, online community and decision support for quantitative acid-base medicine. http://www.acidbase.org.
Kerry Brandis. Anesthesia Education Website. http://www.anaesthesiamcq.com.
James Figge. Human acid base physiology. http://www.figge-fencl.org.
Kellum JA. Determinants of plasma acid–base balance. Crit Care Clin. 2005;21(2):329–46.

Kellum JA, Elbers PWG, editors. Stewarts textbook of acid–base. Amsterdam: 2009. www.acid-base.org.

Ring T, Frische S, Nielsen S. Clinical review: renal tubular acidosis–a physicochemical approach. Crit Care. 2005;9(6):573–80.

Rodríguez Soriano J. Renal tubular acidosis: the clinical entity. J Am Soc Nephrol. 2002;13:2160.

Rose B, Post T, editors. Clinical physiology of acid–base and electrolyte disorders. New York: McGraw-Hill; 2000.

Stewart PA. How to understand acid base balance. A quantitative acid–base primer for biology and medicine. New York: Elsevier; 1981.

Stewart PA. Modern quantitative acid–base chemistry. Can J Physiol Pharmacol. 1983;61: 1444–61.

Story DA. Bench-to-bedside review: a brief history of clinical acid–base. Crit Care. 2004;8(4): 253–8.

Story DA, Morimatsu H, Bellomo R. Strong ions, weak acids and base excess: a simplified Fencl-Stewart approach to clinical acid–base disorders. Br J Anaesth. 2004;92(1):54–60.

# Kidney-Organ Interaction

**6**


Sean M. Bagshaw, Frederik H. Verbrugge, Wilfried Mullens, Manu L.N.G. Malbrain, and Andrew Davenport


## 6.1 Introduction

The practice of critical care nephrology demands an intimate understanding of the interactions and "crosstalk" that occurs between the kidney and multiple organ systems, in particular the heart, lung, gut, and brain. Accumulating evidence suggests that acute injury and dysfunction to the kidney can incite and propagate cardiac, pulmonary, gastrointestinal, and neurologic injury and dysfunction through a host of mechanisms.

Among patients hospitalized with acute kidney injury (AKI), the therapeutic options to mitigate kidney injury and loss of function once established are relatively limited and largely represent enhanced surveillance and measures to avoid iatrogenic complications and harm. AKI has a high attributable risk of morbidity and mortality.


S.M. Bagshaw, MD, MSc (✉)
Division of Critical Care Medicine, Faculty of Medicine and Dentistry, University of Alberta, Edmonton, Canada
e-mail: bagshaw@ualberta.ca

F.H. Verbrugge, MD
Department of Cardiology, Ziekenhuis Oost-Limburg, Genk, Belgium

Doctoral School for Medicine and Life Sciences, Hasselt University, Diepenbeek, Belgium

W. Mullens, MD, PhD
Department of Cardiology, Ziekenhuis Oost-Limburg, Genk, Belgium

Faculty of Medicine and Life Sciences, Biomedical Research Institute, Hasselt University, Diepenbeek, Belgium

Manu L.N.G. Malbrain, MD, PhD
ICU and High Care Burn Unit, Ziekenhuis Netwerk Antwerpen, ZNA Stuivenberg/St-Erasmus, Antwerp, Belgium
e-mail: manu.malbrain@skynet.be

A. Davenport, MD
University College London Centre for Nephrology, Royal Free Hospital, London, UK
e-mail: andrewdavenport@nhs.net



© Springer International Publishing 2015
H.M. Oudemans-van Straaten et al. (eds.), *Acute Nephrology for the Critical Care Physician*, DOI 10.1007/978-3-319-17389-4_6

Indeed, the hazard of major morbid complications after AKI, including incident chronic kidney disease (CKD) and accelerated progression to end-stage kidney disease (ESKD), along with increased susceptibility to infections/sepsis, malignancy, and fractures and excessive mortality remain elevated long after the initial episode of AKI. This attributable morbidity and mortality may be partially explained by AKI contributing to extrarenal injury/dysfunction to distant organs [1].

Our understanding of the pathophysiological mechanisms underlying this kidney-organ "crosstalk" remains incompletely understood; however, it is likely a complex interaction of patient-specific susceptibilities (i.e., genetic, comorbid disease), acute illness severity, and the extent of organ injury; host responses to injury including dysfunctional inflammatory cascades, oxidative stress, activation of pro-apoptotic pathways, altered molecular expression, and leukocyte trafficking; and the impact of therapeutic interventions aimed to treat critical illness. This chapter will provide a broad overview of the fundamentals of kidney-organ interactions.

## 6.2 The Kidney and the Heart

The prevalence of cardiac and kidney disease is high and increasing concomitantly with population demographic transition. Importantly, cardiac and kidney disease frequently coexist and together can synergistically modify the risk of major morbidity and premature death and translate into excessive health services use. The "cardiorenal syndrome" is generally characterized by the presence of pathophysiological organ "crosstalk" between the heart and the kidneys, whereby an acute or chronic injury or decompensation in the function of one organ can precipitate injury or dysfunction to the other. A large body of literature from observational studies and clinical trials has clearly shown that acute/chronic heart disease can directly contribute to and/or accelerate acute/chronic worsening of kidney function and vice versa. Recently, a consensus definition and classification scheme for the cardiorenal syndrome was proposed to help standardize its nomenclature with the aim to better understand its underlying pathophysiological mechanisms, epidemiology, and therapeutic approaches. This classification scheme proposed five distinct "cardiorenal" syndrome subtypes (Table 6.1). These subtypes are characterized by important heart-kidney interactions that share a pathophysiological basis, however, have unique discriminating features, in terms of predisposing or precipitating events, risk identification, natural history, and outcomes. In this section, we will focus on the two subtypes of cardiorenal syndrome most likely to be encountered in critical care.

### 6.2.1 Type I Cardiorenal Syndrome

This subtype is commonly encountered and is characterized by an acute cardiac event or disorder that precipitates AKI. The prototypical conditions contributing to type I CRS are acute decompensated heart failure (ADHF) and acute myocardial infarction (AMI).

**Table 6.1** Diagnostic and classification scheme for cardiorenal syndrome

| Cardiorenal syndrome (CRS) | A complex pathophysiological disorder of the heart and kidneys whereby acute or chronic dysfunction in one organ may induce acute or chronic dysfunction in the other organ |
|---|---|
| CRS type I (acute cardiorenal syndrome) | Abrupt worsening of cardiac function (e.g., ACS or ADHF) leading to AKI or acute worsening of kidney function |
| CRS type II (chronic cardiorenal syndrome) | Chronic abnormalities in cardiac function (e.g., chronic congestive heart failure) contributing to progressive and permanent chronic kidney disease |
| CRS type III (acute renocardiac syndrome) | AKI or abrupt worsening of kidney function contributing to acute cardiac disorder or decompensation |
| CRS type IV (chronic renocardiac syndrome) | Chronic kidney disease (e.g., diabetic nephropathy) contributing to decreased cardiac function, cardiac hypertrophy, fibrosis, and/or increased risk of adverse cardiovascular events |
| CRS type V (secondary cardiorenal syndrome) | Systemic condition (e.g., sepsis) contributing to both cardiac and/or kidney injury |

*ACS* acute coronary syndrome, *ADHF* acute decompensated heart failure

The pathophysiological mechanisms contributing to AKI in ADHF and AMI are numerous and complex, however, likely involve alterations to myocardial performance, cardiac output, and systemic and central venous hemodynamics that compromise kidney perfusion and coupled with maladaptive and compensatory neuro-hormonal activation (i.e., activation of the sympathetic nervous system, increased activity of renin-angiotensin-aldosterone, and non-osmotic release of arginine vasopressin). These mechanisms will be further modified not only by the severity of the inciting event but also by preexisting susceptibilities including baseline cardiac and kidney function and presence of chronic kidney disease (CKD). Observational data have confirmed that persistent AKI in ADHF is more likely among those with baseline CKD and diminished renal reserve [2].

In both ADHF and AMI, the development of AKI is associated with worse outcomes, higher rehospitalization rates, and increased health-care costs [3, 4]. Moreover, there appears to be a biological gradient between the severity of AKI and risk of death [5, 6]. Among patients reperfused following AMI, those developing AKI tended to have higher plasma norepinephrine, B-natriuretic peptide, and interleukin-6 levels in the 2 weeks after reperfusion compared to those without AKI. Those with AKI show higher risk of in-hospital death and major adverse cardiac events, including greater changes in LV remodeling during recovery. Even small acute changes in serum creatinine modify the risk of death following AMI [6]. Among those developing AKI, greater risk of cardiovascular events such as congestive heart failure (CHF), recurrent AMI, and stroke and need for rehospitalization have been shown [6]. Moreover, patients with AMI complicated by AKI have increased risk of development of incident CKD and accelerated progression to ESKD [7].

## 6.2.2 Type III Cardiorenal Syndrome

This subtype is characterized by AKI that contributes to the development of acute cardiac injury and/or dysfunction (i.e., AMI, CHF, arrhythmias). While any episode of AKI may predispose to acute cardiac dysfunction and type III CRS, the most common conditions encountered include contrast-induced AKI (CI-AKI), drug-induced nephropathies, AKI after major noncardiac surgery, AKI after cardiac surgery, post-infectious glomerulonephritis, and rhabdomyolysis. The pathophysiological mechanisms of how AKI contributes to acute cardiac injury and/or dysfunction are incompletely understood. An episode of AKI may have effects that depend both on the severity and duration of AKI and that both directly and indirectly predispose to an acute cardiac event. Moreover, baseline patient susceptibility will modify the subsequent risk for cardiac events associated with AKI (i.e., preexisting risk factors and cardiac disease).

Experimental data suggest that cardiac injury may be directly induced by inflammatory mediators release, oxidative stress, apoptosis, and activation of neuroendocrine systems early after AKI [1, 8]. Likewise, AKI may be associated with physiological derangements (i.e., extracellular volume expansion, retention of uremic [cardiotoxic] compounds, metabolic acidosis, electrolyte abnormalities [i.e., hyperkalemia, hypocalcemia]), alterations to coronary vasoreactivity, and ventricular remodeling and fibrosis that indirectly exert negative effects on cardiac performance. AKI may also adversely impact cardiac function by contributing to alternations in drug pharmacokinetics and pharmacodynamics.

CI-AKI serves as a prototypical example of type III CRS. CI-AKI remains a leading cause of iatrogenic kidney injury following diagnostic and interventional procedures and portends adverse effects on prognosis, progression of CKD, and consumption of health resources. While AKI is most often attributable to the administration of radiocontrast media, additional susceptibilities and confounding factors in the population undergoing the procedure are also likely to be contributory (i.e., atheroembolic disease, kidney hypoperfusion, concomitant nephrotoxins). The reported incidence is highly variable depending on the population at risk being evaluated and the type of procedure performed (i.e., emergent, intravascular, type, and volume of contrast media). The natural history of CI-AKI in many patients may follow an asymptomatic rise in serum creatinine with early return to baseline, and these patients would not be expected to fulfill the criteria for type III CRS. However, in an estimated 0.2–1.1 %, AKI progresses to require the initiation of renal replacement therapy (RRT) [9, 10].

In these patients, AKI may be associated with volume overload, retention of uremic solutes, CHF, pulmonary edema, and cardiac arrhythmias. Several factors have been found to independently predict development of more severe AKI after contrast media including older age, preexisting CKD, diabetes mellitus, cerebral vascular disease, heart failure, and volume/dose of contrast media. However, the difficulty in evaluating the epidemiology of type III CRS attributable to CI-AKI or AKI from other causes is that few studies have specifically reported the temporal occurrence of cardiovascular events following AKI.

## 6.3  The Kidney and the Lung

Kidney and lung injury are highly prevalent in critical illness. These two organ systems are intimately interconnected. Injury and/or dysfunction in either or both of these organ systems can directly incite or exacerbate injury and/or impairment in the other.

### 6.3.1  Impact of AKI on Lung Function

The loss of metabolic/fluid homeostasis and excretory function characteristic of AKI is associated with the retention of metabolic waste products (i.e., uremic toxins), nonvolatile acids, and the expansion of extracellular volume. This decrement in kidney function can precipitate clinically important and adverse physiological consequences on the normal function of numerous organ systems, in particular the lung [1]. The accumulation of uremic compounds is known to contribute to lung inflammation and injury and has been termed *uremic pneumonitis*. However, this complication of AKI is rarely seen due to earlier initiation and more intensive application of RRT [11]. Metabolic derangement in AKI, such as abnormalities in serum phosphate and calcium level and metabolic acidosis, may also contribute to respiratory muscle weakness and dysfunction [12]. Perhaps the most common life-threatening pulmonary complication associated with AKI is alveolar edema. Expansion of extracellular volume can contribute to increased pulmonary capillary hydrostatic pressure. This coupled with alterations to pulmonary microvascular permeability and reduced serum oncotic pressure can predispose to rapid increases in extravascular lung water [13]. AKI can also contribute to lowering the threshold for accumulation of extravascular lung water [14] along with impaired clearance of alveolar fluid once present. Indeed, lung injury in AKI can occur in the absence of overt volume overload [15]. This is due, in part, to the downregulation of epithelial sodium transporters (ENaC), sodium-potassium adenosine triphosphatases (Na-K-ATPase), and aquaporins at the alveolar-capillary barrier. In further support of the hypothesis that lung injury in AKI represents more than alveolar edema, experimental models of ischemic-/reperfusion-induced AKI have shown lung injury that is characterized by not only pulmonary vascular congestion and interstitial edema but also focal alveolar hemorrhage and inflammatory cell infiltrate [16]. Indeed, the systemic inflammation incited by AKI, including the release and reduced clearance of proinflammatory mediators, is an important mechanism contributing to acute lung injury. Moreover, the magnitude of AKI, both in terms of severity and duration, can also modify the intensity of lung injury.

Naturally, this organ crosstalk and associated clinical complications may be aggravated in critical illness due to concurrent widespread systemic inflammation (i.e., sepsis, major trauma) and diminished baseline physiological reserve due to preexisting chronic lung, cardiac, or kidney disease and in response to resuscitation (i.e., large-volume resuscitation). Among patients receiving mechanical ventilation, the development of AKI has been associated with impaired or delayed weaning,

**Table 6.2** Potential mechanisms of impaired kidney function associated with mechanical ventilation

| | |
|---|---|
| Alterations to cardiovascular function | Reduced cardiac output |
| | Reduced renal blood flow |
| | Altered distribution of intrarenal blood flow |
| | Elevated inferior vena cava and renal vein pressure |
| Alterations to neuro-hormonal function | Sympathetic nervous system activation |
| | Renin-angiotensin-aldosterone system stimulation |
| | Reduced atrial natriuretic peptide secretion |
| | Increased (non-osmotic) arginine vasopressin secretion |
| Exaggerated effects of mechanical ventilation | Intravascular volume depletion |
| | Impaired baseline myocardial performance |
| | Alterations to pulmonary compliance |
| | Prior chronic kidney disease |
| | Prior chronic pulmonary disease |

higher likelihood of tracheostomy, and prolongation of ICU stay [17]. Those patients developing lung injury and respiratory failure necessitating mechanical ventilation, concurrent with or following an episode of AKI, have worse outcome and increased risk of mortality [18, 19].

## 6.3.2 Impact of Lung Injury on the Kidney

Lung injury, such as acute respiratory distress syndrome (ARDS), can contribute to downstream kidney injury and dysfunction through a number of mechanisms including impaired gas exchange, systemic and regional hemodynamic alterations, systemic inflammation, and the application of mechanical ventilation (Table 6.2).

Abnormalities in gas exchange are common among critically ill patients with lung injury. These patients often receive supplemental oxygen, noninvasive ventilatory support, or invasive mechanical ventilation when respiratory failure ensues, with the aim of correcting hypoxemia and restoring near-normal gas exchange. However, this is often challenging or not possible, and many patients may have residual hypoxemia or hypercapnea in the setting of ARDS and lung-protective ventilation and/or permission hypercapnea. The exact mechanisms by which hypoxemia contributes to AKI are incompletely understood and, however, are likely multifactorial and relate to altered cardiovascular function, renal microcirculatory dysfunction, neuro-hormonal activation, and circulating systemic inflammatory mediators [20]. Small clinical studies have suggested that hypoxemia may impair renal autoregulation and glomerular filtration rate (GFR) and contribute to sodium and water retention, while reversal of hypoxemia may improve renal blood flow (RBF) [21, 22]. Hypercapnea has also been associated with impaired kidney function, attributed to alterations in RBF and renovascular resistance; however, experimental data have been inconsistent [23]. Further, acute hypercapnea can also

**Table 6.3**  Mechanisms of ventilator-induced lung injury (VILI)

| Volutrauma | Ventilation with excessive tidal volume or end-expiratory volumes |
|---|---|
| Barotrauma | Ventilation with excessive end-inspiratory or plateau pressures |
| Atelect-trauma | Ventilation below the lower inflection point on the pressure-volume curve with cyclic opening and closing of alveoli |
| Biotrauma | Local and systemic release of inflammatory mediators in response to mechanical stress and disruption of alveoli |

contribute to or worsen existing acidemia. The combined impact of hypoxemia and hypercapnea may act synergistically to impair kidney function [24].

Lung injury may be the result of primary lung disease (i.e., aspiration, contusion) or a systemic process (i.e., pancreatitis, sepsis); however, the application of mechanical ventilation is well recognized as a potentially important precipitant or exacerbating factor in lung injury. Ventilator-induced lung injury (VILI) is attributable to the use of excessive end-inspiratory pressures and volumes coupled with the added effects of barotrauma, atelect-trauma, and biotrauma (Table 6.3). The mechanical disruption of the alveolar-capillary barrier from excessive pressure-volume loading during positive pressure ventilation can induce the release of local inflammatory mediators into the systemic circulation [25]. This inflammation due to VILI can contribute to downstream end-organ injury, including AKI [26]. In a murine model of lung injury, the application of injurious MV was associated with increased expression of IL-6 in kidney tissue, increased evidence of renal tubular apoptosis, and impaired kidney function [27, 28].

## 6.4    The Kidney in the Abdominal Compartment

The kidneys are encapsulated organs, located in the retroperitoneal space of the abdominal compartment. Therefore, alterations in the abdomen can seriously disturb kidney function. This section discusses the impact of elevated intra-abdominal pressure (IAP), deranged splanchnic and renal hemodynamics, and abdominal organ dysfunction on renal function in critically ill patients.

### 6.4.1   Intra-abdominal Hypertension and Abdominal Compartment Syndrome

There has been increasing focus on the detrimental effects of elevated IAP in AKI [29]. IAP is normally between 5 and 7 mmHg in healthy individuals and $\leq$10 mmHg in critically ill adults, measured supine at end-expiration, zeroed at the level where the midaxillary line crosses the iliac crest [30]. By consensus, intra-abdominal hypertension (IAH) is defined as a sustained increase in IAP $\geq$12 mmHg, and abdominal compartment syndrome (ACS) as a sustained increase >20 mmHg with new organ dysfunction/failure [30]. The most important risk factors for these conditions are shock/hypotension, resuscitation with a large amount of fluids, and worsening respiratory status [31]. Therefore, it should not be surprising that IAH is common among critically ill patients and associated with worse outcome [32]. However, it is less clear whether the relationship between IAH and organ dysfunction represents cause and effect and if prevention/treatment of IAH might improve organ function and prognosis.

## 6.4.2 Elevated Intra-abdominal Pressure and Renal Function

Elevated IAP influences renal function in different ways. First, IAH might lead to a significant decrease in RBF as renal perfusion pressure equals mean arterial pressure minus IAP [33]. Further, higher intrarenal vascular resistance (organ compression) shunts blood away from the kidneys. This is of particular concern for the renal medulla, which receives only ~12 % of the RBF, exacerbated by neurohumoral activation [34]. Indeed, AKI through ischemic tubular necrosis is probably the most common complication in the ICU necessitating RRT. Second, the combination of systemic venous congestion and elevated IAP decreases the glomerular filtration gradient [35]. Because the kidney is an encapsulated organ, a pressure rise in the venous system translates into a higher renal interstitial and Bowman's capsular pressure, directly impeding glomerular filtration [36, 37]. Intriguingly, in advanced heart failure – presumably because of low renal perfusion – the kidneys are extremely sensitive to even small elevations in IAP (8–10 mmHg) [38]. Moreover, decreasing IAP in such cases, through ultrafiltration or paracentesis, can dramatically improve renal function [38]. Extrapolating these findings to the general ICU population, recent evidence suggests that a comprehensive management strategy with appropriate use of an open abdomen in patients at risk significantly improves survival from IAH/ACS [39].

## 6.4.3 Gut Microbiota and the Intestinal Barrier Function

A new area of research is the role of gut microbiota in AKI. It has been clearly established that bacterial fermentation processes in the large intestines are an important source of tightly protein-bound toxins such as p-cresyl sulfate and indoxyl sulfate [40]. Because of this protein binding, such toxins are difficult to clear from the circulation, even by means of hemodialysis [41]. They may accelerate kidney dysfunction, and plasma levels are correlated to all-cause mortality [42, 43]. This offers a strong rationale for targeting gut microbiota and toxin production in the bowel compartment with future therapies.

In normal circumstances, the gut has an important barrier function, preventing entrance of toxins and microorganisms into the systemic circulation. However, especially when abdominal perfusion is impaired, like in advanced heart failure or patients with IAH, this function might become compromised [44]. Indeed, it has been shown that the intestinal morphology, permeability, and function are substantially altered in heart failure [45, 46]. Consequently, leakage of lipopolysaccharides in the systemic circulation may cause further hemodynamic compromise leading to a detrimental vicious cycle [44, 47]. As the ICU clusters, the most vulnerable patients with regard to hemodynamic compromise, kidney and organ dysfunction, this is likely an underrecognized problem and should be an area of further research. Only recently, IAP has been identified as a potential missing link in patients with cardiorenal syndrome, and the term cardio-abdominal-renal syndrome (CARS) was coined [44].

### 6.4.4  Hepatorenal Syndrome

AKI is a fearsome complication in patients with decompensating liver cirrhosis, where it occurs in ~20 %, and is associated with poor outcome [48]. Patients with cirrhosis are susceptible to developing AKI because of the progressive vasodilatory state and reduced effective blood volume. Hepatorenal syndrome is initiated by portal hypertension and may be triggered by bacterial infections, nonbacterial systemic inflammatory reactions, excessive diuresis, gastrointestinal hemorrhage, diarrhea, nephrotoxic agents, or IAH [49]. Orthotopic liver transplantation is the best current treatment and leads to a gradual recovery of renal function in the vast majority of patients.

### 6.4.5  Conclusions

The kidneys are well-perfused organs, located inside the retroperitoneal space of the abdomen. Elevated IAP may seriously disrupt systemic and renal hemodynamics, which might cause renal dysfunction and loss of intestinal barrier function with subsequent entry of toxins into the systemic circulation. A more thorough understanding of kidney-organ interactions in the abdominal compartment may hopefully lead to new therapeutic targets to better preserve renal function in critically ill patients. Within this regard it is important to consider IAP as a missing link in patients with congestive heart failure developing worsening kidney function. This condition has been termed as CARS.

## 6.5  The Kidney and the Brain

The kidney and brain are vital organs protected in health by an autoregulated blood supply. Both organs play a role in regulating sodium and water balance in the body and visceral sympathetic nervous system activity.

### 6.5.1  Hyponatremia

Hyponatremia may occur following acute cerebral damage, with reports of an incidence of 56 % postsubarachnoid hemorrhage, but may also develop posttraumatic brain injury. Mortality increases as serum sodium falls, increasing as serum sodium

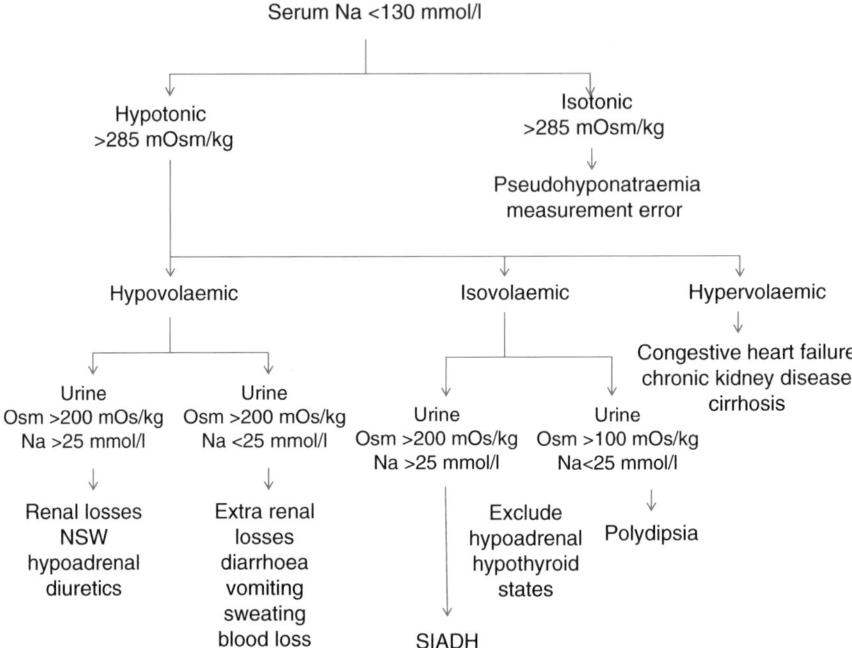



**Fig. 6.1** Investigating hyponatremia in the brain-injured patient. Clinically examine patients and determine volume status, and review daily weights and serial estimations of fluid intake and output charts, then check serum osmolality, hematocrit, urea, creatinine, and urate and urinary osmolality and electrolytes. Measure liver function tests and thyroid, adrenal, and natriuretic hormones as required

falls from <130 to <120 mmol/L from 11 to 25 % [50]. Vasopressin release from the hypothalamus, termed syndrome of inappropriate antidiuretic hormone release (SIADH) and leads to water retention by the kidney, is the most common cause of hyponatremia (60–70 %), but cerebral salt wasting, now termed nephrogenic sodium wasting (NSW), may also develop (6–10 %). Both conditions cause hyponatremia, and although physical examination may help to discriminate between these conditions, with SIADH patients typically being euvolemic [51] and those with NSW having signs of extracellular volume depletion, in clinical practice, it may be difficult to distinguish between these conditions and, in a small proportion of cases, both conditions may be present (5 %). Similarly biochemical investigation may also be unhelpful as both conditions will have a reduced serum osmolality (<285 mOsmo/kg), with a relatively increased urinary sodium (>25 mmol/l) and urinary osmolality (>200 mOsmo/kg) (Fig. 6.1). However, patients with NSW should have increased urea, creatinine, and hematocrit due to intravascular volume depletion, whereas they should be normal or lowered in SIADH due to relative water retention [52]. In both conditions serum urate is typically reduced. It is important to make the correct diagnosis as instituting the standard treatment for SIADH, namely, water restriction and a vasopressin receptor antagonist, can lead to permanent ischemic cerebral damage and mortality in patients with NSW, who require a controlled increase in serum sodium, approximately 8 mmol/day, using hypertonic saline in combination with fludrocortisone [53].

## 6.5.2 Hypernatremia

Cranial diabetes insipidus can develop acutely posttraumatic brain injury, pituitary surgery or infarction, stroke, cerebral tumor, and infection (meningitis or encephalitis), although most cases are idiopathic and are thought to be autoimmune. Initially patients are polyuric, passing a dilute urine (<150 mOsm/kg) due to a failure of vasopressin release but after 4–5 days may then become transiently oliguric due to the release of stored ADH from the hypothalamus, before a chronic state ensues [54]. The conscious patient typically compensates by drinking large volumes of water, but the unconscious patient may develop profound life-threatening hypernatremia.

For patients with acute hypernatremia (<48 h), rapid lowering of serum sodium by 1 mmol/h by the administration of hypotonic fluids does not increase the risk of cerebral edema, whereas those with hypernatremia of unknown or longer duration a slower pace of correction, aiming for around 10 mmol/L/day is important to prevent cerebral edema. As the risk of cerebral edema also depends upon the volume infused, then smaller volumes of more hypotonic fluids are advantageous [55].

$$\text{Water deficit} = \text{Total body water} \times \left( \left( \text{Current serum sodium} / 140 \right) - 1 \right).$$

## 6.5.3 Acute Kidney Injury and the Brain

Acute kidney injury typically leads to systemic inflammation, exacerbated by reduced cytokine clearances. Cytokines and other inflammatory mediators may gain entry to the brain through the fenestrated vascular endothelium in the floor of the third ventricle, leading to appetite suppression and increasing the risk of delirium [56]. Increasing osmolality and inflammation as renal failure progressively leads to the disruption of the blood-brain barrier. In addition, kidney failure leads to the accumulation of the waste products of nitrogen metabolism, with organic acids accumulating in the brain, resulting in changes in both neuronal intracellular osmolality and neurotransmitter levels [57]. So, if untreated, patients become encephalopathic with classic slow wave brain electrical activity (loss of alpha and beta waves, with predominance of theta and delta wave activity) [58] (Fig. 6.2).

Patients with kidney failure are at greater risk of drug-induced encephalopathy, as many drugs are transported from the brain by organic acid transporters, and due to the competition for these transporters, clearance from the brain is delayed leading to accumulation.

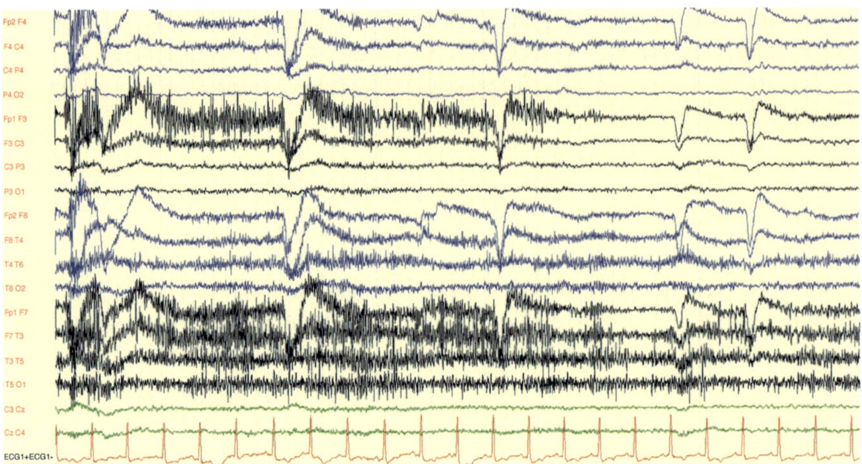

**Fig. 6.2** Electrical encephalography from a patient with uremic encephalopathy showing absent normal faster alpha and beta activity with predominance of slower theta and delta wave activity

Initially kidney transplant recipients may develop an acute psychosis due to high doses of steroids and also an acute encephalopathy due to immunophyllin neurotoxicity (tacrolimus > cyclosporin) [59], and treatment of acute rejection with the newer anti-lymphocyte antibody therapies. Thereafter, continued immunosuppression to maintain kidney transplant function increases the risk of cerebral infections, including viral encephalitis and listerial and fungal meningitis [60].

### 6.5.4 Conditions Affecting Both the Kidney and Brain

The brain and kidney can both be acutely affected by infections (bacterial, leptospirosis; viral, Epstein-Barr virus, human immunodeficiency virus; and protozoal, malaria) and also by systemic vasculitides (polyarteritis nodosa, microscopic polyangiitis). Other conditions including sarcoidosis can cause chronic disease in both organs, and some patients with adult polycystic kidney disease are predisposed to intracerebral aneurysms.

---

**Conclusions**

The kidney interacts with virtually all organ systems in the body. Acute injury to the kidney can clearly contribute to cardiac, pulmonary, gastrointestinal, hepatic, and neurologic injury and/or dysfunction through a host of mechanisms. Likewise, primary injury and/or dysfunction to any of these organ systems can directly and indirectly contribute to kidney injury and impairment.

**Key Messages**

**The Kidney and the Heart**

- Kidney and cardiac diseases commonly coexist. Injury and/or dysfunction in either organ system can synergistically cause injury and/or dysfunction in the other.
- Acute cardiac events (i.e., ADHF, AMI) can contribute to AKI through hemodynamic, neuroendocrine, and inflammation mechanisms.
- AKI can directly and indirectly contribute to acute cardiac events through complications related to loss of kidney excretory function, along with neuro-hormonal activation and systemic inflammation.

**The Kidney and the Lung**

- The kidney and lung are commonly injured in critical illness.
- In AKI, the loss of kidney excretory function expands extracellular volume to increase the risk of pulmonary capillary hydrostatic pressure. This is exacerbated by downregulation of key fluid transport molecules in the alveoli, alterations to microvascular permeability, and reduced serum oncotic pressure, which further lower the threshold for alveolar edema and impair alveolar fluid clearance.
- Mechanical ventilation, through alterations in intrathoracic pressures and systemic hemodynamics and through exacerbation of lung injury, can contribute to AKI and negatively impact kidney function.

**The Kidney and the Abdominal Compartment**

- Normal IAP is ≤10 mmHg in critically ill patients.
- IAH (sustained IAP >12 mmHg) is frequently associated with AKI through multiple pathways (fluid overload, low perfusion, neurohumoral).
- Elevated IAP is considered an important contributor in patients with congestive heart failure and worsening kidney function, and this is termed CARS.
- Gut microbiota and toxins may play a role in the development of AKI and form an area for future research.
- Hepatorenal syndrome needs to be considered in patients with cirrhosis and worsening kidney function.

**The Kidney and the Brain**

- Nephrogenic sodium wasting is a potential cause of hyponatremia in patients with acute brain injury and infections and must not be confused with SIADH.
- Cranial diabetes insipidus may develop acutely following acute brain injury and pituitary surgery, causing hypernatremia.

- Renal transplant patients are at increased risk of drug-induced encephalopathy and psychotic reactions during the first weeks post transplantation.
- In the longer-term renal transplant, patients are immunocompromised and remain at risk of cerebral infections.

## References


1. Grams ME, Rabb H. The distant organ effects of acute kidney injury. Kidney Int. 2012;81(10): 942–8.
2. Aronson D, Burger AJ. The relationship between transient and persistent worsening renal function and mortality in patients with acute decompensated heart failure. J Card Fail. 2010;16(7):541–7.
3. Krumholz HM, Chen YT, Vaccarino V, Wang Y, Radford MJ, Bradford WD, et al. Correlates and impact on outcomes of worsening renal function in patients > or =65 years of age with heart failure. Am J Cardiol. 2000;85(9):1110–3.
4. Metra M, Nodari S, Parrinello G, Bordonali T, Bugatti S, Danesi R, et al. Worsening renal function in patients hospitalised for acute heart failure: clinical implications and prognostic significance. Eur J Heart Fail. 2008;10(2):188–95.
5. Smith GL, Vaccarino V, Kosiborod M, Lichtman JH, Cheng S, Watnick SG, et al. Worsening renal function: what is a clinically meaningful change in creatinine during hospitalization with heart failure? J Card Fail. 2003;9(1):13–25.
6. Jose P, Skali H, Anavekar N, Tomson C, Krumholz HM, Rouleau JL, et al. Increase in creatinine and cardiovascular risk in patients with systolic dysfunction after myocardial infarction. J Am Soc Nephrol. 2006;17(10):2886–91.
7. Newsome BB, Warnock DG, McClellan WM, Herzog CA, Kiefe CI, Eggers PW, et al. Long-term risk of mortality and end-stage renal disease among the elderly after small increases in serum creatinine level during hospitalization for acute myocardial infarction. Arch Intern Med. 2008;168(6):609–16.
8. Kelly KJ. Distant effects of experimental renal ischemia/reperfusion injury. J Am Soc Nephrol. 2003;14(6):1549–58.
9. Weisbord SD, Hartwig KC, Sonel AF, Fine MJ, Palevsky P. The incidence of clinically significant contrast-induced nephropathy following non-emergent coronary angiography. Catheter Cardiovasc Interv. 2008;71(7):879–85.
10. Weisbord SD, Mor MK, Resnick AL, Hartwig KC, Sonel AF, Fine MJ, et al. Prevention, incidence, and outcomes of contrast-induced acute kidney injury. Arch Intern Med. 2008; 168(12):1325–32.
11. Hopps HC, Wissler RW. Uremic pneumonitis. Am J Pathol. 1955;31(2):261–73.
12. Bush A, Gabriel R. The lungs in uraemia: a review. J R Soc Med. 1985;78(10):849–55.
13. National Heart L, Blood Institute Acute Respiratory Distress Syndrome Clinical, Trials N, Wiedemann HP, Wheeler AP, Bernard GR, Thompson BT, et al. Comparison of two fluid-management strategies in acute lung injury. N Engl J Med. 2006;354(24):2564–75.
14. Slutsky RA, Day R, Murray M. Effect of prolonged renal dysfunction on intravascular and extravascular pulmonary fluid volumes during left atrial hypertension. Proc Soc Exp Biol Med. 1985;179(1):25–31.
15. Kramer AA, Postler G, Salhab KF, Mendez C, Carey LC, Rabb H. Renal ischemia/reperfusion leads to macrophage-mediated increase in pulmonary vascular permeability. Kidney Int. 1999;55(6):2362–7.

16. Hassoun HT, Grigoryev DN, Lie ML, Liu M, Cheadle C, Tuder RM, et al. Ischemic acute kidney injury induces a distant organ functional and genomic response distinguishable from bilateral nephrectomy. Am J Physiol Renal Physiol. 2007;293(1):F30–40.
17. Vieira Jr JM, Castro I, Curvello-Neto A, Demarzo S, Caruso P, Pastore Jr L, et al. Effect of acute kidney injury on weaning from mechanical ventilation in critically ill patients. Crit Care Med. 2007;35(1):184–91.
18. Chertow GM, Levy EM, Hammermeister KE, Grover F, Daley J. Independent association between acute renal failure and mortality following cardiac surgery. Am J Med. 1998;104(4): 343–8.
19. Metnitz PG, Krenn CG, Steltzer H, Lang T, Ploder J, Lenz K, et al. Effect of acute renal failure requiring renal replacement therapy on outcome in critically ill patients. Crit Care Med. 2002;30(9):2051–8.
20. Aksu U, Demirci C, Ince C. The pathogenesis of acute kidney injury and the toxic triangle of oxygen, reactive oxygen species and nitric oxide. Contrib Nephrol. 2011;174:119–28.
21. Howes TQ, Deane CR, Levin GE, Baudouin SV, Moxham J. The effects of oxygen and dopamine on renal and aortic blood flow in chronic obstructive pulmonary disease with hypoxemia and hypercapnia. Am J Respir Crit Care Med. 1995;151(2 Pt 1):378–83.
22. Reihman DH, Farber MO, Weinberger MH, Henry DP, Fineberg NS, Dowdeswell IR, et al. Effect of hypoxemia on sodium and water excretion in chronic obstructive lung disease. Am J Med. 1985;78(1):87–94.
23. Anderson RJ, Rose Jr CE, Berns AS, Erickson AL, Arnold PE. Mechanism of effect of hypercapnic acidosis on renin secretion in the dog. Am J Physiol. 1980;238(2):F119–25.
24. Rose Jr CE, Kimmel DP, Godine Jr RL, Kaiser DL, Carey RM. Synergistic effects of acute hypoxemia and hypercapnic acidosis in conscious dogs. Renal dysfunction and activation of the renin-angiotensin system. Circ Res. 1983;53(2):202–13.
25. Chiumello D, Pristine G, Slutsky AS. Mechanical ventilation affects local and systemic cytokines in an animal model of acute respiratory distress syndrome. Am J Respir Crit Care Med. 1999;160(1):109–16.
26. Meduri GU, Headley S, Kohler G, Stentz F, Tolley E, Umberger R, et al. Persistent elevation of inflammatory cytokines predicts a poor outcome in ARDS. Plasma IL-1 beta and IL-6 levels are consistent and efficient predictors of outcome over time. Chest. 1995;107(4):1062–73.
27. Gurkan OU, O'Donnell C, Brower R, Ruckdeschel E, Becker PM. Differential effects of mechanical ventilatory strategy on lung injury and systemic organ inflammation in mice. Am J Physiol Lung Cell Mol Physiol. 2003;285(3):L710–8.
28. Imai Y, Parodo J, Kajikawa O, de Perrot M, Fischer S, Edwards V, et al. Injurious mechanical ventilation and end-organ epithelial cell apoptosis and organ dysfunction in an experimental model of acute respiratory distress syndrome. JAMA. 2003;289(16):2104–12.
29. Malbrain ML, Chiumello D, Pelosi P, Bihari D, Innes R, Ranieri VM, et al. Incidence and prognosis of intraabdominal hypertension in a mixed population of critically ill patients: a multiple-center epidemiological study. Crit Care Med. 2005;33(2):315–22.
30. Kirkpatrick AW, Roberts DJ, De Waele J, Jaeschke R, Malbrain ML, De Keulenaer B, et al. Intra-abdominal hypertension and the abdominal compartment syndrome: updated consensus definitions and clinical practice guidelines from the World Society of the Abdominal Compartment Syndrome. Intensive Care Med. 2013;39(7):1190–206.
31. Holodinsky JK, Roberts DJ, Ball CG, Blaser AR, Starkopf J, Zygun DA, et al. Risk factors for intra-abdominal hypertension and abdominal compartment syndrome among adult intensive care unit patients: a systematic review and meta-analysis. Crit Care. 2013;17(5):R249.
32. Vidal MG, Ruiz Weisser J, Gonzalez F, Toro MA, Loudet C, Balasini C, et al. Incidence and clinical effects of intra-abdominal hypertension in critically ill patients. Crit Care Med. 2008;36(6):1823–31.
33. Wauters J, Claus P, Brosens N, McLaughlin M, Malbrain M, Wilmer A. Pathophysiology of renal hemodynamics and renal cortical microcirculation in a porcine model of elevated intra-abdominal pressure. J Trauma. 2009;66(3):713–9.

34. Janssen WM, Beekhuis H, de Bruin R, de Jong PE, de Zeeuw D. Noninvasive measurement of intrarenal blood flow distribution: kinetic model of renal 123I-hippuran handling. Am J Physiol. 1995;269(4 Pt 2):F571–80.
35. Dupont M, Mullens W, Tang WH. Impact of systemic venous congestion in heart failure. Curr Heart Fail Rep. 2011;8(4):233–41.
36. Maxwell MH, Breed ES, Schwartz IL. Renal venous pressure in chronic congestive heart failure. J Clin Invest. 1950;29(3):342–8.
37. Gottschalk CW, Mylle M. Micropuncture study of pressures in proximal tubules and peritubular capillaries of the rat kidney and their relation to ureteral and renal venous pressures. Am J Physiol. 1956;185(2):430–9.
38. Mullens W, Abrahams Z, Francis GS, Taylor DO, Starling RC, Tang WH. Prompt reduction in intra-abdominal pressure following large-volume mechanical fluid removal improves renal insufficiency in refractory decompensated heart failure. J Card Fail. 2008;14(6):508–14.
39. Cheatham ML, Safcsak K. Is the evolving management of intra-abdominal hypertension and abdominal compartment syndrome improving survival? Crit Care Med. 2010;38(2):402–7.
40. Evenepoel P, Meijers BK, Bammens BR, Verbeke K. Uremic toxins originating from colonic microbial metabolism. Kidney Int Suppl. 2009;114:S12–9.
41. Meyer TW, Leeper EC, Bartlett DW, Depner TA, Lit YZ, Robertson CR, et al. Increasing dialysate flow and dialyzer mass transfer area coefficient to increase the clearance of protein-bound solutes. J Am Soc Nephrol. 2004;15(7):1927–35.
42. Bammens B, Evenepoel P, Keuleers H, Verbeke K, Vanrenterghem Y. Free serum concentrations of the protein-bound retention solute p-cresol predict mortality in hemodialysis patients. Kidney Int. 2006;69(6):1081–7.
43. Niwa T, Nomura T, Sugiyama S, Miyazaki T, Tsukushi S, Tsutsui S. The protein metabolite hypothesis, a model for the progression of renal failure: an oral adsorbent lowers indoxyl sulfate levels in undialyzed uremic patients. Kidney Int Suppl. 1997;62:S23–8.
44. Verbrugge FH, Dupont M, Steels P, Grieten L, Malbrain M, Tang WH, et al. Abdominal contributions to cardiorenal dysfunction in congestive heart failure. J Am Coll Cardiol. 2013;62(6):485–95.
45. Arutyunov GP, Kostyukevich OI, Serov RA, Rylova NV, Bylova NA. Collagen accumulation and dysfunctional mucosal barrier of the small intestine in patients with chronic heart failure. Int J Cardiol. 2008;125(2):240–5.
46. Magnusson M, Magnusson KE, Sundqvist T, Denneberg T. Impaired intestinal barrier function measured by differently sized polyethylene glycols in patients with chronic renal failure. Gut. 1991;32(7):754–9.
47. Charalambous BM, Stephens RC, Feavers IM, Montgomery HE. Role of bacterial endotoxin in chronic heart failure: the gut of the matter. Shock. 2007;28(1):15–23.
48. Hartleb M, Gutkowski K. Kidneys in chronic liver diseases. World J Gastroenterol. 2012;18(24):3035–49.
49. Kramer L, Horl WH. Hepatorenal syndrome. Semin Nephrol. 2002;22(4):290–301.
50. Wright WL. Sodium and fluid management in acute brain injury. Curr Neurol Neurosci Rep. 2012;12(4):466–73.
51. Esposito P, Piotti G, Bianzina S, Malul Y, Dal Canton A. The syndrome of inappropriate antidiuresis: pathophysiology, clinical management and new therapeutic options. Nephron Clin Pract. 2011;119(1):c62–73; discussion c73.
52. Maesaka JK, Imbriano LJ, Ali NM, Ilamathi E. Is it cerebral or renal salt wasting? Kidney Int. 2009;76(9):934–8.
53. Yee AH, Burns JD, Wijdicks EF. Cerebral salt wasting: pathophysiology, diagnosis, and treatment. Neurosurg Clin N Am. 2010;21(2):339–52.
54. Di Iorgi N, Napoli F, Allegri AE, Olivieri I, Bertelli E, Gallizia A, et al. Diabetes insipidus–diagnosis and management. Horm Res Paediatr. 2012;77(2):69–84.
55. Chanson P, Salenave S. Treatment of neurogenic diabetes insipidus. Ann Endocrinol. 2011;72(6):496–9.

56. Liu M, Liang Y, Chigurupati S, Lathia JD, Pletnikov M, Sun Z, et al. Acute kidney injury leads to inflammation and functional changes in the brain. J Am Soc Nephrol. 2008;19(7): 1360–70.
57. Palkovits M, Sebekova K, Gallatz K, Boor P, Sebekova Jr K, Klassen A, et al. Neuronal activation in the CNS during different forms of acute renal failure in rats. Neuroscience. 2009; 159(2):862–82.
58. Adachi N, Lei B, Deshpande G, Seyfried FJ, Shimizu I, Nagaro T, et al. Uraemia suppresses central dopaminergic metabolism and impairs motor activity in rats. Intensive Care Med. 2001;27(10):1655–60.
59. Mammoser A. Calcineurin inhibitor encephalopathy. Semin Neurol. 2012;32(5):517–24.
60. Senzolo M, Ferronato C, Burra P. Neurologic complications after solid organ transplantation. Transpl Int. 2009;22(3):269–78.

# Acute Kidney Injury in Pregnancy

Marjel van Dam and Sean M. Bagshaw

## 7.1 Introduction

Acute kidney injury (AKI) in pregnancy may contribute to maternal and fetal morbidity and mortality, in particular in developing countries. Any disorders leading to kidney injury in the general population, such as ischemic or nephrotoxic injury or antibody-mediated glomerulonephritis, can cause AKI in pregnancy. This chapter will focus on pregnancy-associated complications, typical of each trimester that can result in severe AKI. In the early pregnancy most common problems are prerenal disease due to hyperemesis gravidarum or azotemia caused by hemorrhage. Later in pregnancy several different, pregnancy-specific disorders may contribute to AKI including preeclampsia/HELLP syndrome, thrombotic microangiopathies, acute fatty liver of pregnancy (AFLP), and renal cortical necrosis, related to infection, urinary tract obstruction, or nephrolithiasis.

## 7.2 Epidemiology

Over the past decades the incidence of pregnancy-related AKI in the developed world has decreased [1]. Advancement of prenatal care, improved availability of safe and legal abortion, and more widespread and aggressive antibiotic use (leading to a decreased incidence of septic abortion) are responsible for this decrease.

M. van Dam, MD (✉)
Department of Intensive Care, University Medical Center Utrecht,
P.O. Box 85500, Utrecht 3508 GA, The Netherlands
e-mail: M.J.vanDam@umcutrecht.nl

S.M. Bagshaw, MD MSc
Division of Critical Care Medicine, Faculty of Medicine and Dentistry,
University of Alberta, Edmonton, AB, Canada

© Springer International Publishing 2015
H.M. Oudemans-van Straaten et al. (eds.), *Acute Nephrology for the Critical Care Physician*, DOI 10.1007/978-3-319-17389-4_7

The incidence of pregnancy-related AKI in developed countries is estimated at 1 in 20,000 pregnancies [1]. Different definitions of AKI, especially in the older literature, hamper direct comparisons. Accurate data on pregnancy-related AKI in developing countries is not readily available due to the fact that many patients have limited access to health care, and different regional data collection techniques, both responsible for underreporting [2]. A study performed by Prakash in Eastern India shows that late pregnancy-related AKI occurs in about 1 in 56 births, with an overall mortality of 20 % [3]. Earlier the same group showed that the incidence of pregnancy-related AKI in their region declined from 15 % in 1982–1991 to 10 % in 1992–2002 [4]. Higher mortality in the past was attributed to late referral, frequent sepsis, and high incidence of bilateral diffuse cortical necrosis.

Etiology of pregnancy-related AKI in developed countries is different from the etiology in developing countries. Pregnancy-related AKI in developed countries is caused by largely by preeclampsia, HELLP syndrome, thrombotic microangiopathy, sepsis, and hemorrhage by abruptio placentae. While in the developing countries pregnancy-related AKI is most commonly caused by abruptio placentae, infectious causes such as puerperal sepsis and septic abortion, and postpartum hemorrhage [1].

## 7.3    Physiological Changes in Pregnancy

During normal pregnancy the kidneys increase in length approximately 1–1.5 cm, and the volume of the kidneys augments by 30 %. More than 90 % of pregnant women develop physiologic hydronephrosis of pregnancy during the second trimester which is characterized by dilatation of the collecting system of the kidneys (right more than left) which disappears in a few months postpartum [5]. The increased capacity of the dilated urinary collecting systems is caused by a combination of direct hormonal influence of estrogen and progesterone, inhibition of ureteral peristalsis by prostaglandin E2, mechanical obstruction of the ureters caused by the growing uterus, and increased glomerular filtration rate (GFR), urine formation rate, and urine flow [6].

Soon after conception blood pressure falls as a result of peripheral vasodilatation, mediated by increased nitric oxide synthesis, which also mediates vasodilatation through relaxin produced by the placenta, and reduced vascular responsiveness to angiotensin II. Peripheral vasodilation may show as palmar erythema and spider telangiectasia. This is accompanied by increase in cardiac output and renal plasma flow elevating the GFR by 50 % of baseline, and as a consequence the normal plasma creatinine levels are lowered to <44 μmol/L (0.5 mg/dL) [6].

The blood volume increases by about 50 % in pregnancy. With a disproportionate increase of plasma compared to red blood cells, physiologic anemia of pregnancy develops. Decreased peripheral vascular resistance stimulates sodium retention (500–900 mmol) and causes increased extracellular fluid volume, weight gain, and "benign" edema of the lower extremities. Potassium metabolism is unchanged by pregnancy despite a cumulative retention of about 350 mmol,

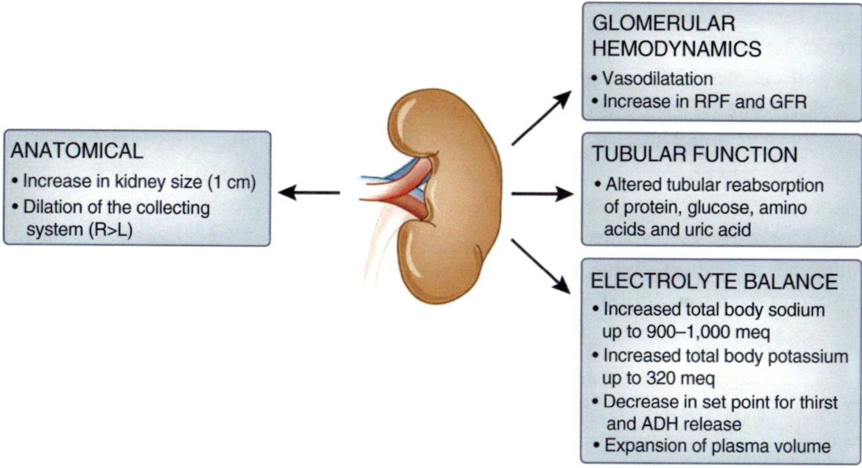


**Fig. 7.1** Summary of renal hemodynamic and metabolic adaptations to normal human pregnancy (*RPF* renal plasma flow, *ADH* antidiuretic hormone) (From Odutayo et al. [10])

necessary for fetal–placental development and expansion of the maternal red blood cell mass and the increased aldosterone levels [6].

In addition, filtered glucose load augmentation leads to renal glucosuria in the absence of hyperglycemia. Increases in GFR and the glomerular permeability to albumin combine to raise the fractional excretion of protein to <300 mg/day [7]. Thirst and a downward setting of the osmotic threshold for arginine vasopressin lower the serum osmolarity (average 10 mOsmol/L) and serum sodium concentration (approximately 5 mmol/L) [6]. Elevated circulating progesterone causes relative hyperventilation (primarily via an increase in tidal volume) and mild respiratory alkalosis, with a decrease in bicarbonate of approximately 4 mmol/L [8]. Although prothrombotic changes, including elevated plasma concentrations of fibrinogen, von Willebrand factor, and factor VIII, occur with normal pregnancy, there is also in activity in Von Willebrand factor cleaving protease (ADAMTS13) [9]. Physiologic changes peak at the end of the second trimester and then begin to trend toward pre-pregnancy levels, whereas anatomical changes may persist up to 3 months postpartum.

Figure 7.1 summarizes the renal hemodynamic and metabolic adaptations to normal human pregnancy.

## 7.4  Laboratory Testing

Laboratory testing of the kidney function in pregnancy requires alertness from the clinician. Serum creatinine is in itself a late marker for AKI, and normal values for the general population are considered high for pregnant women due to higher GFR and hemodilution. Normal plasma creatinine for pregnant women with a previous undisturbed kidney function falls to $40 \pm 11.5$ μmol/L and is significantly lower than in the general population. Novel biomarkers for the diagnosis of AKI, such as neutrophil gelatinase-associated lipocalin (NGAL) in urine and serum, serum cystatin C, urine kidney injury molecule-1 (KIM-1), have not been appropriately investigated in this population. Proteinuria increases with normal pregnancy (up to 300 mg/day) and may not indicate significant kidney injury or pathology [11]. GFR in pregnancy is difficult to measure: the Modification of Diet in Renal Disease (MDRD) and Cockcroft-Gault formulas have been examined and found inaccurate during pregnancy. The creatinine clearance in 24-h urine collection is still considered the gold standard for estimating GFR during pregnancy [12, 13].

## 7.5 Pathophysiology

As in the general adult population, AKI related to pregnancy can be categorized into prerenal, renal, and postrenal. Timing of onset during pregnancy is an important indicator in the differential diagnosis (Table 7.1).

### 7.5.1 First Trimester

Prerenal azotemia during the first trimester of pregnancy is commonly caused by hyperemesis gravidarum and hemorrhage. Hyperemesis gravidarum is diagnosed with the following criteria: persistent vomiting accompanied by weight loss >5 % of pregnancy body weight and ketonuria unrelated to other causes [14]. Hyperemesis patients can present with AKI, metabolic alkalosis, and hypokalemia. Laboratory findings may include increased hematocrit (due to hemoconcentration), mildly elevated aminotransferases, and mild hyperthyroidism [15], possibly caused by the thyroid stimulating hormonal activity of human chorionic gonadotropin [16]. Supportive treatment with antiemetic drugs and intravenous fluid will generally correct the acid-base, electrolyte, and kidney abnormalities.

**Table 7.1** Common risk factors for pregnancy-related AKI

|  | Developed countries | Developing countries |
| --- | --- | --- |
| First trimester | Hyperemesis gravidarum | Hyperemesis gravidarum |
|  |  | Septic abortion |
| Second/third trimester | Preeclampsia/HELLP | Abruptio placentae |
|  | Thrombotic microangiopathy | Infectious causes<br>Puerperal sepsis<br>Septic abortion |
|  | Sepsis | Postpartum hemorrhage |
|  | Postpartum hemorrhage |  |
|  | H1N1 influenza (2009) |  |

Hemorrhage in the first trimester of pregnancy usually is associated with ectopic pregnancy, miscarriage, or abnormal pathology of the genital tract (e.g., polyps, infection). This may lead to hypovolemia and subsequent prerenal azotemia. Treatment of the underlying pathology to prevent further damage is warranted.

## 7.5.2  Second and Third Trimester

### 7.5.2.1 Preeclampsia and Hemolysis, Elevated Liver Enzymes, and Low Platelets (HELLP) Syndrome

Preeclampsia is a pregnancy-specific condition generally defined as the new onset of persistent hypertension (diastolic blood pressure ≥90 mmHg) and proteinuria (≥300 mg in a 24-h urine collection) at or after 20 weeks' gestation [17]. It is hypothesized that a disturbance in the placental function in early pregnancy causes preeclampsia, with a particular role for the impaired remodeling of the spiral artery [18]. Preeclampsia can be asymptomatic, especially in the early stages or with mild disease, but symptoms can include epigastric and right upper quadrant pain (40–90 %), headache, visual changes, nausea, and vomiting [19]. Severe preeclampsia and the HELLP syndrome account for about 40 % of cases of AKI in pregnancy [20]. Although preeclampsia is one of the most important causes of pregnancy-related AKI, the majority of preeclamptic patients do not develop severe AKI. Otherwise, severe preeclampsia, characterized by multiple organ involvement (i.e., pulmonary edema, oliguria [<500 mL/24 h], and thrombocytopenia [platelet count <100,000 μL]) has a higher risk for AKI. The incidence of overt renal failure in severe preeclampsia is estimated at 1.5–2 % based on two case series [21, 22].

Severe preeclampsia is a progressive condition requiring prompt attention of the clinician. Women at term diagnosed with preeclampsia are best managed by induction of labor. After giving birth the symptoms usually resolve, but in some women the symptoms worsen during the first 48 h postpartum. These women are particularly at risk for pulmonary edema, AKI, HELLP syndrome, and stroke [18].

The HELLP syndrome can occur in 4–14 % of cases of preeclampsia. Characteristic laboratory abnormalities of HELLP syndrome include microangiopathic hemolysis (anemia, decreased haptoglobin, increased lactate dehydrogenase [LDH], and a peripheral blood smear with signs of red cell destruction), elevated liver enzymes, and low platelet count. The platelet count is a marker of the severity of the disease and coincides with liver impairment [23].

### 7.5.2.2 Thrombotic Microangiopathies

Thrombotic microangiopathies (TMA) are defined by the occurrence of thrombi of fibrin and/or platelets in the microcirculation of multiple organs. TMA during pregnancy are very uncommon cause for AKI. Pregnancy-related TMA used to be subtyped as thrombotic thrombocytopenic purpura (TTP) and hemolytic uremic syndrome (HUS). Recently TMA has been reclassified into four subtypes, and pregnancy is considered only a precipitating factor [24].

Treatment of TMA should be aimed at treating the underlying pathogenic mechanism in a multidisciplinary approach, which can be either fresh frozen plasma infusions with or without plasma exchange or inhibition of complement activation by eculizumab, as recently advocated by Fakhouri [24].

It can be a diagnostic challenge to differentiate TMA and preeclampsia/HELLP because thrombocytopenia and microangiopathic hemolytic anemia can present in both syndromes. Historical features such as the time of onset (after 20 weeks of gestation), earlier reported proteinuria, elevated liver enzymes, and/or hypertension support a diagnosis of preeclampsia/HELLP.

### 7.5.2.3 Acute Fatty Liver of Pregnancy

Acute fatty liver of pregnancy (AFLP) is a rare complication, with reported incidence of between 1 in 7,000 and 1 in 20,000 pregnancies [25, 26]. AFLP is characterized by acute liver failure and coagulopathy with sudden onset during the third trimester. The severity of liver involvement is variable, ranging from moderate isolated hepatic transaminase elevations to fulminant liver failure with encephalopathy [25]. Other features include elevated bilirubin, prolonged partial thromboplastin time, thrombocytopenia, hypoglycemia, and anemia [27]. Acute (typically nonoliguric) kidney dysfunction is common and seen in approximately 60 % of patients. Renal recovery typically follows delivery and dialysis is rarely needed [25, 27]. Early diagnosis, supportive measures, and prompt delivery are critical in the management. Clinical clues help to distinguish AFLP and HELLP syndrome, although the distinction is academic since the appropriate treatment of both conditions is prompt delivery.

### 7.5.2.4 Renal Cortical Necrosis

Renal cortical necrosis (RCN) is a rare condition in the developed world. In the developing world reported RCN has become more infrequent over the last decades [28]. In a prospective cohort study of over 4,500 late pregnancy-related AKI, Prakash et al. found AKI occurred in 1 in 56 live births (85 cases), of which only two were attributed to RCN [3]. RCN presents characteristically on ultrasound or CT-scan with hypoechoic or hypodense areas in the renal cortex. Calcifications are a late finding, usually occurring after 1–2 months. Treatment is supportive, with a significant chance for persistent loss of kidney function and need for renal replacement therapy.

### 7.5.2.5 Infectious Complications Contributing to AKI during Pregnancy

Pregnant patients are at risk for four specific infectious complications: urinary tract infections, chorioamnionitis (including septic abortion), endometritis (often post Caesarean section), and pneumonia. Progression to sepsis and septic shock is extraordinary, but poses significant mortality for mother and child. Urinary tract infections and sepsis may cause AKI.

## Urinary Tract Infections

Asymptomatic bacteriuria is present in 2–10 % of women, both in the general population and in pregnant women. In diabetics and patients with sickle cell trait as well as women from a lower socioeconomic status the percentage is higher. Approximately 40 % of this group will develop cystitis or pyelonephritis. Urine sediment and culture will help in selecting directed therapy to prevent development of sepsis or severe sepsis with multiple organ failure. Symptomatic urinary tract infections are usually caused by Escherichia coli bacteria. Resistant bacteria may cause perinephric abscess, kidney carbuncle, or cortical abscess, although rare.

## Sepsis/Multiple Organ Failure

Sepsis is an infrequent cause of severe AKI in pregnancy. In 2009 the H1N1 influenza unexpectedly caused severe illness and death in pregnant and postpartum women. During the influenza season, evaluation and antiviral treatment of influenza-like illnesses should be considered early in this patient population [29].

### 7.5.2.6  Urinary Tract Obstruction and Nephrolithiasis

The physiologic hydronephrosis of pregnancy seldom promotes ureteral obstruction due to the growing uterus or polyhydramnios. Stenting of the ureters may be indicated if delivery is not yet recommended. Obstruction may be induced by kidney stones, but is usually unilateral and presents with acute flank pain, hematuria and not with AKI.

## 7.6    Prevention

Care for pregnant women with AKI requires a multidisciplinary approach including maternal–fetal medicine, nephrology, critical care, and neonatal care specialists. Renal replacement therapy may be indicated in a select group of women. There is little evidence in the literature for optimal modality selection. The choice of modality should largely be predicated on the hemodynamic profile of the patient and its availability. There is also a paucity of literature describing the RRT utilization rates for pregnancy-related AKI and outcomes for either mother or baby. Maternal preexisting hypertension and kidney disease are considered risk factors for incident chronic kidney disease and progression to long-term renal replacement therapy [30].

**Key Messages**
- Pregnancy-related acute kidney injury (AKI) is an unusual clinical challenge and requires a multidisciplinary approach
- Pregnancy-related AKI is associated with significant maternal and fetal morbidity and mortality
- Physiological changes hamper normal laboratory testing of kidney function

## References


1. Stratta P, Besso L, Canavese C, Grill A, Todros T, Benedetto C, Hollo S, Segoloni GP. Is pregnancy-related acute renal failure a disappearing clinical entity? Ren Fail. 1996;18(4): 575–84.
2. Lameire NH, Bagga A, Cruz D, De Maeseneer J, et al. Acute kidney injury: an increasing global concern. Lancet. 2013;382(9887):170–9.
3. Prakash J, Niwas SS, Parekh A, Pandey LK, Sharatchandra L, Arora P, Mahapatra AK. Acute kidney injury in late pregnancy in developing countries. Ren Fail. 2010;32(3):309–13.
4. Prakash J, Kumar H, Sinha DK, Kedalaya PG, Pandey LK, Srivastava PK, Raja R, Usha. Acute renal failure in pregnancy in a developing country: twenty years of experience. Ren Fail. 2006;28(4):309–13.
5. Rasmussen PE, Nielsen FR. Hydronephrosis during pregnancy: a literature survey. Eur J Obstet Gynecol Reprod Biol. 1988;27(3):249–59.
6. Krane NK, Hamrahian M. Pregnancy: kidney diseases and hypertension. Am J Kidney Dis. 2007;49(2):336–45.
7. Jeyabalan A, Conrad KP. Renal function during normal pregnancy and preeclampsia. Front Biosci. 2007;12:2425–37.
8. Wolfe LA, Kemp JG, Heenan AP, Preston RJ, Ohtake PJ. Acid-base regulation and control of ventilation in human pregnancy. Can J Physiol Pharmacol. 1998;76:815–27.
9. Sánchez-Luceros A, Farías CE, Amaral MM, Kempfer AC, Votta R, Marchese C, Salviú MJ, Woods AI, Meschengieser SS, Lazzari MA. von Willebrand factor-cleaving protease (ADAMTS13) activity in normal non-pregnant women, pregnant and post-delivery women. Thromb Haemost. 2004;92:1320–6.
10. Odutayo A, Hladunewich M. Obstetric nephrology: renal hemodynamic and metabolic physiology in normal pregnancy. Clin J Am Soc Nephrol. 2012;7:2073–80.
11. Higby K, Suiter CR, Phelps JY, Siler-Khodr T, Langer O. Normal values of urinary albumin and total protein excretion during pregnancy. Am J Obstet Gynecol. 1994;171(4):984–9.
12. Smith MC, Moran P, Ward MK, Davison JM. Assessment of glomerular filtration rate during pregnancy using the MDRD formula. BJOG. 2008;115(1):109–12.
13. Alper AB, Yi Y, Rahman M, Webber LS, Magee L, von Dadelszen P, Pridjian G, Aina-Mumuney A, Saade G, Morgan J, Nuwayhid B, Belfort M, Puschett J. Performance of estimated glomerular filtration rate prediction equations in preeclamptic patients. Am J Perinatol. 2011;28(6):425–30.
14. Goodwin TM. Hyperemesis gravidarum. Clin Obstet Gynaecol. 1998;41:597–605.
15. Abell TL, Riely CA. Hyperemesis gravidarum. Gastroenterol Clin North Am. 1992;21: 835–49.
16. Goodwin TM, Montoro M, Mestman JH, Pekary AE, Hershman JM. The role of chorionic gonadotropin in transient hyperthyroidism of hyperemesis gravidarum. J Clin Endocrinol Metab. 1992;75(5):1333–7.
17. Milne F, Redman C, Walker J, Baker P, Bradley J, Cooper C, de Swiet M, Fletcher G, Jokinen M, Murphy D, Nelson-Piercy C, Osgood V, Robson S, Shennan A, Tuffnell A, Twaddle S, Waugh J. The pre-eclampsia community guideline (PRECOG): how to screen for and detect onset of pre-eclampsia in the community. BMJ. 2005;330(7491):576–80.
18. Steegers EA, von Dadelszen P, Duvekot JJ, Pijnenborg R. Pre-eclampsia. Lancet. 2010; 376(9741):631–44.
19. Sibai BM. Diagnosis, controversies, and management of the syndrome of hemolysis, elevated liver enzymes, and low platelet count. Obstet Gynecol. 2004;103(5 Pt 1):981–91.
20. Kuklina EV, Ayala C, Callaghan WM. Hypertensive disorders and severe obstetric morbidity in the United States. Obstet Gynecol. 2009;113:1299–306.
21. Drakeley AJ, Le Roux PA, Anthony J, Penny J. Acute renal failure complicating severe pre-eclampsia requiring admission to an obstetric intensive care unit. Am J Obstet Gynecol. 2002; 186(2):253–6.

22. Sibai BM, Villar MA, Mabie BC. Acute renal failure in hypertensive disorders of pregnancy. Pregnancy outcome and remote prognosis in thirty-one consecutive cases. Am J Obstet Gynecol. 1990;162(3):777–83.
23. Martin Jr JN, Rinehart BK, May WL, Magann EF, Terrone DA, Blake PG. The spectrum of severe preeclampsia: comparative analysis by HELLP (hemolysis, elevated liver enzyme levels, and low platelet count) syndrome classification. Am J Obstet Gynecol. 1999;180(6 Pt 1): 1373–84.
24. Fakhouri F, Vercel C, Frémeaux-Bacchi V. Obstetric nephrology: AKI and thrombotic micro-angiopathies in pregnancy. Clin J Am Soc Nephrol. 2012;7(12):2100–6.
25. Castro MA, Fassett MJ, Reynolds TB, Shaw KJ, Goodwin TM. Reversible peripartum liver failure: a new perspective on the diagnosis, treatment and cause of acute fatty liver of pregnancy, based on 28 consecutive cases. Am J Obstet Gynecol. 1999;181:389–95.
26. Knight M, Nelson-Piercy C, Kurinczuk JJ, Spark P, Brocklehurst P. A prospective national study of acute fatty liver of pregnancy in the UK. Gut. 2008;57:951–6.
27. Fesenmeier MF, Coppage KH, Lambers DS, Barton JR, Sibai BM. Acute fatty liver of pregnancy in 3 tertiary care centers. Am J Obstet Gynecol. 1932;2005:1416–9.
28. Prakash J, Vohra R, Wani IA, Murthy AS, Srivastva PK, Tripathi K, Pandey LK, Usha, Raja R. Decreasing incidence of renal cortical necrosis in patients with acute renal failure in developing countries: a single-centre experience of 22 years from Eastern India. Nephrol Dial Transplant. 2007;22(4):1213–7.
29. Louie JK, Acosta M, Jamieson DJ, Honein MA, California Pandemic (H1N1) Working Group. Severe 2009 H1N1 influenza in pregnant and postpartum women in California. N Engl J Med. 2010;362:27–35.
30. Jeyabalan A, Conrad RP. Renal physiology and pathophysiology in pregnancy. In: Schrier RW, editor. Renal and electrolyte disorders. 7th ed. Philadelphia: Lippincott Williams & Wilkins; 2010. p. 418–74.

# Part II

# Diagnosis of AKI

# Classical Biochemical Work Up of the Patient with Suspected AKI

**8**

Lui G. Forni and John Prowle

## 8.1 Introduction

The presentation of acute kidney injury (AKI) is dependent on the cause as the patient is often asymptomatic and the AKI is discovered on subsequent investigation. Whilst AKI is defined by temporal changes in serum creatinine concentration as well as urine output these changes provide no information regarding the underlying cause of the AKI and where possible a likely cause should be sought [1, 2]. The aim of testing renal function is to approximate the glomerular filtration rate (GFR) which can be viewed as the best global measure of kidney excretory function reflecting the sum of the filtration rates for all functioning nephrons. The baseline GFR is affected by many factors including age, sex, race, diet and muscle mass and also demonstrates significant variation within individuals, while the normal values quoted are in the range of 120 (±25) ml/min/1.73 $m^2$ of body surface area, GFR tends to decline from a median value at age 20 of 120 ml/min/1.73 $m^2$ by 0.5–1 per year of age over 20. Plasma creatinine is excreted from bloodstream predominantly by glomerular ultrafiltration and thus as GFR decreases – creatinine will accumulate. However to understand the meaning of baseline creatinine and its acute

L.G. Forni (✉)
Department of Intensive Care Medicine, Royal Surrey County Hospital NHS
Foundation Trust, Surrey Perioperative Anaesthesia Critical Care Collaborative Research
Group (SPACeR) and Faculty of Health Care Sciences,
University of Surrey, Guildford, UK
e-mail: l.forni@nhs.net

J. Prowle
Adult Critical Care Unit, The Royal London Hospital, Barts Health NHS Trust,
Whitechapel Road, London E1 1BB, UK

Department of Renal Medicine and Transplantation, The Royal London Hospital, Barts
Health NHS Trust, Whitechapel Road, London E1 1BB, UK

© Springer International Publishing 2015
H.M. Oudemans-van Straaten et al. (eds.), *Acute Nephrology for the Critical
Care Physician*, DOI 10.1007/978-3-319-17389-4_8

alterations requires an understanding of the steady state and dynamic kinetics of creatinine generation and excretion. Similarly urine low output can reflect a well-functioning kidney in the context of hypovolaemia or significant reduction in GFR in advanced acute or chronic kidney disease. The use of creatinine and urine output in consensus criteria for the diagnosis of AKI is considered in an accompanying chapter, here we consider the basis for the traditional clinical use of these parameters for assessment of renal function in individuals.

## 8.2 Biochemical Work Up

### 8.2.1 Creatinine and the Assessment of Renal Function

Creatinine is a spontaneously formed cyclical derivative of *creatine* degradation in the tissues. Creatine is synthesised in the liver and to a lesser extent the kidney and enters cells through a membrane transporter system whereby it is utilised to replenish ATP stores via phosphocreatine production [3]. Skeletal muscle is the major body reservoir creatine and consequently is the source of the majority of plasma creatinine. As a small (113 Da) basic molecule it is freely filtered in the glomerulus and appears unaltered in the urine with the addition of a small additional contribution from active tubular secretion. As renal excretion is so efficient, extra-renal creatinine excretion is also negligible in most conditions. The basis of use of creatinine for assessment of renal function thus relies on its rate of excretion being approximately proportional to GFR. Consequently creatinine excretion approximates to GFR (rate of plasma filtered into the urine) multiplied by the concentration of creatinine in the plasma. At steady state (constant plasma creatinine) excretion will equal creatinine generation (Eq. 8.1) so that the GFR is proportional to the reciprocal of plasma creatinine concentration.

$$\text{GFR} \times \left[ \text{Creat} \right]_{p} = G \tag{8.1}$$

Where $[\text{Creat}]_P$ is the plasma concentration of creatinine (in μmol/ml) and $G$ the creatinine generation rate in μmol/min.

Thus at steady state a lower GFR will be associated with an higher plasma creatinine following the relationship: GFR $\alpha$ 1/[Creat]$_P$ – so that, assuming a steady state has been achieved and that G is constant, a halving of GFR will be accompanied by a doubling of plasma creatinine. This relationship forms the basis of the use of fold increase in creatinine from baseline to define severity of AKI in consensus definitions based on the original RIFLE criteria as this would reflect fold decrease in GFR.

While changes in plasma creatinine define AKI there are significant limitations to its use, particularly in the critically ill [4, 5]. Firstly, use of plasma creatinine as an indirect measure of the GFR is unreliable outside the steady-state, after an acute change in GFR creatinine will rise or fall until achieving a new steady-state where plasma creatinine reflects the new GFR, this process will take a period of time that is dependent on both the magnitude of change in GFR and the underlying creatinine generation rate. With large falls in GFR many days may pass before steady-state is achieved and until then creatinine will underestimate severity of renal dysfunction. Secondly, changes in creatinine *production* can alter measured plasma creatinine concentration as much as changes in excretion (GFR). For example, creatinine production will fall if there is a reduction in lean body mass, if there is a fall in the dietary intake of creatine, or in the presence of liver disease [6]. As these are all common scenario's in the intensive care unit and the degree of renal dysfunction may be underestimated in the critically ill if one is solely guided by the creatinine concentration and, similarly, renal recovery after AKI may be significantly overestimated [7, 8]. Importantly, sepsis is associated with reduced creatinine production which may account for the seemingly slow rise in creatinine often observed in patients with septic AKI [4]. However, despite these limitations creatinine is still almost universally employed given the fact that assay is cheap, relatively easy and quick.

### 8.2.2  Clearance Measurements

Despite the limitations of plasma creatinine, acutely, direct measurement of GFR is not normally performed. GFR can be estimated through the calculation of the clearance of a molecule such as creatinine that is freely filtered from the plasma in the glomerulus and excreted unchanged into the urine (Eq. 8.2)

$$\mathrm{GFR}\left(\mathrm{ml}\,/\,\mathrm{min}\right) \cong \frac{\left[\mathrm{Creat}\right]_{\mathrm{U}}}{\left[\mathrm{Creat}\right]_{\mathrm{P}}} \times Q_{\mathrm{U}} \tag{8.2}$$

Where $[\mathrm{Creat}]_{\mathrm{U}}$ & $[\mathrm{Creat}]_{\mathrm{P}}$ are the urinary and plasma concentrations of creatinine respectively and $Q_{\mathrm{u}}$ is the urine flow rate in ml/min.

Although creatinine clearance is often used to estimate GFR, creatinine is by no means an ideal marker for this purpose. The ideal marker would not only be sensitive and specific in detecting small, early, changes in GFR, but would also not be secreted, metabolised or reabsorbed by tubular cells. Furthermore, it would be easily measured and would not be influenced by exogenous compounds. Tubular secretion of plasma creatinine can cause creatinine clearance to over-estimate GFR by 10–20 % or more, however competing substances for tubular secretion including some drugs can abolish this effect. The difference between Creatinine Clearance and true GFR has become more apparent since the adoption of more accurate Isotope-Dilution Mass-Spectroscopy (IDMS)-traceable laboratory standards and more accurate and precise enzymatic creatinine assays, as previous measurements un-standardised colorimetric assays tended to over-estimate plasma, but not urinary creatinine by detection of non-creatinine plasma chromogens. As an alternative to creatinine exogenous substances without tubular secretion such as inulin, EDTA (ethylenediaminetetraacetic acid) and iohexol are used to measure GFR occasionally, however these are impractical in the everyday acute clinical arena.

### 8.2.3   Alternatives to Creatinine: Cystatin C and Urea

Urea is a water-soluble low molecular weight by product of protein metabolism, which, like creatinine, exhibits a reciprocal relationship with the GFR. However, as a measure of GFR urea clearance has been superseded principally due to the greater variety of factors which influence both its renal clearance and endogenous production [9]. The main drawback with using urea as a GFR marker is that the rate of renal clearance is not constant. Under steady-state conditions approximately 50 % of urea is reabsorbed by proximal renal tubular cells so that the urea clearance is around 50 % of GFR, however, in hypovolaemic states, enhanced tubular reabsorption of sodium and water together accompanied by urea may decrease urea clearance as a proportion of GFR giving rise to a misleading disproportionate rise in the observed urea concentration. Conversely in advanced chronic or acute kidney disease, or in the presence of diuretic agents, urea clearance may rise as a proportion of GFR, so that increase in urea concentration could somewhat blunted. Urea production has also highly variable rates as these may be increased such as in high protein intake, catabolic states and gastrointestinal haemorrhage, but may also be reduced in acute or chronic malnutrition and liver disease. Therefore, plasma urea and urea clearance is not recommended for GFR estimation particularly under non-steady state conditions.

Cystatin C is a low molecular weight cysteine proteinase inhibitor synthesised at a relatively constant rate by all nucleated cells and released into plasma [10]. The main catabolic site of the Cystatin C are the proximal renal tubular cells following the almost complete (>99 %) filtration by the glomerulus [11]. Therefore, little or no Cystatin C is present in the urine. As a consequence, the urinary clearance of Cystatin C cannot be determined but any fall in GFR correlates well with a rise in serum Cystatin C concentration and excellent correlation with radionuclide derived measurements of GFR [12]. However the lack of a standardised method for measurement has prevented widespread adoption into clinical practice. This is coupled with the observation that the accuracy of measurement is affected by older age, sex, smoking status and raised CRP levels as well as abnormal thyroid function and the use of corticosteroids. Nevertheless, confounders of Cystatin C are likely to be less marked than those of creatinine during acute illness and availability of a standardised assay at an acceptable cost may lead to more widespread uptake of Cystatin c measurement in the future.

### 8.2.4   Mathematical Estimation of GFR

Several equations have been developed and validated for the estimation of the GFR or Creatinine Clearance. These include the Cockcroft-Gault equation, the four variable MDRD (Modification of Diet in Renal Disease Study Group equations Study Equation), the CKD-EPI Creatinine Equation, the CKD-EPI Cystatin C Equation and the CKD-EPI Creatinine-Cystatin C Equation. Many laboratories now quote an eGFR value together with serum creatinine. Although useful it must be remembered that, these estimated GFRs are derived values and not measured variables. At heart these equations are dependent on the reciprocal relationship between GFR and plasma creatinine at steady state transforming this into a direct GFR estimate by providing what is essentially an estimate of creatinine generation normalised to body surface area for individuals of a given age, sex and racial background. They are thus dependent on a patient firstly, being in steady state between GFR and plasma creatinine and, secondly, having a typical creatinine production for the out-patient populations used to generate these estimates. As neither of these are the case in most of critically ill patients, these formulae are not recommended for use in the acute setting, but rather as a tool for managing chronic kidney disease.

> **Key Messages**
> - The basis of use of creatinine for assessment of renal function relies on its rate of excretion being approximately proportional to GFR.
> - Creatinine levels will, initially, significantly underestimate the severity of renal dysfunction following a significant fall in GFR until steady-state is achieved.
> - Changes in creatinine production can alter measured plasma creatinine concentration as much as changes in excretion and this is of particular relevance in the critically ill.
> - Cystatin C, a low molecular weight cysteine proteinase inhibitor is synthe-sised at a relatively constant rate by all nucleated cells and almost exclu-sively filtered at the glomerulus.
> - Although confounders of Cystatin measurement are probably less than cre-atinine, there is at present a lack of a standardised Cystatin C method of measurement.

## 8.3  Urinalysis in AKI

### 8.3.1  Urine Analysis

Standard urine analysis involves assessment of urine colour, pH, specific gravity and the presence of glycosuria and/or proteinuria. Further information may be determined from microscopy of the urine. Under normal conditions urine colour is dependant on concentration however under certain pathological states urine colour may aid in diagnosis. For example, a red supernatant may point to myoglobulinae-mia or haemoglobinuria and hence lead to further focused investigation. With regard to the intensive care unit, green urine may be observed as a consequence of intrave-nous propofolol infusion. Although pH and specific gravity may be of use in stable patients, they add little to diagnosis within the ICU. However, the presence of hae-maturia particularly in the presence of proteinuria should alert the clinician to the possibility of parenchymal renal disease. Indeed the presence of proteinuria may complicate AKI particularly in the presence of sepsis although this is often tubular in origin reflecting incomplete reabsorption of low molecular weight proteins by proximal tubular cells. Glomerular proteinuria reflects leakage of larger molecular weight proteins such as albumin across the glomerular capillary wall and this may reflect acute injury such as glomerulonephritis but may also have been present prior to admission [13, 14]. The presence of premorbid proteinuria has significant prognostic implications. For all these reasons, a simple urinary dipstick analysis should be undertaken in all patients and where necessary proteinuria may be quantified either by timed collection or through a urinary protein: creatinine ratio.

## 8.3.2  Urine Microscopy

The assessment of the urinary sediment is often overlooked in the intensive care unit but can yield important information regarding the cause of the AKI. For example, frank haematuria may suggest underlying renal tract pathology whereas the presence of dysmorphic red cells imply glomerular injury. Similarly, casts, which appear cylindrical in nature due to the development within the renal tubule, may signify significant injury. Cellular casts consisting of either epithelial cells, erythrocytes or leukocytes are associated with significant renal damage. White cell casts are seen both in infection and with tubulointerstitial damage whereas red cell casts are seen in glomerulonephritis in the presence of vasculitis. Epithelial cell casts reflect cell necrosis and desquamation and classically are thought to reflect acute tubular cell necrosis. Although these findings have been described, they are not routinely employed due to the lack of consistency between the findings seen on urinary microscopy and correlation with biochemical values. Several attempts have been made to correlate findings with diagnosis and prediction of outcome but so far these have proved far from perfect and are rarely employed in clinical practice [15]. Crystals may also be seen in the urine, though are rarely of significance in the critically ill.

> **Key Messages**
> - Simple urinary dipstick analysis should be undertaken in all patients where possible.
> - Proteinuria may complicate AKI particularly in the presence of sepsis.
> - The presence of premorbid proteinuria has significant prognostic implications.
> - Haematuria particularly in the presence of proteinuria should alert the clinician to the possibility of parenchymal renal disease.

## 8.4  Urine Chemistry

There are many potential tests which may be performed on the urine but in practice few are applied to the patient with AKI. Principally these involve the fractional excretion of sodium and urea as well as urinary estimation of creatinine. Although

**Table 8.1** Classical urinary indices in AKI due to pre-renal causes and intrinsic disease

| Urinary indices | Pre-renal AKI | Intrinsic AKI |
| --- | --- | --- |
| UNa | <20 mmol/l | >40 mmol/l |
| FeNa | <1 % | >2 % |
| FeU | <35 % | >50 % |

Where *UNA* urinary sodium, *FeNa* fractional excretion of sodium and *FeU* fractional excretion of urea

historically measures such as the urine:plasma creatinine ratio and the serum urea:creatinine ratio have been used to try to differentiate between AKI secondary to volume deplete states and intrinsic disease results are inconsistent and these techniques are now rarely employed. In fact while elevated urea proportional to creatinine could reflect dehydration and reversible renal dysfunction, in critical illness, reduction in creatinine generation and increase in urea generation during active muscle wasting may lead to elevated urea:creatinine ratios that are in fact associated with more severe illness and adverse outcomes [16], illustrating the difficulty in meaningfully interpreting these measurements.

## 8.4.1  Urinary Sodium

The urinary sodium is used by some as an indicator of a 'pre-renal' aetiology for renal dysfunction given the avid sodium reabsorption by the renal tubules in volume deplete states. Thus a urinary sodium value of 10–20 mmol/l is suggestive of a haemodynamically reversible cause of renal dysfunction whereas a value of >40 mmol/l is classically referred to as being indicative of established, not rapidly reversible, tubular injury (Table 8.1). However, despite the dogma that such biochemical values can translate directly into a diagnostic test for a pathological diagnosis, there is little to substantiate this in the literature particularly within the critically ill. Indeed, the currently available data suggests that measurement of the urinary sodium has little or no diagnostic or prognostic utility within this population [17].

## 8.4.2  Fractional Excretion of Sodium (FeNa)

The fractional excretion of sodium measures the percentage of filtered sodium that is excreted in the urine and is given by:

$$FeNa(\%) = \left( \frac{Urinary\,Sodium \times Serum\,Creatinine}{Serum\,Sodium \times Urinary\,Creatinine} \right) \times 100 \tag{8.3}$$

As with the urinary sodium estimation the fractional excretion of sodium is thought to provide differentiation between pre-renal AKI and intrinsic AKI, which is predominantly referred to as acute tubular necrosis. Given the resorptive power of the renal tubules in volume deplete states a FeNa of <1 % is associated significantly active $Na^+$ resorption whereas in established AKI the FeNa is >1 %. However, the utility of the FeNa is also subject to numerous proviso's, particularly in the critically ill. For example, the use of loop diuretics is, unsurprisingly, associated with an FeNa in excess of 1 % regardless of volume state. Furthermore, values of <1 % have been observed in many conditions associated with parenchymal renal disease, also single measurements of serum creatinine may not provide an accurate estimate of the GFR as pointed out before. Furthermore, the FeNa may be >1 % when pre-renal disease is present in sodium wasting states such as in chronic kidney disease or diuretics as noted. As such it is of little use in isolation and even in clinical context, interpretation should be cautiously undertaken.

### 8.4.3 Fractional Excretion of Urea (FeU)

Calculated in a similar fashion the FeU advocates of this analysis promote its superiority over FeNa as a means of identifying pre-renal AKI particularly in the early stages of the condition, and where diuretics may have been administered, with a FeU <35 % indicative of a pre-renal cause. Although some evidence does point to it being superior to FeNa for differentiating pre-renal from renal causes of AKI, it is still subject to much criticism and many confounders making the interpretation difficult [18].

> **Key Messages**
> - The fractional excretion of sodium is of little use in isolation particularly in the critically ill.
> - The fractional excretion of urea may be superior to sodium in determining a pre-renal cause but is subject to many confounders

## 8.5 Non-biochemical Investigations and Renal Biopsy in AKI

### 8.5.1 Further Investigations

Where glomerular disease is suspected from urinalysis or the history, then the further investigation including serological testing should be considered. In the absence of an active urinary sediment it is unlikely that an intrinsic cause is present, however, where suspected, the cause should be investigated as this may change the immediate management of the patient. However, it is worth remembering that although further investigation may point to a particular diagnosis often nephrology colleagues may also require histological confirmation. This is particularly relevant when lupus nephritis is considered, where the positive serology does not provide information as to the degree of renal involvement. Also serological tests may not be entirely diagnostic nor do not prove that the cause of the positive serology is causing

**Table 8.2**  Further investigation for AKI where appropriate

| Proteinuria | Possible systemic disease | Investigation |
|---|---|---|
| Nephrotic range | SLE/CTD | ANA, dsDNA, C3/C4 |
|  | Amyloid | Serum free light chains |
|  | Hepatitis B | Hep B serology |
|  | Hepatitis C | Hep C serology, cryoglobulins |
|  | HIV | Anti-HIV Ab |
| Non-nephrotic range | GPA/EGPA | ANCA (Pr3 +/−) |
|  | Small vessel vasculitides | ANCA (MPO +) |
|  | SLE/CTD | ANA, dsDNA, C3/C4 |
|  | Bacterial endocarditis | Blood cultures |
|  | Anti GBM | Anti GBM antibodies |
|  | Cryoglobulinaemia | Cryoglobulins |

the underlying renal disease. As with all investigations these results must be taken in clinical context.

## 8.5.2  Serological Testing and Biopsy

Several tests may point to a specific cause for the observed AKI and depend in part on the degree of proteinuria. Assuming the standard tests outlined above have been performed, then various systemic disorders could account for the AKI depending on the degree of proteinuria. Appropriate further investigations will include viral serology as well as serological analysis as outlined in Table 8.2 [19]. Under certain circumstances further evaluation may be necessary and require histological confirmation. However, percutaneous renal biopsy is rare in the critically ill which is in stark contrast to the management of AKI outside the ICU environment where the renal biopsy is an essential tool in patient management. Percutaneous biopsy does carry both a morbidity and mortality risk and significant complications include haemorrhage, infection and arteriovenous fistula formation [19]. Alternative approaches include open renal biopsy, although in modern practice this is rarely performed, or laparoscopic renal biopsy. Transjugular renal biopsy (TJRB) has been used successfully to obtain renal tissue in high risk patients with results and complication rates comparable to conventional renal biopsy, but this technique has rarely been used in the ICU setting [20].

> **Key Messages**
> - In the absence of an active urinary sediment it is unlikely that an intrinsic renal cause for AKI is present.
> - Native renal biopsy may be performed in the ICU but does carry a morbidity and mortality risk.

## 8.6    Oliguria in AKI

The accurate measurement of the urine output is rare outside critical care but is integral in the definition of AKI as well as providing dynamic insight into kidney function. Although AKI implies a reduction in GFR this does not always equate to oliguria and in some patients urine outputs may be preserved through variations in GFR or the rate of tubular reabsorption. Given that a healthy adult with typical GFR of 100 ml/min can make less than 1,000 ml of urine a day without developing renal problems, tubular reabsorption can lead to less than 1 % of the filtrated volume appearing as urine. Thus, in healthy adults subjected to water deprivation urine output falls to a physiological minimum as hormonal mechanisms (principally the renin/angiotensin/aldosterone system (RAAS) and the hypothalamic-pituitary antidiuretic hormone (ADH) axis) act to maintain plasma osmolality and extracellular volume. If water deprivation is maintained, maximal urinary concentrating capacity results in an obligatory minimum urine output of around 500 ml/day [21, 22]. Urine output below this level therefore implies that a reduction in GFR must have occurred. Severe oliguria, indicated by a sustained urine output of approximately <15 ml/h or 0.3–0.4 ml/kg/h is therefore necessarily associated with renal dysfunction. However, less profound oliguria can be triggered by pain, surgical stress, venodilation and hypovolaemia – causing salt and water retention, by neurohormonal mechanisms, even when cardiac output and blood pressure are maintained. With more severe illness, or in the presence of co-morbid conditions, the patient's cardiovascular reserve may become exhausted and GFR may decrease further contributing to oliguria, in the context of ADH, sympathetic and RAAS mediated urinary concentration. Crucially, however, the ability to excrete maximally concentrated urine is dependent on intact tubular function – in the setting of acute or chronic kidney disease or diuretic therapy urine volume may be maintained until GFR has reduced to a very low level. Thus oliguria in the presence of biochemical renal dysfunction has traditionally been regarded as indicative of the most severe kidney injury, associated with greater need for renal replacement therapy and higher risk of death [23, 24]. In summary, oliguria can be regarded either as an early sign of haemodynamic instability and a healthy kidney or a late sign of severity of renal dysfunction in an acutely or chronically injured kidney, a dual role that can confuse the clinical interpretation of urine output. Consequently, urine output suffers from a lack of sensitivity and specificity with regard to the aetiology and prognosis of AKI, particularly in the absence of haemodynamic change or the need for vasopressors [25]. Importantly, the presence of oliguria may be a portent to poor outcomes not only through the presence of AKI but also the fact that this may be associated with fluid overload. This observation has been made in several multicenter studies with the consistent message that AKI in the presence of volume overload implies a worse prognosis [26].

> **Key Messages**
> - The accurate measurement of the urine output is integral to the definition of AKI and provides dynamic insight into kidney function.
> - A measured reduction in GFR does not always equate to oliguria as urine output may be preserved through variations in GFR or the rate of tubular reabsorption.
> - Oliguria may be a portent to poor outcomes not only due to AKI but also the fact that this may be associated with fluid overload.

# References


1. Kidney Disease: Improving Global Outcomes (KDIGO) Acute Kidney Injury Work Group. KDIGO Clinical Practice Guideline for Acute Kidney Injury. Kidney Int Suppl. 2012;2:1–138.
2. Joannidis M, et al. Prevention of acute kidney injury and protection of renal function in the intensive care unit. Intensive Care Med. 2010;36(3):392–411.
3. Walker JB. Creatine: biosynthesis, regulation, and function. Adv Enzymol Relat Areas Mol Biol. 1979;50:177–242.
4. Waikar SS, Bonventre JV. Creatinine kinetics and the definition of acute kidney injury. J Am Soc Nephrol. 2009;20(3):672–9.
5. Doi K, et al. Reduced production of creatinine limits its use as marker of kidney injury in sepsis. J Am Soc Nephrol. 2009;20(6):1217–21.
6. Cocchetto DM, Tschanz C, Bjornsson TD. Decreased rate of creatinine production in patients with hepatic disease: implications for estimation of creatinine clearance. Ther Drug Monit. 1983;5:161–8.
7. Schetz M, Gunst J, Van den Berghe G. The impact of using estimated GFR versus creatinine clearance on the evaluation of recovery from acute kidney injury in the ICU. Intensive Care Med. 2014;40(11):1709–17.
8. Prowle JR, et al. Serum creatinine changes associated with critical illness and detection of persistent renal dysfunction after AKI. Clin J Am Soc Nephrol. 2014;9(6):1015–23.
9. Group, K.D.I.G.O.K.C.W. KDIGO 2012 clinical practice guideline for the evaluation and management of chronic kidney disease. Kidney Int. 2013(3):1–150.
10. Bagshaw SM, Bellomo R. Cystatin C in acute kidney injury. Curr Opin Crit Care. 2010;16(6):533–9.
11. Perrone RD, Madias NE, Levey AS. Serum creatinine as an index of renal function: new insights into old concepts. Clin Chem. 1992;38(10):1933–53.
12. Shlipak MG, Mattes MD, Peralta CA. Update on cystatin C: incorporation into clinical practice. Am J Kidney Dis. 2013;62(3):595–603.
13. Parikh CR, et al. Tubular proteinuria in acute kidney injury: a critical evaluation of current status and future promise. Ann Clin Biochem. 2010;47(Pt 4):301–12.
14. Han SS, Ahn SY, Ryu J, Baek SH, Chin HJ, Na KY, Chae DW, Kim S. Proteinuria and hematuria are associated with acute kidney injury and mortality in critically ill patients: a retrospective observational study. BMC Nephrol. 2014;15:93.

15. Wald R, et al. Interobserver reliability of urine sediment interpretation. Clin J Am Soc Nephrol. 2009;4(3):567–71.
16. Rachoin JS, et al. The fallacy of the BUN:creatinine ratio in critically ill patients. Nephrol Dial Transplant. 2012;27(6):2248–54.
17. Pons B, et al. Diagnostic accuracy of early urinary index changes in differentiating transient from persistent acute kidney injury in critically ill patients: multicenter cohort study. Crit Care. 2013;17(2):R56.
18. Darmon M, et al. Diagnostic performance of fractional excretion of urea in the evaluation of critically ill patients with acute kidney injury: a multicenter cohort study. Crit Care. 2011;15(4):R178.
19. Amery CE, Forin LG. Renal disease presenting as acute kidney injury: the diagnostic conundrum on the intensive care unit. Curr Opin Crit Care. 2014;20(6):606–12.
20. Augusto JF, et al. Safety and diagnostic yield of renal biopsy in the intensive care unit. Intensive Care Med. 2012;38(11):1826–33.
21. Javaid MM, Johnston M, Kalsi N, Venn RM, Forni LG. Acute kidney injury on the intensive care unit – the use of transjugular renal biopsy in aiding diagnosis. Neth J Crit Care. 2010;15(2):61–5.
22. Gamble JL. Physiological information gained from studies of the life raft ration. Harvey Lect. 1946;42:247–78.
23. Chesley LC. Renal excretion at low urine volumes and the mechanism of oliguria. J Clin Invest. 1938;17(5):591–7.
24. Morgan DJ, Ho KM. A comparison of nonoliguric and oliguric severe acute kidney injury according to the risk injury failure loss end-stage (RIFLE) criteria. Nephron Clin Pract. 2010;115(1):c59–65.
25. Teixeira C, et al. Fluid balance and urine volume are independent predictors of mortality in acute kidney injury. Crit Care. 2013;17(1):R14.
26. Prowle JR, et al. Oliguria as predictive biomarker of acute kidney injury in critically ill patients. Crit Care. 2011;15(4):R172.
27. Prowle JR, et al. Fluid balance and acute kidney injury. Nat Rev Nephrol. 2010;6(2):107–15.

# Acute Kidney Injury Biomarkers

**9**

Marlies Ostermann, Dinna Cruz, and Hilde H.R. De Geus

## 9.1    Introduction

Clinicians caring for patients with a raised serum creatinine face several questions which impact decision making and management: Has acute kidney injury (AKI) occurred? If yes, what is the aetiology and how severe is it? What is the prognosis? Will kidney function recover?

The diagnosis of AKI is based on an acute rise in serum creatinine, fall in urine output or both. Although these tests are easily available at little cost, they are neither renal specific nor indicative of the exact aetiology or prognosis. Furthermore, after a renal insult, the rise of serum creatinine is often delayed by 24–36 h, and AKI is not recognised in its early phase.

To overcome some of the shortcomings of serum creatinine, traditional tests like urine microscopy and oliguria have been re-discovered and re-evaluated with some encouraging results (see Chap. 8). However, there is general agreement that additional new biomarkers are needed to improve risk assessment, early detection, differential diagnosis and prognostication of AKI [1]. Numerous molecules and proteins have been identified and tested in different experimental and clinical scenarios with mixed results [1–3]. For these tests to be incorporated into routine

M. Ostermann (✉)
Department of Critical Care, Guy's and St Thomas Hospital,
London, United Kingdom
e-mail: Marlies.Ostermann@gstt.nhs.uk

D. Cruz
Department of Nephrology Dialysis and Transplantation,
San Bortolo Hospital, Vicenza, Italy
e-mail: dinnacruzmd@yahoo.com

H.H.R. De Geus
Department of Intensive Care Medicine, Erasmus Medical Centre,
Doctor Molewaterplein 50-60, Rotterdam, The Netherlands
e-mail: geushrhde@yahoo.com

© Springer International Publishing 2015
H.M. Oudemans-van Straaten et al. (eds.), *Acute Nephrology for the Critical Care Physician*, DOI 10.1007/978-3-319-17389-4_9

**Table 9.1** Expectations of novel AKI biomarkers

| |
| --- |
| Provision of information above and beyond serum creatinine and/or urine output |
| Non-invasive test using easily accessible samples |
| Results rapidly available |
| Specific cut-off values to distinguish between normal and abnormal renal function |
| Ability to differentiate between AKI and chronic kidney disease |
| Ability to differentiate between intrinsic AKI and pre-renal fluid responsive azotemia |
| Reliability in the setting of common comorbidities |
| Correlation with severity of AKI |
| Prognostication of important outcomes (i.e. need for renal replacement therapy, mortality) |
| Differentiation between different aetiologies of AKI |
| Indication of duration of AKI |
| Tool to guide clinical management and allow monitoring |

*Abbreviations*: *AKI* acute kidney injury

clinical practice, it is essential that they provide information which is above and beyond serum creatinine and urine output (Table 9.1).

## 9.2    Types of Biomarkers

Biomarkers of AKI vary in their origin, function, distribution and time of release following renal injury (Table 9.2 and Fig. 9.1). They can be broadly divided into:

(a) Markers of glomerular function: small molecular weight proteins that are present in the systemic circulation and undergo glomerular filtration (i.e. serum creatinine, cystatin C)
(b) Markers of tubular function: molecules that are filtered and undergo tubular reabsorption (i.e. retinol-binding protein)
(c) Markers of tubular injury, damage or repair: molecules that are released as a result of direct renal cell damage, inflammatory activation or following gene upregulation [i.e. Kidney Injury Molecule 1 (KIM-1) or Interleukin 18 (IL 18)]

Biomarkers of kidney damage (NGAL, KIM-1 or IL 18) can be utilized to describe the nature, severity and site of renal injury. They may also provide information related to the underlying pathogenesis and prognosis. In contrast, functional biomarkers (i.e. creatinine, cystatin C) represent changes in renal function independent of site of damage. Most biomarkers are either damage or functional markers but some fulfil both roles (i.e. NGAL).

**Table 9.2** AKI biomarkers in human studies

| AKI biomarker | Production/origin | Handling by the kidney | Detection time after renal injury | Confounding factors |
|---|---|---|---|---|
| Alanine aminopeptidase (AAP) Alkaline phosphatase (ALP) γ-glutamyl transpeptidase (γ-GT) | Enzymes located on the brush border villi of the proximal tubular cells | Released from brush border after damage to proximal tubular cells | Within <12 h | |
| Calprotectin (activator of the innate immune system) | Cytosolic calcium-binding complex of two proteins of the S100 group (S100A8/S100A9) and derived from neutrophils and monocytes | Measure of local inflammatory activity; detectable in urine following intrinsic AKI | Within <12 h | Inflammatory bowel disease Urinary tract infection Probably CKD |
| Cystatin C | 13 kDa cysteine protease inhibitor produced by all nucleated human cells and released into plasma at constant rate | Freely filtered in glomeruli and completely reabsorbed and catabolized by proximal tubular cells; no tubular secretion | 12–24 h post-renal injury | Systemic inflammation Malignancy Thyroid disorders Glucocorticoid disorder Smoking Hyperbilirubinaemia Hypertriglyceridaemia |
| α glutathione S-transferase (α GST) | 47–51 kDa cytoplasmic enzyme produced in proximal tubule | Released into urine following tubular injury | Within 12 h | |
| π glutathione S-transferase (π GST) | 47–51 kDa cytoplasmic enzyme produced in distal tubules | Released into urine following tubular injury | Within 12 h | |
| Hepatocyte growth factor (HGF) | Antifibrotic cytokine produced by mesenchymal cells and involved in renal tubular cell regeneration after AKI | | Within <12 h | |

(continued)

**Table 9.2** (continued)

| AKI biomarker | Production/origin | Handling by the kidney | Detection time after renal injury | Confounding factors |
| --- | --- | --- | --- | --- |
| Hepcidin | 2.78 kDa peptide hormone produced in hepatocytes and other tissues; renoprotective role during ischaemia/reperfusion injury | Freely filtered with significant tubular uptake and catabolism (fractional excretion 2 %); higher levels in patients without AKI | Within 12–24 h | Systemic inflammation |
| Insulin-like growth factor binding protein-7 (IGFBP-7) and Tissue metalloproteinase-2 (TIMP-2) | Metalloproteinases involved in cell cycle arrest | Released into urine after tubular epithelial injury | Within 12 h | |
| Interleukin-18 (IL-18) | 18 kDa proinflammatory cytokine | Released into urine from proximal tubular cells following injury | 6–24 h after renal injury | Inflammation Sepsis Heart failure |
| Kidney Injury Molecule–1 (KIM-1) | Transmembrane glycoprotein produced by proximal tubular cells after ischaemic or nephrotoxic injury | Released into urine following ischaemic or nephrotoxic tubular damage | 12–24 h after renal injury | Renal cell carcinoma Chronic proteinuria Chronic kidney disease Sickle cell nephropathy |
| Liver-type fatty acid-binding protein (L-FABP) | 14 kDa intracellular lipid chaperone produced in proximal tubular cells and hepatocytes | Freely filtered in glomeruli and reabsorbed in proximal tubular cells; increased urinary excretion after tubular cell damage | 1 h after ischaemic tubular injury | Chronic kidney disease Polycystic kidney disease Liver disease Sepsis |
| MicroRNA | Endogenous single-stranded molecules of non-coding nucleotides | Upregulated following tubular injury and detectable in plasma and urine | Within <20 h post-renal insult | Sepsis |
| Monocyte chemoattractant peptide-1 (MCP-1) | Peptide expressed in renal mesangial cells and podocytes | Released into urine | ? | Variety of primary renal diseases |

| N-acetyl-β-D-glucosaminidase (NAG) | >130 kDa lysosomal enzyme; produced in proximal and distal tubular cells (and non-renal cells) | Too large to undergo glomerular filtration; released into urine after tubular damage | 12 h | Diabetic nephropathy |
|---|---|---|---|---|
| Neutrophil gelatinase-associated lipocalin (NGAL) also known as oncogene 24p3 | 25 kDa glycoprotein produced by epithelial tissues throughout the body | Plasma NGAL is excreted via glomerular filtration and undergoes complete reabsorption in healthy tubular cells NGAL is also produced in distal tubular segments and released into urine following tubular damage | Within 2–4 h | Sepsis Malignancy Chronic kidney disease Pancreatitis COPD Endometrial hyperplasia |
| Netrin-1 | Laminin-related molecule, minimally expressed in proximal tubular epithelial cells of normal kidneys | Highly expressed in injured proximal tubules | Within 2–6 h | |
| Retinol binding protein (RBP) | 21 kDa single-chain glycoprotein; specific carrier for retinol in the blood (delivers retinol from the liver to peripheral tissues) | Totally filtered by the glomeruli and reabsorbed but not secreted by proximal tubules; minor decrease in tubular function leads to excretion of RBP in urine | Within 12 h | Type II diabetes Obesity Acute critical illness |

*Abbreviations*: *AKI* acute kidney injury, *GFP* glomerular filtration rate, *COPD* chronic obstructive pulmonary disease, *CKD* chronic kidney disease

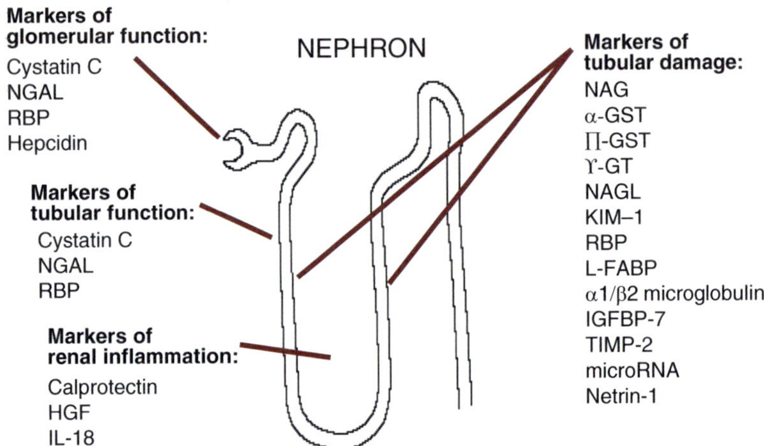


**Fig. 9.1** Origin and function of novel AKI biomarkers (Modified from Ref. [3]). *Abbreviations*: *AKI* acute kidney injury, *NGAL* neutrophil gelatinase-associated lipocalin, *NAG* N-acetyl-β-D-glucosaminidase, *GST* glutathione S-transferase, *γ-GT* γ-glutamyl transpeptidase, *KIM-1* Kidney Injury Molecule-1, *IL-18* interleukin 18, *RBP* retinol binding protein, *L-FABP* liver-type fatty acid-binding protein, *IGFBP-7* insulin-like growth factor binding protein-7, *TIMP-2* tissue metalloproteinase–3, *HGF* hepatocyte growth factor

In theory, these new biomarkers have great potential, especially when used in combination and measured sequentially. They have been studied in adult and paediatric patients with and without co-morbidities and in various clinical scenarios [Intensive Care Unit (ICU), emergency department, post-contrast exposure, following transplantation and after cardiac surgery]. Some studies were performed in well-defined settings where the exact timing of renal injury was known (i.e. after surgery), whereas others were undertaken in patient cohorts with a less defined onset of AKI, for instance in patients with sepsis. These differences account for some of the discrepant findings.

## 9.3　Novel AKI Biomarkers in Clinical Practice

### 9.3.1　Diagnosis of Early AKI

Although the risk factors for AKI are well known, the early diagnosis of AKI in high-risk patients remains a challenge. The most commonly encountered comorbidities associated with AKI are age, diabetes, hypertension, obesity, liver disease, congestive heart failure, vascular disease and chronic kidney disease (CKD), and the most common renal insults include sepsis, hypotension, nephrotoxic agents and cardiopulmonary bypass surgery [4].

Following a definite renal injury, serum creatinine rise lags by 24–36 h. As a result, the early stage of AKI often remains unnoticed. Many studies have focussed on the ability of biomarkers to diagnose AKI before a detectable serum creatinine rise in different clinical settings.

### 9.3.1.1 Subclinical AKI

Recent studies identified a unique cohort of patients with a transient elevation in urinary and plasma NGAL levels without detectable changes in serum creatinine [5, 6]. Affected patients had a greater risk of complications, a longer stay in ICU and a higher risk of dying compared to patients without elevated NGAL levels. These results imply the existence of a state of "subclinical AKI" where renal injury has occurred but glomerular function is still preserved. Whether this phase of AKI represents a golden window for effective therapeutic interventions will need to be investigated in future studies.

### 9.3.1.2 In the Emergency Department

The identification of patients with early AKI at a time when serum creatinine is still in the normal range may be particularly useful in patients presenting to the emergency department. However, existing data are conflicting. A study in emergency patients with suspected sepsis showed that a plasma NGAL (pNGAL) >150 ng/ml had a sensitivity of >80 % for predicting AKI but specificity was poor at 51 % [7].

A different study was performed in 635 patients who were admitted to hospital from the emergency department. It concluded that a single measurement of urinary NGAL (uNGAL) helped to distinguish acute renal injury from normal function, prerenal azotemia and CKD and was also highly predictive of clinical outcomes, including nephrology consultation, need for renal replacement therapy (RRT) and admission to the ICU [8]. However, the mean serum creatinine of those with AKI was already elevated at 495 μmol/L (standard deviation 486) at presentation in the emergency department.

A study in 207 consecutive patients presenting to the emergency department with acute heart failure demonstrated that after control for pre-existing chronic cardiac or kidney disease, serum creatinine but not pNGAL was an independent predictor of AKI [9]. In contrast, a multi-centre study in 665 patients admitted to hospital from the emergency department showed that adding serial pNGAL results to clinical judgement improved the prediction of AKI [10]. Results of further studies are awaited to decide how best to utilise novel AKI biomarkers in the emergency setting.

### 9.3.1.3 Post-cardiac Surgery

The most studied AKI biomarkers after cardiac surgery are those that reflect an inflammatory process (such as IL-18) or markers which are released by tubular cells following renal injury (such as NGAL and KIM-1). Studies have focussed on the ability to diagnose early AKI and to predict outcomes, including progression to more severe AKI, need for RRT and mortality [11–14]. The majority of studies concluded that NGAL, IL-18, cystatin C, KIM-1 and liver-type fatty acid-binding protein (L-FABP) indicated AKI earlier than serum creatinine. For instance, urine

IL-18 and urine and plasma NGAL peaked within 6 h after admission to ICU which was well before a serum creatinine rise at 24–72 h [15]. In a different study, the addition of urine IL-18 and pNGAL results to a clinical risk model based on age, gender, ethnicity, diabetes, hypertension, preoperative renal function and cardiopulmonary bypass time increased the area under the curve to predict AKI from 0.69 to 0.76 and 0.75, respectively [14].

Other studies focussed on the performance of new AKI biomarkers as indicators of severity and progression of renal injury. Measurement of 32 different biomarkers in 95 patients with AKI stage 1 after cardiac surgery showed that IL-18 was the best predictor for worsening AKI or death, followed by L-FABP, NGAL and KIM-1 [12]. A different study showed that π glutathione S-transferase (π GST) was best at predicting the progression to AKI stage 3 in patients with a raised serum creatinine after cardiac surgery, followed by NGAL, cystatin C, hepatocyte growth factor and KIM-1 [13]. Of note, IL-18 was not measured. Markers of cell cycle arrest have also shown promising results [16]. In high-risk patients after cardiac surgery, serial levels of urinary tissue inhibitor of metalloproteinases-2 (TIMP-2) and insulin-like growth factor-binding protein 7 (IGFBP7) performed well in predicting early AKI and also renal recovery.

However, despite promising results in the research setting, it remains unclear how to use these new AKI biomarkers effectively after cardiac surgery.

### 9.3.1.4 During Critical Illness

AKI is common during critical illness, especially in patients with sepsis. There have been numerous studies investigating the performance of biomarkers in diagnosing early and progressive AKI in critically ill patients in the ICU [5, 17–35]. Studies evaluating cystatin C, urine IL-18, uNGAL and pNGAL have shown mixed results, mainly as a result of heterogenous patient populations and differences in timing and frequency of measurements. Furthermore, results may be confounded by sepsis per se (Table 9.2).

Some studies have evaluated biomarker panels rather than individual markers. For instance, in a diverse population of 420 critically ill patients, the combination of urinary [TIMP-2] and [IGFBP7] identified patients at risk for imminent AKI (sensitivity 92 %) [35]. The decision how to utilise novel biomarkers in critically ill patients remains a challenge, in particular in light of a dynamic disease process and the presence of confounding factors.

### 9.3.2 Prediction of Outcome in AKI

### 9.3.2.1 Need for RRT

Some AKI biomarkers have the capacity, either alone or in combination with traditional renal function tests and clinical judgement to predict the need for RRT [26]. Higher biomarker concentrations are often associated with need for RRT, in particular plasma cystatin C, urinary KIM-1 and N-acetyl-β-D-glucosaminidase (NAG) [3]. However, most studies were confounded by the fact that the precise indications for RRT were not provided. There is also insufficient evidence that biomarkers can indicate the optimal time for initiating RRT. In some studies, the use of a novel biomarker was only marginally better than prediction based on clinical parameters [36]. Finally, there are no data showing that AKI biomarkers are able to indicate when sufficient renal recovery has occurred and RRT can be discontinued.

### 9.3.2.2 Renal Recovery

There is increasing recognition that AKI survivors are at risk of developing CKD and end-stage renal failure even if renal function initially recovers. The underlying cellular and physiologic mechanisms that determine renal prognosis after AKI are not well understood [37]. Epidemiologic studies suggest that advanced age and pre-existing CKD are significant risk factors for non-recovery.

It is hoped that novel biomarkers may be able to identify those patients who are at high risk of poor long-term outcomes so that appropriate follow-up arrangements can be made. Results from the "Biological Markers of Recovery for the Kidney" study showed that decreasing levels of uNGAL and urinary hepatocyte growth factors in patients receiving RRT were associated with greater odds of renal recovery but results of further studies are awaited [38].

### 9.3.2.3 Prediction of Mortality

There is good evidence that some novel AKI biomarkers are predictive of mortality, in particular when used in critically ill patients. The most widely studied biomarker is NGAL but others have also demonstrated an association with hospital mortality, for instance cystatin C and IL-18 [3]. There is some evidence that AKI biomarker may also predict outcome beyond hospital discharge. A study in 528 ICU patients showed that levels of urinary NGAL, IL-18 and KIM-1 were associated with mortality at 1 year [39]. The Translational Research in Biomarker Endpoints in AKI programme even concluded that there was an independent association between urinary IL-18 and KIM-1 measured in the immediate period post-cardiac surgery and 3-year mortality [9]. The mechanisms that underlie the association between elevated urinary AKI biomarkers and long-term mortality are not clear. It is possible that AKI biomarkers reflect not only renal damage but also correlate with risk of CKD and secondary effects on non-renal organs.

## 9.3.3  Prediction of Renal Function After Transplantation

In the field of transplantation, the identification of early non-invasive biomarkers to monitor graft status and accurately predict transplant outcome is an increasingly important research area. However, existing data are variable and conflicting. A study in 99 consecutive deceased kidney donors in the ICU (176 recipients) found that increased donor uNGAL levels but not pNGAL levels predicted histological changes in subsequent donor kidney biopsies, a higher risk of delayed graft function (DGF) beyond 14 days and worse 1-year graft survival [40]. In contrast, a study in

41 deceased kidney donors concluded that pNGAL was better in predicting DGF [41]. Finally, a study in 53 organ donors demonstrated that after adjusting for age, gender, ethnicity, urine output and cold ischemia time, both uNGAL and urinary IL-18 on day 0 predicted the trend in serum creatinine in the post-transplant period and had a role as early biomarkers of DGF [42].

In liver transplant recipients, uNGAL detected AKI at 4 h and pNGAL at 8 h after transplantation whereas glutathione S-transferase (GST) and KIM-1 failed to detect AKI [43]. In another study, serum creatinine, cystatin C, serum IL-6, and IL-8 and urine IL-18, NGAL, IL-6, and IL-8 were measured before and within 24 h after liver transplantation [44]. In patients who developed AKI, all markers apart from cystatin C and serum IL-6 were elevated within the first 24 h following surgery.

To date, these novel biomarkers remain research tools and have not been incorporated into routine clinical practice following transplant surgery.

## 9.4    Adjunctive Roles

Over the last decade, the search for novel AKI biomarkers has significantly improved our understanding of AKI. Molecules which are released early in AKI have revealed some important biological pathways in the pathogenesis of AKI.

Some of these biomarkers also have the potential to facilitate the development of new drugs by indicating renal injury earlier than conventional methods. Collaborations between international centres and major pharmaceutical companies, the US Food and Drug Administration (FDA) and the European Medicines Agency (EMEA) have begun and rodent urinary and plasma biomarkers have been accepted as surrogates for renal histology for initial evaluation and monitoring of nephrotoxicity in drug development [45, 46]. Finally, there is some hope that some of the novel molecules not only serve as diagnostic tools but also as potential therapeutic targets for the treatment of AKI.

## 9.5    Unmet Needs

While biomarkers appear to perform in the research setting, their role in routine clinical practice is influenced by patient case mix, comorbidities, aetiology of AKI, timing of renal insult, timing of biomarker measurement and the selected thresholds for diagnosis [1, 33, 47, 48]. Furthermore, their performance is compared with serum creatinine, a poor marker of renal function. Biomarker studies have generally not included new imaging techniques, like Doppler ultrasound or Magnetic resonance imaging [1].

One of the difficulties is to identify those patients who would benefit most from the use of biomarkers. Indiscriminate biomarker testing in patients at low risk of AKI is not cost-effective. Research studies have repeatedly shown that novel renal biomarkers perform best in patients without co-morbidities and in settings with a well-defined renal insult. The results are less robust in heterogeneous patient groups and a less defined time of onset, like patients with sepsis. It is unlikely that a single biomarker will be useful in all settings. Instead, it is more likely that a panel of functional and damage biomarkers in combination with traditional markers of renal function and clinical judgement will provide best results. Finally, evidence that the use of novel biomarkers influences decision making and improves patients' outcomes is still lacking.

## References


1. Murray PT, Mehta RL, Shaw A, Ronco C, Endre Z, Kellum JA, Chawla LS, Cruz D, Ince C, Okusa MD. Potential use of biomarkers in acute kidney injury: report and summary of recommendations from the 10th Acute Dialysis Quality Initiative consensus conference. Kidney Int. 2014;85:513–21.
2. Coca SG, Yaavarthy R, Concato J, Parikh CR. Biomarkers for the diagnosis and risk stratification of acute kidney injury: a systematic review. Kidney Int. 2008;73(9):1008–16.
3. Ostermann M, Philips BJ, Forni LG. Clinical review: biomarkers of acute kidney injury: where are we now? Crit Care. 2012;16:233.
4. Cartin-Ceba R, Kashiouris M, Plataki M, Kor DJ, Gajic O, Casey ET. Risk factors for development of acute kidney injury in critically ill patients: a systematic review and meta-analysis of observational studies. Crit Care Res Pract. 2012;2012:691013.
5. Haase M, Devarajan P, Haase-Fielitz A, et al. The outcome of neutrophil gelatinase-associated lipcalin-positive subclinical acute kidney injury: a multicenter pooled analysis of prospective studies. J Am Coll Cardiol. 2011;57:1752–61.
6. Haase M, Kellum JA, Ronco C. Subclinical AKI–an emerging syndrome with important consequences. Nat Rev Nephrol. 2012;8:735–9.
7. Shapiro NI, Trzeciak S, Hollander JE, et al. The diagnostic accuracy of plasma neutrophil gelatinase-associated lipocalin in the prediction of acute kidney injury in emergency department patients with suspected sepsis. Ann Emerg Med. 2010;56:52–9.
8. Nickolas TL, Schmidt-Ott KM, Canetta P, et al. Diagnostic and prognostic stratification in the emergency department using urinary biomarkers of nephron damage a multicenter prospective cohort study. J Am Coll Cardiol. 2012;59:246–55.
9. Breidthardt T, Socrates T, Drexler B, et al. Plasma neutrophil gelatinase-associated lipocalin for the prediction of acute kidney injury in acute heart failure. Crit Care. 2012;16:R2.
10. Di Somma S, Magrini L, De Berardinis B, et al. Additive value of blood neutrophil gelatinase-associated lipocalin to clinical judgement in acute kidney injury diagnosis and mortality prediction in patients hospitalized from the emergency department. Crit Care. 2013;17:R29.
11. Coca SG, Garg AX, Thiessen-Philbrook H, et al. Urinary biomarkers of AKI and mortality 3 years after cardiac surgery. J Am Soc Nephrol. 2014;25:1063–71.
12. Arthur JM, Hill EG, Alge JL, et al. Evaluation of 32 urine biomarkers to predict the progression of acute kidney injury after cardiac surgery. Kidney Int. 2014;85:431–8.
13. Koyner JL, Vaidya VS, Bennett MR, et al. Urinary biomarkers in the clinical prognosis and early detection of acute kidney injury. Clin J Am Soc Nephrol. 2010;5:2154–65.
14. Koyner JL, Parikh CR. Clinical utility of biomarkers of AKI in cardiac surgery and critical illness. Clin J Am Soc Nephrol. 2013;8:1034–42.
15. Parikh CR, Devarajan P, Zappitelli M, et al. Postoperative biomarkers predict acute kidney injury and poor outcomes after adult cardiac surgery. J Am Soc Nephrol. 2011;22:1748–57.
16. Meersch M, Schmidt C, Van Aken H, et al. Urinary TIMP-2 and IGFBP7 as early biomarkers of acute kidney injury and renal recovery following cardiac surgery. PLoS One. 2014;9, e93460.

17. DeGeus HRH, Woo JG, Wang Y, et al. Urinary NGAL measured on admission to the Intensive Care Unit accurately discriminates between sustained and transient acute kidney injury in adult critically ill patients. Nephron Extra. 2011;1:9–23.
18. Cruz DN, de Cal M, Garzotto F, et al. Plasma neutrophil gelatinase-associated lipcalin is an early biomarker for acute kidney injury in an adult ICU population. Intensive Care Med. 2010;36:444–51.
19. Constantin JM, Futier E, Perbet S, et al. Plasma neutrophil gelatinase-associated lipocalin is an early marker of acute kidney injury in adult critically ill patients: a prospective study. J Crit Care. 2010;25:176e1–e6.
20. De Geus HR, Bakker J, Lesaffre EM, le Noble JL. Neutrophil gelatinase-associated lipocalin at ICU admission predicts for acute kidney injury in adult patients. Am J Respir Crit Care Med. 2011;183:907–14.
21. Zhang Z, Lu B, Sheng X, Jin N. Cystatin C in prediction of acute kidney injury: a systemic review and meta-analysis. Am J Kidney Dis. 2011;58:356–65.
22. Royakkers AA, Korevaar JC, van Suijlen JD, et al. Serum and urine cystatin C are poor biomarkers for acute kidney injury and renal replacement therapy. Intensive Care Med. 2011;37:493–501.
23. Doi K, Negishi K, Ishizu T, et al. Evaluation of new acute kidney injury biomarkers in a mixed intensive care unit. Crit Care Med. 2011;39:2464–9.
24. Nejat M, Pickering JW, Walker RJ, Endre ZH. Rapid detection of acute kidney injury by plasma cystatin C in the intensive care unit. Nephrol Dial Transplant. 2010;25:3283–9.
25. Cruz DN, De Geus HR, Bagshaw SM. Biomarker strategies to predict need for renal replacement therapy in acute kidney injury. Semin Dial. 2011;24:124–31.
26. Siew ED, Ware LB, Gebretsadik T, et al. Urine neutrophil gelatinase-associated lipocalin moderately predicts acute kidney injury in critically ill adults. J Am Soc Nephrol. 2009;20: 1823–32.
27. Bagshaw SM, Bennett M, Haase M, et al. Plasma and urine neutrophil gelatinase-associated lipocalin in septic versus non-septic acute kidney injury in critical illness. Intensive Care Med. 2010;36:452–61.
28. Martensson J, Bell M, Oldner A, et al. Neutrophil gelatinase-associated lipocalin in adult septic patients with and without acute kidney injury. Intensive Care Med. 2010;36:1333–40.
29. Kumpers P, Hafer C, Lukasz A, et al. Serum neutrophil gelatinase-associated lipocalin at inception of renal replacement therapy predicts survival in critically ill patients with acute kidney injury. Crit Care. 2010;14:R9.
30. Villa P, Jimenez M, Soriano MC, Manzanares J, Casasnovas P. Serum cystatin concentration as a marker of acute renal dysfunction in critically ill patients. Crit Care. 2005;9:R139–43.
31. Makris K, Markou N, Evodia E, et al. Urinary neutrophil gelatinase-associated lipocalin (NGAL) as an early marker of acute kidney injury in critically ill multiple trauma patients. Clin Chem Lab Med. 2009;47:79–82.
32. Kashani K, Al-Khafaji A, Ardiles T, et al. Discovery and validation of cell cycle arrest biomarkers in human acute kidney injury. Crit Care. 2013;17:R25.
33. Vanmassenhove J, Vanholder R, Nagler E, Van Biesen W. Urinary and serum biomarkers for the diagnosis of acute kidney injury: an in-depth review of the literature. Nephrol Dial Transplant. 2013;28:254–73.
34. Bihorac A, Chawla LS, Shaw AD, et al. Validation of cell-cycle arrest biomarkers for acute kidney injury using clinical adjudication. Am J Respir Crit Care Med. 2014;189:932–9.
35. Matsa R, Ashley E, Sharma V, Walden AP, Keating L. Plasma and urine neutrophil gelatinase associated lipocalin in the diagnosis of new onset acute kidney injury in critically ill patients. Crit Care. 2014;18:R137.
36. Liangos O, Perianayagam MC, Vaidya VS, et al. Urinary N-acetyl-beta-(D)-glucosaminidase activity and kidney injury molecule-1 level are associated with adverse outcomes in acute renal failure. J Am Soc Nephrol. 2007;18:904–12.
37. Goldstein SL, Chawla L, Ronco C, Kellum JA. Renal recovery. Crit Care. 2014;18:301.

38. Srisawat N, Wen X, Lee M, et al. Urinary biomarkers and renal recovery in critically ill patients with renal support. Clin J Am Soc Nephrol. 2011;6:1815–23.
39. Ralib AM, Pickering JW, Shaw GM, et al. Test characteristics of urinary biomarkers depend on quantitation method in acute kidney injury. J Am Soc Nephrol. 2012;23:322–33.
40. Hollmen ME, Kyllonen LE, Inkinen KA, Lalla ML, Merenmies J, Salmela KT. Deceased donor neutrophil gelatinase-associated lipocalin and delayed graft function after kidney transplantation: a prospective study. Crit Care. 2011;15:R121.
41. Bataille A, Abbas S, Semoun O, Bourgeois E, Marie O, Bonnet F, et al. Plasma neutrophil gelatinase-associated lipocalin in kidney transplantation and early renal function prediction. Transplantation. 2011;92:1024–30.
42. Parikh CR, Jani A, Mishra J, et al. Urine NGAL and IL-18 are predictive biomarkers for delayed graft function following kidney transplantation. Am J Transplant. 2006;6:1639–45.
43. Dedeoglu B, de Geus HR, Fortrie G, Betjes MG. Novel biomarkers for the prediction of acute kidney injury in patients undergoing liver transplantation. Biomark Med. 2013;7:947–57.
44. Sirota JC, Walcher A, Faubel S, Jani A, McFann K, Devarajan P, Davis CL, Edelstein CL. Urine IL-18, NGAL, IL-8 and serum IL-8 are biomarkers of acute kidney injury following liver transplantation. BMC Nephrol. 2013;14:17.
45. Dieterle F, Sistare F, Goodsaid F, et al. Renal biomarker qualification submission: a dialog between the FDA-EMEA and predictive safety testing consortium. Nat Biotechnol. 2010;28: 455–62.
46. Sistare FD, DeGeorge JJ. Promise of new translational safety biomarkers in drug development and challenges to regulatory qualification. Biomark Med. 2011;5:497–514.
47. Bagshaw SM, Zappitelli M, Chawla LS. Novel biomarkers of AKI: the challenges of progress 'Amid the noise and the haste'. Nephrol Dial Transplant. 2013;28:235–8.
48. Shao X, Tian L, Xu W, et al. Diagnostic value of urinary Kidney Injury Molecule 1 for acute kidney injury: a meta-analysis. PLoS One. 2014;9, e84131.

Matthieu M. Legrand and Michael Darmon


Acute kidney injury (AKI) is a common issue in hospitalized patients, especially in critically ill patients or in the perioperative setting. Because AKI has been associated with an increased risk of mortality and high costs, strategies to decrease its incidence or hasten recovery are mandatory. Among strategies to prevent AKI or to limit its progression, treatment of the aetiology and correction of contributors such as nephrotoxic or hemodynamic optimization are central. In this line, renal imaging plays a key role both in identifying the causal mechanism of the syndrome and, more recently, in evaluating renal hemodynamics. While excessive fluid loading may be associated with important side effects and a positive fluid balance with a poor clinical outcome, development of tools to better estimate renal perfusion in response to treatment appears of paramount importance. Tools have been developed to assess kidney perfusion or renal vasculature. In this chapter, we describe different renal imaging tools used to assess the cause of kidney failure and clinical value to image the kidney. We also discuss techniques to assess renal perfusion and function.


M.M. Legrand (✉)
Department of Anesthesiology and Critical Care,
Hôpital Européen Georges Pompidou Assistance Publique- Hopitaux de Paris,
20 Rue Leblanc, Paris 75015, France
e-mail: matthieu.m.legrand@gmail.com

M. Darmon
Medical Intensive Care Unit, Hôpital Saint Louis,
1 Avenue Claude Vellefaux, Paris 75010, France
e-mail: michael.darmon@sls.aphp.fr



© Springer International Publishing 2015

H.M. Oudemans-van Straaten et al. (eds.), *Acute Nephrology for the Critical Care Physician*, DOI 10.1007/978-3-319-17389-4_10

## 10.1 Renal Echography

### 10.1.1 Brightness Mode (B-Mode)

Renal ultrasonography is often the first-line imaging technique due to wide availability, safety, non-invasiveness and low cost. Two-dimensional grey-scale ultrasound is the most commonly used technique in the initial assessment of patients with AKI and findings derived from this technique can greatly influence diagnostics and management [1, 2].

Using the brightness mode (B-mode), a grey-scale image is produced when the high-frequency sound waves are generated and then received by the ultrasonography transducer, in which returning echoes are represented as bright dots. The two basic things provided by B mode ultrasonography of the kidney include kidney size and echogenicity. Brightness of the dots represents the strength of the reflected echoes. Brighter structures are therefore structures reflecting more ultrasounds. Normal kidneys appear as bright as normal liver or spleen tissue. Therefore, brighter renal parenchyma will therefore be brighter than normal liver or spleen.

The longitudinal length of the kidney is mostly used to determine kidney size due to reproducibility and easy measurement.

The size of the kidney can provide evidence for underlying chronic disease or for some causes of renal failure. For instance, enlarged kidneys in patients with AKI suggest infiltrative diseases, renal vein thrombosis or acute rejection in transplants kidneys while smaller kidneys suggest underlying chronic kidney disease. This enlargement includes thickness of the renal parenchyma (including the cortex and the medulla which is about 1.5 cm thick). Renal cortex and medulla appear with very close echogenicity. However, because of presence of fat tissue, the caliceal system appears hypoechogenic. In the same line, because the medullary pyramids contain urine in parallel tubules, they appear hypoechogenic compared to the cortex. In pathology, although echogenicity is not specific, results of renal echography can provide useful information.

While most infiltrative disease (e.g. lymphoma, monoclonal gammapathies), inflammatory states (e.g. acute proliferative glomerulonephritis, acute tubular necrosis, acute interstitial nephritis, HIV nephropathy) are associated with increased echogenicity of the renal parenchyma, renal oedema leads to hypoechogenic aspect of the kidney. Acute tubular necrosis can be associated with normal, increased or decreased parenchymal echogenicity. Of note, chronic kidney disease is often associated with increased brightness since fibrous tissue (e.g. glomerulosclerosis, interstitial fibrosis) increases echogenicity. On the other hand, cortical necrosis leads to cortical oedema and hypoechogenicity of the cortex. Therefore, echogenicity cannot be used to differentiate AKI from chronic kidney disease. However, if the kidneys are small and echogenic, this strongly suggests chronic kidney disease. Table 10.1 summarizes renal echography characteristics of several pathological processes.

Of note, chronic kidney disease can lead to decrease in cortical thickness although this sign lacks sensitivity and no clear cut-off exists. Several kidney diseases are

**Table 10.1** Ultrasound characteristics of specific kidney disease in B-mode

|                            | Echogenicity          | Size                          |
| -------------------------- | --------------------- | ----------------------------- |
| Diabetic nephropathy       | Normal                | Normal or increased           |
| Obesity                    | Normal                | Increased                     |
| Acromegaly                 | Normal                | Increased                     |
| Lymphoma/leukaemia         | Normal                | Increased                     |
| Glomerulonephritis         | Normal or increased   | Increased                     |
| Vasculitis                 | Normal or increased   | Increased                     |
| Tubulointerstitial disease | Normal or increased   | Increased                     |
| Amyloid                    | Normal or increased   | Increased                     |
| Multiple myeloma           | Normal or increased   | Increased                     |
| HIV nephropathy            | Normal or increased   | Increased                     |
| Pre-eclampsia              | Normal or increased   | Increased                     |
| Pyelonephritis             | Normal or decreased   | Increased (often unilateral)  |
| Renal vein thrombosis      | Normal or decreased   | Increased (often unilateral)  |
| Urinary tract obstruction  | Normal or decreased   | Increased (often unilateral)  |
| Medullary nephrocalcinosis | Increased (medulla)   | Normal                        |
| Urate nephropathy          | Increased (medulla)   | Normal                        |
| Sickle cell disease        | Increased (medulla)   | Normal or decrease            |
| Sjögen syndrome            | Increased (medulla)   | Normal or decrease            |
| Medullary sponge kidney    | Increased (medulla)   | Normal                        |
| Oedema                     | Decreased (cortex)    | Increased                     |
| Acute cortical necrosis    | Decreased (cortex)    | Normal or decrease            |

*HIV* human immunodeficiency virus

more specifically associated with changes in medulla echogenicity. Nephrocalcinosis is characterized by increased medullary echogenicity due to calcium deposit, as well as sickle cell disease and gout.

While normal kidney length is about 11 cm (the left kidney being about 0.3 mm longer than the right kidney), there is an expected atrophy with ageing. It should be mentioned as well that height and weight also positively correlate with kidney size.

A goal of ultrasonography examination in B-mode is also to detect urinary tract obstruction as the cause of AKI. Urinary tract obstruction is involved in 1–15 % of cases of AKI, although it remains a relative rare cause of AKI in ICU patients. It should be especially suspected when a clinical suspicion exists (such as flank pain, urolithiasis, neurogenic bladder, benign prostatic hyperplasia, pelvic cancer, single functional kidney, pelvic surgery), or when the clinical course of AKI is not rapidly favourable despite treatment. While caliceal dilatation suggests urinary tract obstruction, false-negative findings on echo can be observed especially in hypovolemic patients or in patients with retroperitoneal tumours or fibrosis or with early obstruction. Repeated exams can help in detecting such patients especially after volume repletion (except for retroperitoneal fibrosis or tumours in which alternative methods must be used, i.e. CT scan or MRI).

False-positive findings include pregnancy, diabetes insipidus, vesicoureteral reflux, after relief of obstruction, megacystic-megaureter syndrome, full bladder, urinary tract infection. All these conditions are often associated with caliceal dilation.

Finally, ultrasound examination with Doppler can be used by experienced laboratory personnel to screen for renal artery stenosis or to detect vascular abnormalities (arterial stenosis or vein thrombosis), e.g. in renal transplants recipients.

## 10.1.2 Doppler-Based Resistive Index (RI)

Renal Doppler has also been suggested as a useful tool in evaluating intra-renal perfusion in various settings [2–8]. Hence, intra-renal Doppler-based renal resistive index (RI) has been tested to assess renal allograft status [9, 10] and changes in renal perfusion in critically ill patients [11–13] and for predicting the reversibility of an acute kidney injury (AKI) [14, 15].

### 10.1.2.1 Methods

Although 2- to 5-MHz transducers are optimal to measure RI [16, 17], various transducers may be successfully used for this purpose, including small phased array transducer. The first step is a B-mode US with a postero-lateral approach allowing location of the kidneys and detection of signs of chronic renal damage. Subsequently, colour Doppler or power Doppler US allows vessels' localization (Fig. 10.1a) [16] and may allow a semi-quantitative evaluation of renal perfusion (Table 10.2) [18].

Either the arcuate arteries or the interlobar arteries are then insonated with pulsed wave Doppler using a Doppler gate as low as possible between 2- and 5-mm [16, 17]. In order to obtain repeatable measures, the waveforms should be optimized for the measurements using the lowest pulse repetition frequency (usually 1.2–1.4 kHz) without aliasing (to maximize waveform size), the highest gain without obscuring background noise, and the lowest wall filter [16, 17]. A spectrum is considered optimal when three to five consecutive similar-appearing waveforms are noted [16, 17]. To characterize the intra-renal Doppler waveform, most investigators have used the resistive index (RI) so-called Pourcelot Index (Fig. 10.1b).

Three to five reproducible waveforms are obtained, and RIs from these waveforms are averaged to compute the mean RI for each kidney. This easily calculated parameter is defined as:

$$RI = [\text{peak systolic shift} - \text{minimum diastolic shift}]/\text{peak systolic shift}$$

Renal pulsatility index may also be calculated:

$$PI = [\text{peak systolic velocity} - \text{minimum diastolic velocity}]/\text{mean velocity}$$

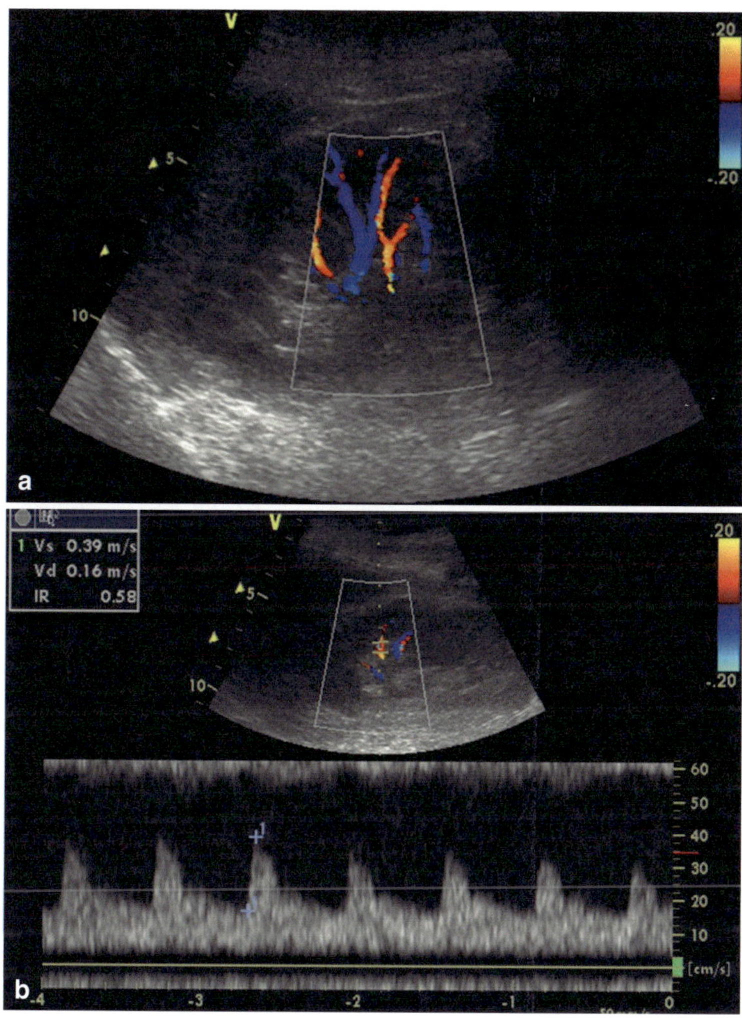

**Fig. 10.1**  Results of a renal colour Doppler ultrasonography showing renal vascularization (**a**). RI measurement using pulsed wave Doppler (**b**)

**Table 10.2**  Colour Doppler for a semi-quantitative evaluation of intra-renal vascularisation [18]

| Stage | Quality of renal perfusion by colour Doppler |
|---|---|
| 0 | Unidentifiable vessels |
| 1 | Few vessels in the vicinity of the hilum |
| 2 | Hilar and interlobar vessels in most of the renal parenchyma |
| 3 | Renal vessels identifiable until the arcuate arteries in the entire field of view |

RI might however be more adapted to the study of high-resistance vascular territories. In addition, RI and pulsatility index are closely correlated ($r=0.92$; $P<0.001$) [11]. Last, pulsatility index has been shown to be subject to wider variations than RI (reproducibility 9–22 % vs. 4–7 %) [19].

### 10.1.2.2 Normal Values, Feasibility and Reproducibility

RI can theoretically range from 0 to 1. RI is normally lower than 0.70. In several studies, mean RI (±SD) in healthy subjects ranged from 0.58 (±0.05) to 0.64 (±0.04) [20, 21]. The normal RI range is, however, age dependent. Thus, RI values greater than 0.70 have been described in healthy children younger than 4 years [22] and in individuals older than 60 years and considered healthy [23]. When the RI is measured for both kidneys, the side-to-side difference is usually less than 5 % [24].

Renal RI is a simple and non-invasive tool easy to use at the patient bedside. Feasibility of the measure has been showed to be good, even in the settings of critically ill patients. A recent study suggested a half-day course to be sufficient to allow inexperienced operators in successfully measuring RI [25]. Inter-observer reproducibility of RI measurement by senior radiologist or senior intensivist is considered excellent [14, 26]. In critically ill patients, the inter-observer reproducibility between senior and inexperienced operator is good and measures seem accurate (absence of systematic bias) although associated with a lack of precision (wide 95 % confidence interval of ±0.1) [25].

### 10.1.2.3 Significance and Usual Confounders

Both physiological and clinical significance of the RI remains debated. Initially considered an indicator of renal vascular resistance and blood flow [7], both experimental and clinical studies have demonstrated correlation of RI with vascular resistance and blood flow to be weak [27, 28]. Thus, observed RI changes in response to supra-physiological pharmacologically induced changes in renal vascular resistance are modest (RI changes of 0.047 IU (±0.008) per logarithmic increase in renal resistances) [29]. Both in vitro and ex-vivo studies however demonstrated a strong relationship between vascular compliance (vascular distensibility) and RI [27–29]. This strong relationship between vascular compliance and RI has been confirmed in a recent large cohort of renal allograft [10]. In this line, age-related arterial stiffening may explain the progressive increase in RI with age [30]. Similarly, elevated RI observed in several pathological states such as diabetes mellitus and hypertension may also be related to the influence of these diseases on arterial stiffness and to sub-clinical vascular changes related to the underlying disease [31, 32].

Macrovascular hemodynamic changes also influence RI. Hence, pulse pressure index [(systolic pressure − diastolic pressure/systolic pressure)] had direct and dramatic effects on RI values [29]. Additionally, since RI depends in part on the minimum diastolic shift, it may be influenced by the heart rate [33]. According to observations performed by Mostbeck and colleagues regarding RI changes as consequences of heart rate variations, a formula has been developed to correct the RI value for heart rate: [Corrected RI=observed RI −0.0026×(80-heart rate)] [33]. This formula has, however, never been validated in clinical studies.

In addition to these factors, both oxygen and carbon dioxide levels can affect RI. Several studies have demonstrated that RI varies according to $P_aO_2$ and $P_aCO_2$

levels [34–36]. These studies performed in healthy subjects, patients with chronic obstructive respiratory disease, renal transplant recipients or patients with acute respiratory distress syndrome suggest that hypoxemia and hypercapnia may increase RI [34–36].

Besides vascular and hemodynamic factors, kidney interstitial pressure has been shown to be associated with RI in ex vivo studies [28]. An increase in interstitial pressure reduces the transmural pressure of renal arterioles, thereby diminishing arterial distensibility and, consequently, decreasing overall flow and vascular compliance. Similarly, intra-abdominal pressure may affect RI via the same mechanisms. Thus, incremental changes in intra-abdominal pressure correlated linearly with RI in a porcine model [37], and reduction in intra-abdominal pressure with paracentesis was followed by a decrease in RI in cirrhotic patients with tense ascites [38]. Finally, ureteral pressure, likely acting via interstitial pressure, also affects RI [6].

These numerous confounders suggest RI to be an integrative parameter rather than reliable tool to assess renal perfusion or a substitute for renal biopsy.

### 10.1.2.4 Clinical Relevancy in ICU

Doppler-based RI has been suggested to monitor renal perfusion in critically ill patients, detect early renal dysfunction in severe sepsis patients or in assessing prognosis of AKI.

Renal Doppler has also been proposed to monitor renal perfusion in critically ill patients [12]. In recent studies, RI was used to assess the impact on renal perfusion of low-dose dopamine infusion and gradual changes in mean arterial pressure in response to norepinephrine infusion in critically ill patients [11, 13]. Despite significant results, the observed RI variations were modest and their real impact on renal perfusion and moreover on renal function remains unclear. Assuming that RI may reflect renal perfusion, it was recently proposed for the early detection of occult hemorrhagic shock in a small study conducted in normotensive trauma patients [39]. If patients with occult hemorrhagic shock had higher RI, they also had higher lactate levels and lower base excess. Although these findings are promising, the exact significance remains uncertain. Hence, as mentioned above, RI is influenced not only by vascular resistance but also by many other parameters such as age, heart rate, mean arterial pressure, changes in renal perfusion, vascular compliance, and renal interstitial oedema and interstitial pressure [27–29]. A study is currently ongoing in way to more clearly underline potential interest of Doppler-based RI in assessing renal perfusion (DORESEP; NCT01473498).

Additionally, several studies assessed interest of Doppler-based RI in detecting early renal dysfunction or in predicting short-term reversibility of AKI [14, 15, 25, 40, 41]. In a study conducted in septic critically ill patients, RI measured at admission was higher in patients who developed subsequently AKI [14]. This finding was recently confirmed in the post-operative setting of cardiopulmonary bypass [42]. Additionally, several cohort studies suggest Doppler-based RI to be differentiating transient from persistent AKI in selected critically ill patients [15, 41, 43]. Interestingly, semi-quantitative renal perfusion assessment seems to be correlated with Doppler-based RI and associated with reversibility of renal dysfunction [25]. Despite these promising results, most of these studies were performed in limited patient samples which may have overestimated diagnostic performance [15, 43–45].

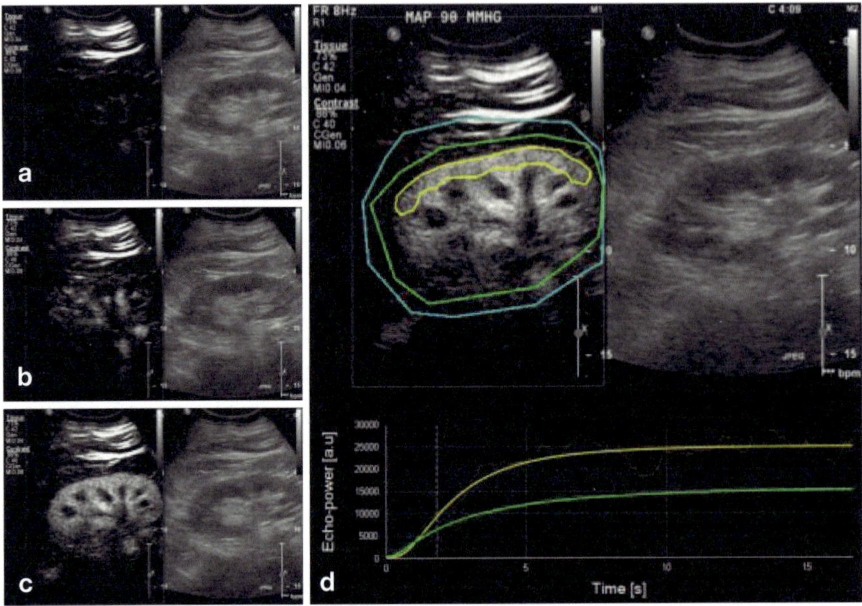

**Fig. 10.2** Illustration of contrast-enhanced ultrasonography. During continuous infusion of the contrast agent, microbubble destruction is obtained by applying pulses at high mechanical index (high ultrasound intensity). Microcirculation replenishment is then observed. All images represent renal contrast-enhanced ultrasonography (CEUS), the left part of the image shows contrast-image mode imaging and the right part the standard (B-mode) image. (**a**) Immediately after the flash; (**b**) during replenishment (2 s after the flash); (**c**) at full replenishment (6 s after the flash); (**d**) sequence analysis with Sonotumor®: a region of interest was drawn (*yellow line*) in the largest possible area of renal cortex closer to the ultrasound probe. The software generates a time intensity curve. This curve is used to generate CEUS-derived parameters (Reproduced from Schneider et al. *Crit Care* 2013 [50] with permission)

Additionally, a recent study has identified discrepant results regarding RI diagnostic performance in this setting [44]. Therefore despite the promising preliminary reports, we still lack adequately powered study validating performance of RI in both early detection of renal insult or AKI prognostic assessment.

## 10.1.3 Contrast-Enhanced Ultrasonography

Contrast-enhanced US (CEUS) relies on the intravascular injection of specific contrast agents that create a signal of high echogenicity thus allowing macro and microvascular structure visualization when using specific imaging techniques. These specific contrast agents consist in gas-filled microbubbles that oscillate in response to US waves therefore creating a non-linear signal of high echogenicity (Fig. 10.2) [46]. This technique is believed to allow an accurate quantification of regional and global renal blood flow [47]. It has been validated in humans to evaluate coronary blood flow [48], and its safety has been largely documented in this context [49]. When adding this technique to recently developed softwares, this technique is believed to allow an accurate quantification of regional blood flow, such as renal blood flow [47]. A recent study has confirmed feasibility of this technique in cardiac surgery patients [50]. The clinical interest of this technique remains however theoretical and validation studies are needed. A recent study raised doubt regarding the interest of CEUS in estimating renal perfusion [51]. Hence, in this study, noradrenaline-induced increases in mean arterial pressure were not associated with a change in overall CEUS derived mean perfusion indices [51]. Additionally, an important heterogeneity in responses was noted among the 12 included patients. Additional studies are ongoing and should help in more clearly assessing input of this technique in clinical setting and reliability of CEUS in assessing renal perfusion.

## 10.2    Computerized Tomography

Computerized tomography (CT) scan remains the most accurate examination for ruling out stone disease and provides information on the location of the stone, detection of underlying renal or abdominal abnormalities in patients with AKI (e.g. polycysts, renal carcinoma, aortic aneurysms) and detection of hydronephrosis without contrast media injection (Fig. 10.3). CT scan with intravascular contrast media is also indicated for search of intra-abdominal inflammatory or infectious process, which can be the cause of AKI in septic patients [52]. The CT scan indication should of course be guided by clinical presentation and physical examination. Likewise, CT scan is the preferred technique for detecting complication of pyelonephritis such as renal abscesses, perinephric abscess or emphysematous pyelonephritis. Ultrasound examination remains poorly sensitive to detect parenchymal alterations in pyelonephritis and can miss subtle parenchyma abnormalities in

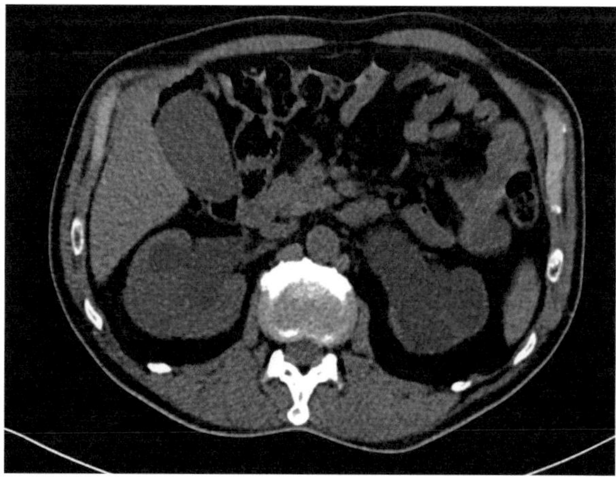

**Fig. 10.3** Example of acute bilateral hydronephrosis detected with non-enhanced absominal CT scan. No stone was observed and the cause was found to be a full bladder

uncomplicated pyelonephritis. However, echography remains the first-line diagnostic technique because it is non-invasive, not expansive, widely available and allow detection of urinary obstruction detection or a single kidney diagnosis when pyelonephritis is suspected or proven. Furthermore, US examination accuracy increases with the use of ultrasound contrast agent to detect parenchyma abnormalities. Therefore, ultrasound examination is sufficient as a first-line examination in uncomplicated pyelonephritis with favourable course (e.g. apyrexia within 48 h of treatment). In other cases (unfavourable evolution, patients with shock or uncontrolled infection,) CT scan should be considered early in the course of the infection.

Significant advances in CT technology have allowed better definition and reconstructing high-resolution 3D reconstruction. CT angiography therefore now allows accurate detection of aortic and renal vascular abnormalities in patients for whom intravascular contrast media injection is considered safe [53, 54].

Finally, last generation CT scan if triphasic helical CT, also known as functional CT, can allow assessment of glomerular filtration rate and renal blood flow [55] but routine indication in critically ill patients are probably to be reserved to suspicion of severe renal stenosis or thrombosis with inconclusive echo Doppler examinations.

## 10.3 Magnetic Resonance Imaging

Magnetic resonance imaging (MRI) techniques allow assessment of parenchymal abnormities such as tumours, pyelonephritis, evaluation and detection of genitourinary tract abnormalities, detection of hydronephrosis or evaluation renal arteries stenosis. MRI is non-invasive and is especially useful in patients for whom contrast-enhanced CT-scan should be avoided for evaluation of renal artery diameter and renal stenosis detection in patients with altered renal function.

Gadolinium-enhanced MRI must be considered carefully in patients with severe renal dysfunction. The American college of radiology, however, underlines the risk of nephrogenic systemic fibrosis (NSF) associated with gadolinium infusion in patients with terminal renal failure [56, 57]. NSF is a disorder with a scleroderma-like presentation, which appears with the administration of gadolinium-based contrast agents in patients with severe renal dysfunction (patients on dialysis mostly and rarely in patients with glomerular filtration rate <30 mL/min/1.73 m$^2$). The pathophysiology and predictive factors remain, however, mostly unknown and require further research.

MR angiography (MRA) using ultra-small particles of iron oxide (small molecules not filtered by the glomeruli) could be used for assessing renal blood flow and can be used for vascular enhancement in patients with chronic kidney disease [58]. Furthermore ultra-small particles of iron oxide can help in detecting inflammatory process due to late uptake by macrophages at the site of inflammation. Phase contrast angiography (PCA)-MRI has been used to determine renal blood flow velocities in transplant-kidney patients and in ICU patients with acute kidney injury [59]. It, however, remains a research tool not being used for routine assessment of renal blood flow. Blood oxygen level dependent (BOLD) MR imaging allows assessment of tissue oxygen tension using deoxyhaemoglobin as an endogenous contrast agent [60, 61]. Interpretation remains however difficult due to multiplicity of factor affecting deoxyhaemoglobin and BOLD MRI is also mainly a research tool.

> **Conclusion**
>
> Renal imaging provides important information on the cause of acute kidney injury and may therefore guide treatment. While echography remains the first-line exam for most conditions, providing easy and non-invasive insights into the process of AKI, other techniques such as CT scan and MRI can be considered based on the clinical and biological presentation or evolution of the syndrome. Finally, renal Doppler and CEUS may hold promise in estimating renal perfusion and may allow individualized treatment. The techniques remains however to be validated in large unselected population of patients. Other techniques to assess renal function and renal perfusion have mostly remained research tools although their use may help in providing interesting insight into the pathophysiological mechanisms involved in renal injury.

# References


1. Granata A, Fiorini F, Andrulli S, Logias F, Gallieni M, Romano G, Sicurezza E, Fiore CE. Doppler ultrasound and renal artery stenosis: an overview. J Ultrasound. 2009;12:133–43.
2. Faubel S, Patel NU, Lockhart ME, Cadnapaphornchai MA. Renal relevant radiology: use of ultrasonography in patients with AKI. Clin J Am Soc Nephrol. 2014;9:382–94.
3. Krumme B, Blum U, Schwertfeger E, Flügel P, Höllstin F, Schollmeyer P, et al. Diagnosis of renovascular disease by intra- and extrarenal Doppler scanning. Kidney Int. 1996;50: 1288–92.
4. Buckley AR, Cooperberg PL, Reeve CE, Magil AB. The distinction between acute renal transplant rejection and cyclosporine nephrotoxicity: value of duplex sonography. AJR Am J Roentgenol. 1987;149:521–5.
5. Patriquin HB, O'Regan S, Robitaille P, Paltiel H. Hemolytic-uremic syndrome: intrarenal arterial Doppler patterns as a useful guide to therapy. Radiology. 1989;172:625–8.
6. Platt JF. Duplex Doppler evaluation of native kidney dysfunction: obstructive and nonobstructive disease. AJR Am J Roentgenol. 1992;158:1035–42.
7. Platt JF, Rubin JM, Ellis JH, DiPietro MA. Duplex Doppler US of the kidney: differentiation of obstructive from nonobstructive dilatation. Radiology. 1989;171:515–7.
8. Allen KS, Jorkasky DK, Arger PH, Velchik MG, Grumbach K, Coleman BG, et al. Renal allografts: prospective analysis of Doppler sonography. Radiology. 1988;169:371–6.
9. Radermacher J, Mengel M, Ellis S, Stuht S, Hiss M, Schwarz A, et al. The renal arterial resistance index and renal allograft survival. N Engl J Med. 2003;349:115–24.
10. Naesens M, Heylen L, Lerut E, Claes K, De Wever L, Claus F, et al. Intrarenal resistive index after renal transplantation. N Engl J Med. 2013;369:1797–806.
11. Deruddre S, Cheisson G, Mazoit J-X, Vicaut E, Benhamou D, Duranteau J. Renal arterial resistance in septic shock: effects of increasing mean arterial pressure with norepinephrine on the renal resistive index assessed with Doppler ultrasonography. Intensive Care Med. 2007;33:1557–62.
12. Duranteau J, Deruddre S, Vigue B, Chemla D. Doppler monitoring of renal hemodynamics: why the best is yet to come. Intensive Care Med. 2008;34:1360–1.

13. Lauschke A, Teichgräber UKM, Frei U, Eckardt K-U. "Low-dose" dopamine worsens renal perfusion in patients with acute renal failure. Kidney Int. 2006;69:1669–74.
14. Lerolle N, Guérot E, Faisy C, Bornstain C, Diehl J-L, Fagon J-Y. Renal failure in septic shock: predictive value of Doppler-based renal arterial resistive index. Intensive Care Med. 2006;32: 1553–9.
15. Darmon M, Schortgen F, Vargas F, Liazydi A, Schlemmer B, Brun-Buisson C, et al. Diagnostic accuracy of Doppler renal resistive index for reversibility of acute kidney injury in critically ill patients. Intensive Care Med. 2011;37:68–76.
16. Platt JF. Doppler ultrasound of the kidney. Semin Ultrasound CT MR. 1997;18:22–32.
17. Schnell D, Darmon M. Renal Doppler to assess renal perfusion in the critically ill: a reappraisal. Intensive Care Med. 2012;38:1751–60.
18. Barozzi L, Valentino M, Santoro A, Mancini E, Pavlica P. Renal ultrasonography in critically ill patients. Crit Care Med. 2007;35:S198–205.
19. Mastorakou I, Lindsell DR, Piepoli M, Adamopoulos S, Ledingham JG. Pulsatility and resistance indices in intrarenal arteries of normal adults. Abdom Imaging. 1994;19:369–73.
20. Keogan MT, Kliewer MA, Hertzberg BS, DeLong DM, Tupler RH, Carroll BA. Renal resistive indexes: variability in Doppler US measurement in a healthy population. Radiology. 1996;199:165–9.
21. Norris CS, Pfeiffer JS, Rittgers SE, Barnes RW. Noninvasive evaluation of renal artery stenosis and renovascular resistance. Experimental and clinical studies. J Vasc Surg. 1984;1:192–201.
22. Bude RO, DiPietro MA, Platt JF, Rubin JM, Miesowicz S, Lundquist C. Age dependency of the renal resistive index in healthy children. Radiology. 1992;184:469–73.
23. Terry JD, Rysavy JA, Frick MP. Intrarenal Doppler: characteristics of aging kidneys. J Ultrasound Med. 1992;11:647–51.
24. El Helou N, Hélénon O, Augusti M, Correas JM, el Rody F, Souissi M, et al. Renal Doppler ultrasonography in the diagnosis of acute obstructions of the upper urinary tract. J Radiol. 1993;74:499–507.
25. Schnell D, Reynaud M, Venot M, Le Maho AL, Dinic M, Baulieu M, et al. Resistive Index or Color-Doppler semi-quantitative evaluation of renal perfusion by inexperienced physicians: results of a pilot study. Minerva Anestesiol. 2014;80(12):1273–81.
26. London NJ, Aldoori MI, Lodge VG, Bates JA, Irving HC, Giles GR. Reproducibility of Doppler ultrasound measurement of resistance index in renal allografts. Br J Radiol. 1993;66:510–3.
27. Bude RO, Rubin JM. Relationship between the resistive index and vascular compliance and resistance. Radiology. 1999;211:411–7.
28. Murphy ME, Tublin ME. Understanding the Doppler RI: impact of renal arterial distensibility on the RI in a hydronephrotic ex vivo rabbit kidney model. J Ultrasound Med. 2000;19(5):303–14.
29. Tublin ME, Tessler FN, Murphy ME. Correlation between renal vascular resistance, pulse pressure, and the resistive index in isolated perfused rabbit kidneys. Radiology. 1999;213: 258–64.
30. Mitchell GF. Effects of central arterial aging on the structure and function of the peripheral vasculature: implications for end-organ damage. J Appl Physiol 1985. 2008;105:1652–60.
31. Derchi LE, Leoncini G, Parodi D, Viazzi F, Martinoli C, Ratto E, et al. Mild renal dysfunction and renal vascular resistance in primary hypertension. Am J Hypertens. 2005;18:966–71.
32. Ohta Y, Fujii K, Arima H, Matsumura K, Tsuchihashi T, Tokumoto M, et al. Increased renal resistive index in atherosclerosis and diabetic nephropathy assessed by Doppler sonography. J Hypertens. 2005;23:1905–11.
33. Mostbeck GH, Gössinger HD, Mallek R, Siostrzonek P, Schneider B, Tscholakoff D. Effect of heart rate on Doppler measurements of resistive index in renal arteries. Radiology. 1990;175:511–3.
34. Sharkey RA, Mulloy EM, O'Neill SJ. The acute effects of oxygen and carbon dioxide on renal vascular resistance in patients with an acute exacerbation of COPD. Chest. 1999;115: 1588–92.

35. Sharkey RA, Mulloy EM, O'Neill SJ. Acute effects of hypoxaemia, hyperoxaemia and hypercapnia on renal blood flow in normal and renal transplant subjects. Eur Respir J. 1998;12(3):653–7.
36. Darmon M, Schortgen F, Leon R, Moutereau S, Mayaux J, Di Marco F, et al. Impact of mild hypoxemia on renal function and renal resistive index during mechanical ventilation. Intensive Care Med. 2009;35:1031–8.
37. Kirkpatrick AW, Colistro R, Laupland KB, Fox DL, Konkin DE, Kock V, et al. Renal arterial resistive index response to intraabdominal hypertension in a porcine model. Crit Care Med. 2007;35:207–13.
38. Umgelter A, Reindl W, Franzen M, Lenhardt C, Huber W, Schmid RM. Renal resistive index and renal function before and after paracentesis in patients with hepatorenal syndrome and tense ascites. Intensive Care Med. 2009;35:152–6.
39. Corradi F, Brusasco C, Vezzani A, Palermo S, Altomonte F, Moscatelli P, et al. Hemorrhagic shock in polytrauma patients: early detection with renal Doppler resistive index measurements. Radiology. 2011;260:112–8.
40. Izumi M, Sugiura T, Nakamura H, Nagatoya K, Imai E, Hori M. Differential diagnosis of prerenal azotemia from acute tubular necrosis and prediction of recovery by Doppler ultrasound. Am J Kidney Dis. 2000;35:713–9.
41. Platt JF, Rubin JM, Ellis JH. Acute renal failure: possible role of duplex Doppler US in distinction between acute prerenal failure and acute tubular necrosis. Radiology. 1991;179:419–23.
42. Bossard G, Bourgoin P, Corbeau JJ, Huntzinger J, Beydon L. Early detection of postoperative acute kidney injury by Doppler renal resistive index in cardiac surgery with cardiopulmonary bypass. Br J Anaesth. 2011;107:891–8.
43. Schnell D, Deruddre S, Harrois A, Pottecher J, Cosson C, Adoui N, et al. Renal resistive index better predicts the occurrence of acute kidney injury than cystatin C. Shock. 2012;38:592–7.
44. Dewitte A, Coquin J, Meyssignac B, Joannes-Boyau O, Fleureau C, Roze H, et al. Doppler resistive index to reflect regulation of renal vascular tone during sepsis and acute kidney injury. Crit Care. 2012;16:R165.
45. Schnell D, Camous L, Guyomarc'h S, Duranteau J, Canet E, Gery P, et al. Renal perfusion assessment by renal Doppler during fluid challenge in sepsis. Crit Care Med. 2013;41:1214–20.
46. Raisinghani A, Rafter P, Phillips P, Vannan MA, DeMaria AN. Microbubble contrast agents for echocardiography: rationale, composition, ultrasound interactions, and safety. Cardiol Clin. 2004;22:171–80.
47. Schneider A, Johnson L, Goodwin M, Schelleman A, Bellomo R. Bench-to-bedside review: contrast enhanced ultrasonography–a promising technique to assess renal perfusion in the ICU. Crit Care. 2011;15:157.
48. Vogel R, Indermühle A, Reinhardt J, Meier P, Siegrist PT, Namdar M, et al. The quantification of absolute myocardial perfusion in humans by contrast echocardiography: algorithm and validation. J Am Coll Cardiol. 2005;45:754–62.
49. Dolan MS, Gala SS, Dodla S, Abdelmoneim SS, Xie F, Cloutier D, et al. Safety and efficacy of commercially available ultrasound contrast agents for rest and stress echocardiography a multicenter experience. J Am Coll Cardiol. 2009;53:32–8.
50. Schneider AG, Goodwin MD, Schelleman A, Bailey M, Johnson L, Bellomo R. Contrast-enhanced ultrasound to evaluate changes in renal cortical perfusion around cardiac surgery: a pilot study. Crit Care. 2013;17:R138.
51. Schneider AG, Goodwin MD, Schelleman A, Bailey M, Johnson L, Bellomo R. Contrast-enhanced ultrasonography to evaluate changes in renal cortical microcirculation induced by noradrenaline: a pilot study. Crit Care. 2014;18:653.
52. Kalantarinia K. Novel imaging techniques in acute kidney injury. Curr Drug Targets. 2009;10:1184–9.
53. Saba L, Caddeo G, Sanfilippo R, Montisci R, Mallarini G. Multidetector-row CT angiography diagnostic sensitivity in evaluation of renal artery stenosis: comparison between multiple reconstruction techniques. J Comput Assist Tomogr. 2007;31:712–6.

54. Wittenberg G, Kenn W, Tschammler A, Sandstede J, Hahn D. Spiral CT angiography of renal arteries: comparison with angiography. Eur Radiol. 1999;9:546–51.
55. Hamed MA. New advances in assessment of the individual renal function in chronic unilateral renal obstruction using functional CT compared to 99mTc-DTPA renal scan. Nucl Med Rev Cent East Eur. 2014;17:59–64.
56. Bhave G, Lewis JB, Chang SS. Association of gadolinium based magnetic resonance imaging contrast agents and nephrogenic systemic fibrosis. J Urol. 2008;180:830–5.
57. Prchal D, Holmes DT, Levin A. Nephrogenic systemic fibrosis: the story unfolds. Kidney Int. 2008;73:1335–7.
58. Nayak AB, Luhar A, Hanudel M, Gales B, Hall TR, Finn JP, Salusky IB, Zaritsky J. High-resolution, whole-body vascular imaging with ferumoxytol as an alternative to gadolinium agents in a pediatric chronic kidney disease cohort. Pediatr Nephrol. 2015;30(3): 515–21.
59. Beierwaltes WH, Harrison-Bernard LM, Sullivan JC, Mattson DL. Assessment of renal function; clearance, the renal microcirculation, renal blood flow, and metabolic balance. Compr Physiol. 2013;3:165–200.
60. Inoue T, Kozawa E, Okada H, Inukai K, Watanabe S, Kikuta T, Watanabe Y, Takenaka T, Katayama S, Tanaka J, Suzuki H. Noninvasive evaluation of kidney hypoxia and fibrosis using magnetic resonance imaging. J Am Soc Nephrol. 2011;22:1429–34.
61. Textor SC, Glockner JF, Lerman LO, Misra S, McKusick MA, Riederer SJ, Grande JP, Gomez SI, Romero JC. The use of magnetic resonance to evaluate tissue oxygenation in renal artery stenosis. J Am Soc Nephrol. 2008;19:780–8.

Part III

Prevention and Protection

# Prevention of AKI and Protection of the Kidney



Michael Joannidis and Lui G. Forni

## 11.1 Introduction

Acute kidney injury (AKI) poses a significant risk to patients resulting in an increase in both mortality and morbidity. As discussed in previous chapters, the major causes of AKI in the ICU include renal hypoperfusion, sepsis and septic shock, heart failure and direct nephrotoxicity although in most cases the aetiology is multifactorial with a combination of events leading to AKI. Major risk factors have been identified which predispose to the development of AKI (Table 11.1). Given the poor outcomes of patients with AKI it is of the highest priority for physicians treating critically ill patients. Given that to-date no single pharmaceutical intervention has proven effective in preventing AKI a more systemic approach should be considered which includes three major issues:

1. Ensuring adequate renal perfusion
2. Modulation of renal physiology
3. Avoiding further, additional renal insult

M. Joannidis, MD (✉)
Division of Intensive Care and Emergency Medicine,
Department of Internal Medicine, Medical University Innsbruck,
Innsbruck A-6020, Austria
e-mail: michael.joannidis@i-med.ac.at

L.G. Forni
Department of Intensive Care Medicine, Royal Surrey County Hospital
NHS Foundation Trust, Surrey Perioperative Anaesthesia Critical Care Collaborative
Research Group (SPACeR) and Faculty of Health Care Sciences,
University of Surrey, Guildford, UK
e-mail: luiforni@nhs.net

© Springer International Publishing 2015
H.M. Oudemans-van Straaten et al. (eds.), *Acute Nephrology for the Critical Care Physician*, DOI 10.1007/978-3-319-17389-4_11

**Table 11.1** Major risk factors for AKI

| Patient factors | Advanced Age<br>Female<br>Black Race |
|---|---|
| Pre-existing co-morbidities | Chronic Kidney Disease (CKD)<br>Liver Disease<br>Respiratory Disease<br>Heart Failure<br>Diabetes: Especially with proteinuria<br>Cancer |
| Current susceptibilities | Volume Depletion<br>Dehydration<br>Hypoalbuminemia |
| Exposures | Critical Illness<br>Sepsis<br>Circulatory Shock<br>Burns |
| Surgery | Cardiac Surgery (especially with CPB)<br>Trauma |
| Drugs | Nephrotoxic Agents<br>Radiocontrast |

Adapted from KDIGO

## 11.2 Ensuring Adequate Kidney Perfusion

According to large cohort studies hypovolemia, sepsis and heart failure have been shown to be the most frequent causes of AKI, it follows that as a consequence reduced renal perfusion is considered a major risk factor as well as a trigger for this syndrome. However, the practicalities of how to provide optimal renal perfusion are far from straightforward but are best achieved by a systematic approach with the main targets being:

(a) Optimizing systemic haemodynamics
(b) Reducing factors compromising renal perfusion and filtration
(c) Selective vasodilation of the renal vascular bed

### 11.2.1 Optimizing Systemic Hemodynamics

Optimisation of systemic hemodynamics is accomplished through enhanced hemodynamic monitoring. Usual targets include adequate oxygen delivery achieved by normalizing the stroke index and arterial oxygen saturation. Central venous saturation and lactate clearance may be additionally included for evaluation but the results must be viewed in context. Detailed recommendations on how to guide hemodynamic management is outside the remit of this chapter but was recently addressed in the recommendations by the European Society of Intensive Care Medicine [1].

### 11.2.1.1 Vasopressors

Vasopressors are the mainstay of therapy in vasodilatory shock: Noradrenalin is the preferred choice over adrenaline or dopamine given they are associated with higher rates of arrhythmias [2, 3]. Vasopressin may be an option in vasoplegic states where noradrenalin use fails to attain target values and some recent studies suggest a lower incidence of AKI stage 1 when vasopressin rather than noradrenalin is used [4].

### 11.2.1.2 Inotropes

Where reduced cardiac output predominates the clinical picture, inotropic agents including inodilators are a reasonable option. Interestingly, recent data indicates that the calcium sensitizers levosimendan may be superior with regard to effects on renal function compared to dobutamine especially in the setting of sepsis [5, 6].

### 11.2.1.3 Volume Therapy

Both relative and overt hypovolaemia contribute to reduced cardiac filling pressures and potentially lead to reduced renal perfusion and therefore timely, appropriate fluid administration is a preventive measure which should be effective both through the restoration of the circulating volume and potentially minimising drug induced nephrotoxicity [7]. Where volume replacement is indicated this should be performed in a controlled fashion directed by hard end points with hemodynamic monitoring [8] as injudicious use of fluids carries its own inherent risk [9] (see below).

Volume replacement may employ 5 % glucose (i.e. free water), crystalloids (isotonic, half isotonic), colloids or a combination thereof. Glucose solutions substitute free water and are mainly used to correct hyperosmolar states. Given free water is distributed throughout the extracellular volume, glucose solutions provide only about half of the effects on volume expansion as compared to crystalloids. Isotonic crystalloids represent the mainstay for correction of extracellular volume depletion. However, increased chloride load resulting from normal saline may result in a hyperchloraemic acidosis and potential renal vasoconstriction as well as altered perfusion of other organs such as the gut [10]. Recent investigations suggest increased risk of AKI and RRT as well as increased mortality associated with use of large volumes of 0.9 % saline as compared to so called 'balanced solutions' which contain significantly lower chloride concentrations [11–13]. However, to-date there are no published randomised controlled studies comparing saline to balanced solutions and the effects on renal function and recent evidence suggest that other cofounders may also play a role in the development of AKI. Whereas crystalloids expand plasma volume by approximately 25 % of the infused volume, colloid infusion results in a greater expansion of plasma volume. The degree of expansion is dependent on concentration, mean molecular weight and (for starches) the degree of molecular substitution. Furthermore, volume effects of colloids are dependent on the integrity of the vascular barrier which is often compromised in the presence of a severe SIRS response as well as sepsis. Artificial colloids used clinically include gelatines, starches and dextrans. Human albumin (HA) is the only naturally occurring colloid with additional pleiotropic properties outside the scope of this chapter.

Hydroxyethyl starches (HES) are highly polymerised non-ionic sugar molecules characterised by molecular weight, grade of substitution, concentration and C2/C6 ratio. Their volume effect is greater than that of albumin especially when larger sized polymers are employed. These molecules degrade through hydrolytic cleavage the products of which undergo renal elimination. However, these degradation products may be reabsorbed and contribute to osmotic nephrosis and possibly medullary hypoxia [14–16]. A further problem with HES may be dose dependant tissue deposition and associated pruritus [17–19] which appear to be characteristic for all preparations of HES independent of molecular size and substitution grade. Recent randomized controlled trials (RCT) have substantiated increased risk for AKI and renal replacement therapy by using starches especially in sepsis [20–22] leading to the recommendation not to use starches in critically ill patients [23, 24]. Gelatines have an average molecular weight of ca. 30 KD and the observed intravascular volume effect is shorter than that observed with HA or HES although potential side effects of there use include the possibility of prion transmission, histamine release and coagulation problems particularly with the use of large volumes [25, 26]. Furthermore, there is a theoretical risk of osmotic nephrosis with gelatine use although data is scarce and studies fail to demonstrate any deleterious effects on renal function as determined by changes in serum creatinine [27–29]. Dextrans are single chain polysaccharides comparable to albumin in size (40–70 kDa) and with a reasonably high volume effect though again anaphylaxis, coagulation disorders and indeed AKI may occur at doses higher than 1.5 g/kg/day [30–33]. Osmotic nephrosis has also been reported for dextrans [16].

HA may appear attractive in hypooncotic hypovolaemia but in some countries is costly [34–36]. A large multicenter RCT comparing 20 % albumin to crystalloid failed to demonstrate any difference in outcomes including renal function, but proved that albumin itself was safe [37]. The most recent trial in patients with sepsis showed improved survival and a better negative fluid balance in patients with septic shock [38]. Importantly, to-date no negative effect on renal function have been reported from RCTs using 20 % albumin.

## 11.2.2 Reducing Factors Compromising Renal Perfusion

According to the currently available data a fluid overload of >10 % has been found to be associated with increased mortality in critically ill patients [39]. Moreover, fluid overload has also been demonstrated to be a significant risk factor for AKI. Volume overload may impair renal function through effects on glomerular filtration through several mechanisms. General organ oedema increases interstitial pressure throughout and in organs which are encapsulated, such as the kidneys, the limited ability to mitigate this change through distension leads to a further rise compromising function. Venous congestion with volume overload reflected by a rise in central venous pressure has been shown to be associated with a reduced glomerular filtration rate (GFR) and increased sodium reabsorption in animal studies. Moreover, recent investigations demonstrate an association between increased central venous pressures (>12 mmHg) and the rate of AKI in critically ill patients [40]. Thirdly, massive fluid overload is a major risk factor for abdominal hypertension which further impairs renal function through its putative effects on renal perfusion. Furthermore, volume overload is associated with lung injury requiring increased ventilation pressures, especially positive endexpiratory pressure (PEEP) which also increases central venous pressure (CVP) and subsequently intrabdominal pressure. Treatment of volume overload includes aggressive pursuit of a negative fluid balance with volume restriction and diuretic usage. Volume overload may lead to the initiation of renal replacement therapy (RRT) if a negative fluid balance cannot be achieved over the desired period and indeed intractable volume overload is considered an absolute indication for commencing renal replacement therapy [41].

## 11.2.3 Selective Renal vasodilation

### 11.2.3.1 Dopamine

*Dopamine* when used at so-called 'renal doses' is still widely used but is ineffective in improving renal function although an increased diuresis on the first day of use has been observed [42]. Indeed, dopamine may worsen renal perfusion in patients with acute kidney injury as determined by change in observed renal resistive indexes [43]. Despite showing promising results in pilot studies on patients at risk of contrast nephropathy [44, 45] and sepsis-associated acute kidney injury [46, 47], selective dopamine $A_1$ agonists such as fenoldopam have failed to demonstrate significant renal protection in larger studies of either early presumed acute tubular necrosis [48, 49] or contrast nephropathy [50].

### 11.2.3.2 Prostaglandins

*Prostaglandins* have been investigated mainly in the setting of contrast nephropathy. Both prostaglandin E1 (PGE1) and PGI (Iloprost) administered intravenously resulted in attenuated rise of serum creatinine after the use of contrast media [51, 52]. However, major adverse events include hypotension as well as flushing and nausea at higher doses thereby limiting their extensive use.

### 11.2.3.3 Natriuretic Peptide

*Natriuretic peptides* improve renal blood flow through afferent glomerular dilation resulting in an increase in both GFR and urinary sodium excretion and, in addition, B-type natriuretic peptides (BNPs) inhibit aldosterone. Atrial natriuretic peptide (ANP) use in human studies has been controversial attenuating rise in serum creatinine in ischemic renal failure [53] or in AKI after liver transplantation but it is ineffective in large RCTs of both non-oliguric [54] and oliguric AKI [55]. A recent study using low-dose BNP (nesiritide) suggested there was some preservation of renal function in patients with chronic kidney disease stage 3 undergoing cardiopulmonary bypass surgery [56].

Currently, the most promising preliminary reports in the intensive care setting do exist for the adenosine antagonist theophylline for either contrast nephropathy [57–59] as well as some types of nephrotoxic AKI like cisplatin associated renal dysfunction [60]. A randomized placebo controlled trial in neonates with perinatal asphyxia showed significant increase in creatinine clearance after a single dose of theophylline within the first hour of birth [61].

## 11.3 Modulation of Renal Physiology

### 11.3.1 Renal Metabolism, Tubular Obstruction

Diuretics, particularly those acting on the loop of Henle, have provided most data regarding the potential pharmacological manipulation of renal metabolism and inhibition of tubular obstruction. Loop diuretics are known to reduce oxygen consumption within the renal medulla and increased oxygen tension in the renal medulla in both animals and healthy volunteers has been observed [62]. However, a randomized controlled trial performed in established renal failure could not demonstrate improvement in outcome. Application of very high doses of furosemide, on the other hand, increases risk of serious adverse events like hearing loss significantly and as such cannot be recommended [63].

### 11.3.2 Oxygen Radical Damage

Several roles have been proposed for reactive oxygen species (ROS) under both normal and pathological conditions, with the NAD(P)H oxidase system pivotal in their formation and instrumental in the development of certain pathophysiological conditions [64, 65]. Under certain circumstances a role for antioxidant supplementation may be proposed with potential candidates including N-acetylcysteine (NAC), selenium and the antioxidant vitamins (vitamin E ($\alpha$-tocopherol) and vitamin C (ascorbic acid)). However, most studies involving antioxidant supplementation suffer from a lack of data regarding optimal dosing as well as timing.

#### 11.3.2.1 N-acetylcysteine

*N-acetylcysteine*, has been investigated in multiple trials particularly in the setting of contrast nephropathy. Despite several reports showing prevention of contrast nephropathy [66, 67] evaluation of this substance by meta–analyses yields controversial results [68]. Furthermore NAC was ineffective in other circumstances where AKI is common such as major cardiovascular surgery or sepsis [69, 70–72].

Finally studies of IV NAC in both human volunteers as well as patients receiving contrast media demonstrate a decrease in serum creatinine not reflected by concomitant changes of cystatin C considered the more sensitive marker of early changes in GFR [73, 74].

#### 11.3.2.2 Mannitol

*Mannitol*, an osmotic diuretic with potential oxygen radical scavenging properties was investigated in randomized trials for the prevention of contrast nephropathy but generally was inferior to general measures such as volume expansion [75]. Some authors favour mannitol for treatment of AKI following crush injuries but controlled trials are still awaited [76].

### 11.3.2.3 Selenium

*Selenium* is an essential component of the selenoenzymes including glutathione peroxidase and thioredoxin reductase. Selenium supplementation reduces oxidative stress, nuclear factor-B translocation, and cytokine formation as well as attenuating tissue damage. Angstwurm et al. performed a small RCT in 42 patients and showed that selenium supplementation decreased the requirement for RRT from 43 to 14 % [77]. This finding was not reproduced in a consequent prospective RCT in septic shock although selenium appeared to reduce 28 days mortality [78].

Cocktails of antioxidants have been investigated in several small studies showing controversial results. In one randomized trial in patients undergoing elective aortic aneurysm repair use of an antioxidant cocktail resulted in an increased creatinine clearance on the second postoperative day but the incidence of renal failure was very low [79].

### 11.3.2.4 Ascorbic Acid

*Ascorbic acid* used in preclinical at high-doses can prevent or restore ROS-induced microcirculatory flow impairment, prevent or restore vascular responsiveness to vasoconstrictors and potentially preserve the endothelial barrier [80]. When given PO 2 h pre-contrast in a single centre trial there appeared to be protection against the development of contrast nephropathy but the rate of AKI in the control group was high and no patients required renal support [81]. A recent meta-analysis on this subject found a renal protective effect of ascorbic acid against contrast-induced AKI [82]. To-date no multicentre randomised control trials have demonstrated any benefit in reducing the rate of AKI by using antioxidant supplementation.

### 11.3.3  Avoiding Additional Nephrotoxic Damage

The use of nephrotoxic drugs can cause or worsen acute kidney injury, or delay recovery of renal function. Moreover when renal function declines, failure to appropriately adjust the doses of medications can cause further adverse effects. The potential for inappropriate drug use in patients with, or at risk of developing, acute kidney injury is high and this is potentially a preventable cause of AKI. Therefore, any assessment of a patient at risk or with AKI must include a thorough review of prescribed medications. Particular agents associated with AKI in the critically ill include aminoglycosides, amphotericin and the angiotensin-converting enzyme inhibitors (ACEI) and angiotensin receptor blockers (ARBs) [8].

### 11.3.3.1 Aminoglycoside

*Aminoglycoside* antimicrobial agents are highly potent, bactericidal antibiotics effective against multiple bacterial pathogens particularly when administered with beta-lactams and other cell-wall active antimicrobial agents. Despite their well documented side effects including nephrotoxicity, and to a lesser degree ototoxicity and neuromuscular blockade there use continues to increase due to progressive antimicrobial resistance to other antimicrobial agents and lack of new alternatives. However, given the potential risks aminoglycosides should be used for as short a period of time as possible and care should be taken in those groups most susceptible to nephrotoxicity. This includes older patients, patients with chronic kidney disease, sepsis (particularly in the presence of intravascular volume depletion), diabetes mellitus and concomitant use of other nephrotoxic drugs. Aminoglycoside demonstrates concentration-dependent bactericidal activity which enables extended interval dosing which optimizes efficacy and minimizes toxicity. This dosing strategy, together with meticulous attention to therapeutic drug monitoring when used for more than a 24 h period may limit the risk of nephrotoxicity.

### 11.3.3.2 Amphotericin B

*Amphotericin B* is a polyene antifungal agent which is insoluble in water and has been the standard of treatment for life threatening systemic mycoses for over 50 years. This is despite its well known and common drug-induced toxicity which includes thrombophlebitis, electrolyte disturbances, hypoplastic anemia and nephrotoxicity the latter of which is associated with higher mortality rates, increased LOS, and increased total costs of health care. An alternative approach is to use, where possible, non-amphotericin B antifungal agents which are better tolerated.

### 11.3.3.3 Angiotensin-Converting Enzyme Inhibitors

*Angiotensin-converting enzyme inhibitors* (ACEI) and angiotensin receptor blockers (ARBs) are widely used in the management of hypertension and heart failure and are often used in patients with CKD particularly in the presence of significant proteinuria. These agents are potentially nephrotoxic medications given that they antagonize the normal physiological response to a reduction in renal blood flow. ACEI and ARBs, cause vasodilation of efferent blood vessels, resulting in AKI in susceptible patients as the body's normal compensatory response to a decreased GFR is impeded. Hence in the critically ill and in those at risk of hypovolaemia they should be withheld unless there is an impelling clinical reason for continuing therapy. It is important to stress that on the patient's recovery the reintroduction of these agents should not be forgotten where continuing therapy is needed.

## References


1. Cecconi M, De BD, Antonelli M, Beale R, Bakker J, Hofer C, et al. Consensus on circulatory shock and hemodynamic monitoring. Task force of the European Society of Intensive Care Medicine. Intensive Care Med. 2014;40(12):1795–815.
2. De BD, Biston P, Devriendt J, Madl C, Chochrad D, Aldecoa C, et al. Comparison of dopamine and norepinephrine in the treatment of shock. N Engl J Med. 2010;362(9):779–89.
3. Dellinger RP, Levy MM, Rhodes A, Annane D, Gerlach H, Opal SM, et al. Surviving Sepsis Campaign: international guidelines for management of severe sepsis and septic shock, 2012. Intensive Care Med. 2013;39(2):165–228.

4. Gordon AC, Russell JA, Walley KR, Singer J, Ayers D, Storms MM, et al. The effects of vasopressin on acute kidney injury in septic shock. Intensive Care Med. 2010;36(1): 83–91.

5. Morelli A, De CS, Teboul JL, Singer M, Rocco M, Conti G, et al. Effects of levosimendan on systemic and regional hemodynamics in septic myocardial depression. Intensive Care Med. 2005;31(5):638–44.

6. Hasslacher J, Bijuklic K, Bertocchi C, Kountchev J, Bellmann R, Dunzendorfer S, et al. Levosimendan inhibits release of reactive oxygen species in polymorphonuclear leukocytes in vitro and in patients with acute heart failure and septic shock: a prospective observational study. Crit Care. 2011;15(4):R166.

7. Badr KF, Ichikawa I. Prerenal failure: a deleterious shift from renal compensation to decompensation. N Engl J Med. 1988;319(10):623–9.

8. Kellum JA, Lameire N. Diagnosis, evaluation, and management of acute kidney injury: a KDIGO summary (Part 1). Crit Care. 2013;17(1):204.

9. Himmelfarb J, Joannidis M, Molitoris B, Schietz M, Okusa MD, Warnock D, et al. Evaluation and initial management of acute kidney injury. Clin J Am Soc Nephrol. 2008;3(4):962–7.

10. Wilkes NJ, Woolf R, Mutch M, Mallett SV, Peachey T, Stephens R, et al. The effects of balanced versus saline-based hetastarch and crystalloid solutions on acid–base and electrolyte status and gastric mucosal perfusion in elderly surgical patients. Anesth Analg. 2001;93(4): 811–6.

11. Yunos NM, Bellomo R, Glassford N, Sutcliffe H, Lam Q, Bailey M. Chloride-liberal vs. chloride-restrictive intravenous fluid administration and acute kidney injury: an extended analysis. Intensive Care Med. 2015;41(2):257–64.

12. Yunos NM, Bellomo R, Hegarty C, Story D, Ho L, Bailey M. Association between a chloride-liberal vs chloride-restrictive intravenous fluid administration strategy and kidney injury in critically ill adults. JAMA. 2012;308(15):1566–72.

13. Shaw AD, Raghunathan K, Peyerl FW, Munson SH, Paluszkiewicz SM, Schermer CR. Association between intravenous chloride load during resuscitation and in-hospital mortality among patients with SIRS. Intensive Care Med. 2014;40(12):1897–905.

14. Legendre C, Thervet E, Page B, Percheron A, Noel LH, Kreis H. Hydroxyethylstarch and osmotic-nephrosis-like lesions in kidney transplantation. Lancet. 1993;342(8865): 248–9.

15. Bernard C, Alain M, Simone C, Xavier M, Jean-Francois M. Hydroxyethylstarch and osmotic nephrosis-like lesions in kidney transplants. Lancet. 1996;348(9041):1595.

16. Dickenmann M, Oettl T, Mihatsch MJ. Osmotic nephrosis: acute kidney injury with accumulation of proximal tubular lysosomes due to administration of exogenous solutes. Am J Kidney Dis. 2008;51(3):491–503.

17. Bork K. Pruritus precipitated by hydroxyethyl starch: a review. Br J Dermatol. 2005;152(1): 3–12.

18. Barron ME, Wilkes MM, Navickis RJ. A systematic review of the comparative safety of colloids. Arch Surg. 2004;139(5):552–63.

19. Wiedermann CJ, Joannidis M. Accumulation of hydroxyethyl starch in human and animal tissues: a systematic review. Intensive Care Med. 2014;40(2):160–70.

20. Gattas DJ, Dan A, Myburgh J, Billot L, Lo S, Finfer S. Fluid resuscitation with 6 % hydroxyethyl starch (130/0.4 and 130/0.42) in acutely ill patients: systematic review of effects on mortality and treatment with renal replacement therapy. Intensive Care Med. 2013;39(4): 558–68.

21. Myburgh JA, Finfer S, Bellomo R, Billot L, Cass A, Gattas D, et al. Hydroxyethyl starch or saline for fluid resuscitation in intensive care. N Engl J Med. 2012;367(20):1901–11.

22. Perner A, Haase N, Guttormsen AB, Tenhunen J, Klemenzson G, Aneman A, et al. Hydroxyethyl starch 130/0.42 versus Ringer's acetate in severe sepsis. N Engl J Med. 2012; 367(2):124–34.

23. Mutter TC, Ruth CA, Dart AB. Hydroxyethyl starch (HES) versus other fluid therapies: effects on kidney function. Cochrane Database Syst Rev. 2013;7, CD007594. doi:10.1002/14651858. CD007594.pub3.:CD007594.

24. Reinhart K, Perner A, Sprung CL, Jaeschke R, Schortgen F, Johan Groeneveld AB, et al. Consensus statement of the ESICM task force on colloid volume therapy in critically ill patients. Intensive Care Med. 2012;38(3):368–83.
25. Mardel SN, Saunders FM, Allen H, Menezes G, Edwards CM, Ollerenshaw L, et al. Reduced quality of clot formation with gelatin-based plasma substitutes. Br J Anaesth. 1998;80(2):204–7.
26. Tabuchi N, de Haan J, Gallandat Huet RC, Boonstra PW, van Oeveren W. Gelatin use impairs platelet adhesion during cardiac surgery. Thromb Haemost. 1995;74(6):1447–51.
27. Beyer R, Harmening U, Rittmeyer O, Zielmann S, Mielck F, Kazmaier S, et al. Use of modified fluid gelatin and hydroxyethyl starch for colloidal volume replacement in major orthopaedic surgery. Br J Anaesth. 1997;78(1):44–50.
28. Schortgen F, Lacherade JC, Bruneel F, Cattaneo I, Hemery F, Lemaire F, et al. Effects of hydroxyethylstarch and gelatin on renal function in severe sepsis: a multicentre randomised study. Lancet. 2001;357(9260):911–6.
29. Thomas-Rueddel DO, Vlasakov V, Reinhart K, Jaeschke R, Rueddel H, Hutagalung R, et al. Safety of gelatin for volume resuscitation–a systematic review and meta-analysis. Intensive Care Med. 2012;38(7):1134–42.
30. Kurnik BR, Singer F, Groh WC. Case report: dextran-induced acute anuric renal failure. Am J Med Sci. 1991;302(1):28–30.
31. Laxenaire MC, Charpentier C, Feldman L. Anaphylactoid reactions to colloid plasma substitutes: incidence, risk factors, mechanisms. A French multicenter prospective study. Ann Fr Anesth Reanim. 1994;13(3):301–10.
32. Mailloux L, Swartz CD, Capizzi R, Kim KE, Onesti G, Ramirez O, et al. Acute renal failure after administration of low-molecular weight dextran. N Engl J Med. 1967;277(21):1113–8.
33. Messmer KF. The use of plasma substitutes with special attention to their side effects. World J Surg. 1987;11(1):69–74.
34. Horstick G, Lauterbach M, Kempf T, Bhakdi S, Heimann A, Horstick M, et al. Early albumin infusion improves global and local hemodynamics and reduces inflammatory response in hemorrhagic shock. Crit Care Med. 2002;30(4):851–5.
35. Inoue M, Okajima K, Itoh K, Ando Y, Watanabe N, Yasaka T, et al. Mechanism of furosemide resistance in analbuminemic rats and hypoalbuminemic patients. Kidney Int. 1987;32(2):198–203.
36. Zhang H, Voglis S, Kim CH, Slutsky AS. Effects of albumin and Ringer's lactate on production of lung cytokines and hydrogen peroxide after resuscitated hemorrhage and endotoxemia in rats. Crit Care Med. 2003;31(5):1515–22.
37. Finfer S, Bellomo R, Boyce N, French J, Myburgh J, Norton R. A comparison of albumin and saline for fluid resuscitation in the intensive care unit. N Engl J Med. 2004;350(22):2247–56.
38. Caironi P, Tognoni G, Masson S, Fumagalli R, Pesenti A, Romero M, et al. Albumin replacement in patients with severe sepsis or septic shock. N Engl J Med. 2014;370(15):1412–21.
39. Prowle JR, Echeverri JE, Ligabo EV, Ronco C, Bellomo R. Fluid balance and acute kidney injury. Nat Rev Nephrol. 2010;6(2):107–15.
40. Legrand M, Dupuis C, Simon C, Gayat E, Mateo J, Lukaszewicz AC, et al. Association between systemic hemodynamics and septic acute kidney injury in critically ill patients: a retrospective observational study. Crit Care. 2013;17(6):R278.
41. Rosner MH, Ostermann M, Murugan R, Prowle JR, Ronco C, Kellum JA, et al. Indications and management of mechanical fluid removal in critical illness. Br J Anaesth. 2014;113(5):764–71.
42. Friedrich JO, Adhikari N, Herridge MS, Beyene J. Meta-analysis: low-dose dopamine increases urine output but does not prevent renal dysfunction or death. Ann Intern Med. 2005;142(7):510–24.
43. Lauschke A, Teichgraber UK, Frei U, Eckardt KU. 'Low-dose' dopamine worsens renal perfusion in patients with acute renal failure. Kidney Int. 2006;69(9):1669–74.
44. Stone GW, McCullough PA, Tumlin JA, Lepor NE, Madyoon H, Murray P, et al. Fenoldopam mesylate for the prevention of contrast-induced nephropathy: a randomized controlled trial. JAMA. 2003;290(17):2284–91.

45. Chu VL, Cheng JW. Fenoldopam in the prevention of contrast media-induced acute renal failure. Ann Pharmacother. 2001;35(10):1278–82.
46. Brienza N, Malcangi V, Dalfino L, Trerotoli P, Guagliardi C, Bortone D, et al. A comparison between fenoldopam and low-dose dopamine in early renal dysfunction of critically ill patients. Crit Care Med. 2006;34(3):707–14.
47. Morelli A, Ricci Z, Bellomo R, Ronco C, Rocco M, Conti G, et al. Prophylactic fenoldopam for renal protection in sepsis: a randomized, double-blind, placebo-controlled pilot trial. Crit Care Med. 2005;33(11):2451–6.
48. Tumlin JA, Finkel KW, Murray PT, Samuels J, Cotsonis G, Shaw AD. Fenoldopam mesylate in early acute tubular necrosis: a randomized, double-blind, placebo-controlled clinical trial. Am J Kidney Dis. 2005;46(1):26–34.
49. Bove T, Zangrillo A, Guarracino F, Alvaro G, Persi B, Maglioni E, et al. Effect of fenoldopam on use of renal replacement therapy among patients with acute kidney injury after cardiac surgery: a randomized clinical trial. JAMA. 2014;312(21):2244–53.
50. Heyman SN, Goldfarb M, Shina A, Karmeli F, Rosen S. N-acetylcysteine ameliorates renal microcirculation: studies in rats. Kidney Int. 2003;63(2):634–41.
51. Koch JA, Plum J, Grabensee B, Modder U. Prostaglandin E1: a new agent for the prevention of renal dysfunction in high risk patients caused by radiocontrast media? PGE1 Study Group. Nephrol Dial Transplant. 2000;15(1):43–9.
52. Spargias K, Adreanides E, Giamouzis G, Karagiannis S, Gouziouta A, Manginas A, et al. Iloprost for prevention of contrast-mediated nephropathy in high-risk patients undergoing a coronary procedure. Results of a randomized pilot study. Eur J Clin Pharmacol. 2006;62(8):589–95.
53. Sward K, Valsson F, Odencrants P, Samuelsson O, Ricksten SE. Recombinant human atrial natriuretic peptide in ischemic acute renal failure: a randomized placebo-controlled trial. Crit Care Med. 2004;32(6):1310–5.
54. Allgren RL, Marbury TC, Rahman SN, Weisberg LS, Fenves AZ, Lafayette RA, et al. Anaritide in acute tubular necrosis. Auriculin Anaritide Acute Renal Failure Study Group. N Engl J Med. 1997;336(12):828–34.
55. Lewis J, Salem MM, Chertow GM, Weisberg LS, McGrew F, Marbury TC, et al. Atrial natriuretic factor in oliguric acute renal failure. Anaritide Acute Renal Failure Study Group. Am J Kidney Dis. 2000;36(4):767–74.
56. Chen HH, Redfield MM, Nordstrom LJ, Horton DP, Burnett Jr JC. Subcutaneous administration of the cardiac hormone BNP in symptomatic human heart failure. J Card Fail. 2004;10(2):115–9.
57. Ix JH, McCulloch CE, Chertow GM. Theophylline for the prevention of radiocontrast nephropathy: a meta-analysis. Nephrol Dial Transplant. 2004;19(11):2747–53.
58. Bagshaw SM, Ghali WA. Theophylline for prevention of contrast-induced nephropathy: a systematic review and meta-analysis. Arch Intern Med. 2005;165(10):1087–93.
59. Huber W, Schipek C, Ilgmann K, Page M, Hennig M, Wacker A, et al. Effectiveness of theophylline prophylaxis of renal impairment after coronary angiography in patients with chronic renal insufficiency. Am J Cardiol. 2003;91(10):1157–62.
60. Benoehr P, Krueth P, Bokemeyer C, Grenz A, Osswald H, Hartmann JT. Nephroprotection by theophylline in patients with cisplatin chemotherapy: a randomized, single-blinded, placebo-controlled trial. J Am Soc Nephrol. 2005;16(2):452–8.
61. Bhat MA, Shah ZA, Makhdoomi MS, Mufti MH. Theophylline for renal function in term neonates with perinatal asphyxia: a randomized, placebo-controlled trial. J Pediatr. 2006;149(2):180–4.
62. Epstein FH, Prasad P. Effects of furosemide on medullary oxygenation in younger and older subjects. Kidney Int. 2000;57(5):2080–3.
63. Ho KM, Sheridan DJ. Meta-analysis of frusemide to prevent or treat acute renal failure. BMJ. 2006;333(7565):420.
64. Evans RG, Fitzgerald SM. Nitric oxide and superoxide in the renal medulla: a delicate balancing act. Curr Opin Nephrol Hypertens. 2005;14(1):9–15.
65. Haugen E, Nath KA. The involvement of oxidative stress in the progression of renal injury. Blood Purif. 1999;17(2–3):58–65.

66. Tepel M, van der GM, Schwarzfeld C, Laufer U, Liermann D, Zidek W. Prevention of radiographic-contrast-agent-induced reductions in renal function by acetylcysteine. N Engl J Med. 2000;343(3):180–4.

67. Marenzi G, Assanelli E, Marana I, Lauri G, Campodonico J, Grazi M, et al. N-acetylcysteine and contrast-induced nephropathy in primary angioplasty. N Engl J Med. 2006;354(26): 2773–82.

68. Bagshaw SM, McAlister FA, Manns BJ, Ghali WA. Acetylcysteine in the prevention of contrast-induced nephropathy: a case study of the pitfalls in the evolution of evidence. Arch Intern Med. 2006;166(2):161–6.

69. Hynninen MS, Niemi TT, Poyhia R, Raininko EI, Salmenpera MT, Lepantalo MJ, et al. N-acetylcysteine for the prevention of kidney injury in abdominal aortic surgery: a randomized, double-blind, placebo-controlled trial. Anesth Analg. 2006;102(6):1638–45.

70. Macedo E, Abdulkader R, Castro I, Sobrinho AC, Yu L, Vieira Jr JM. Lack of protection of N-acetylcysteine (NAC) in acute renal failure related to elective aortic aneurysm repair-a randomized controlled trial. Nephrol Dial Transplant. 2006;21(7):1863–9.

71. Komisarof JA, Gilkey GM, Peters DM, Koudelka CW, Meyer MM, Smith SM. N-acetylcysteine for patients with prolonged hypotension as prophylaxis for acute renal failure (NEPHRON). Crit Care Med. 2007;35(2):435–41.

72. Haase M, Haase-Fielitz A, Bagshaw SM, Reade MC, Morgera S, Seevenayagam S, et al. Phase II, randomized, controlled trial of high-dose N-acetylcysteine in high-risk cardiac surgery patients. Crit Care Med. 2007;35(5):1324–31.

73. Hoffmann U, Fischereder M, Kruger B, Drobnik W, Kramer BK. The value of N-acetylcysteine in the prevention of radiocontrast agent-induced nephropathy seems questionable. J Am Soc Nephrol. 2004;15(2):407–10.

74. Poletti PA, Saudan P, Platon A, Mermillod B, Sautter AM, Vermeulen B, et al. I.v. N-acetylcysteine and emergency CT: use of serum creatinine and cystatin C as markers of radiocontrast nephrotoxicity. AJR Am J Roentgenol. 2007;189(3):687–92.

75. Solomon R, Werner C, Mann D, D'Elia J, Silva P. Effects of saline, mannitol, and furosemide to prevent acute decreases in renal function induced by radiocontrast agents. N Engl J Med. 1994;331(21):1416–20.

76. Abassi ZA, Hoffman A, Better OS. Acute renal failure complicating muscle crush injury. Semin Nephrol. 1998;18(5):558–65.

77. Angstwurm MW, Schottdorf J, Schopohl J, Gaertner R. Selenium replacement in patients with severe systemic inflammatory response syndrome improves clinical outcome. Crit Care Med. 1999;27(9):1807–13.

78. Angstwurm MW, Engelmann L, Zimmermann T, Lehmann C, Spes CH, Abel P, et al. Selenium in Intensive Care (SIC): results of a prospective randomized, placebo-controlled, multiple-center study in patients with severe systemic inflammatory response syndrome, sepsis, and septic shock. Crit Care Med. 2007;35(1):118–26.

79. Wijnen MH, Vader HL, Van Den Wall Bake AW, Roumen RM. Can renal dysfunction after infra-renal aortic aneurysm repair be modified by multi-antioxidant supplementation? J Cardiovasc Surg (Torino). 2002;43(4):483–8.

80. Oudemans-van Straaten HM, Spoelstra-de Man AM, de Waard MC. Vitamin C revisited. Crit Care. 2014;18(4):460.

81. Spargias K, Alexopoulos E, Kyrzopoulos S, Iokovis P, Greenwood DC, Manginas A, et al. Ascorbic acid prevents contrast-mediated nephropathy in patients with renal dysfunction undergoing coronary angiography or intervention. Circulation. 2004;110(18):2837–42.

82. Sadat U, Usman A, Gillard JH, Boyle JR. Does ascorbic acid protect against contrast-induced acute kidney injury in patients undergoing coronary angiography: a systematic review with meta-analysis of randomized, controlled trials. J Am Coll Cardiol. 2013;62(23):2167–75.

# Part IV

# Renal Replacement Therapy

Marlies Ostermann, Ron Wald, Ville Pettilä,
and Sean M. Bagshaw


## 12.1 Introduction

Acute kidney injury (AKI) is a common complication among critically ill patients supported in an intensive care unit (ICU) setting [1]. Recent epidemiologic data indicate the incidence of AKI is increasing and may characterize the ICU course in up to two-thirds of patients [2–5]. Among those with more severe AKI or those with complications attributable to AKI, renal replacement therapy (RRT) is commonly initiated [6, 7].

The decision to initiate RRT is often multi-factorial; however, it clearly results in an escalation in both the complexity and costs of care [8, 9] Epidemiologic data would imply that these critically ill patients are at increased risk of substantial morbidity, including non-recovery of kidney function, long-term dialysis dependence [10], and excess mortality; with case-fatality rates approaching 60 % [4, 6, 7, 11].


M. Ostermann, MD, PhD
Department of Critical Care and Nephrology,
Guy's and St Thomas Hospital, London SE1 9RT, UK

R. Wald, MD
Division of Nephrology, St. Michael's Hospital,
30 Bond Street, Toronto, ON M5B 1 W8, Canada

V. Pettilä, MD, PhD
Intensive Care Units, Division of Anaesthesia and Intensive Care Medicine,
Department of Surgery, Helsinki University Central Hospital,
Box 340, Haartmaninkatu 4, 00290 Helsinki, Finland

S.M. Bagshaw, MD, MSc, FRCPC (✉)
Division of Critical Care Medicine, Faculty of Medicine and Dentistry,
University of Alberta, 2-124E, Clinical Sciences Building,
8440-112 ST NW, EdmontON AB T6G 2B7, Canada
e-mail: bagshaw@ualberta.ca



© Springer International Publishing 2015
H.M. Oudemans-van Straaten et al. (eds.), *Acute Nephrology for the Critical Care Physician*, DOI 10.1007/978-3-319-17389-4_12

**Table 12.1** Benefits and drawbacks of earlier RRT in critically ill patients with AKI

| Benefits | Drawbacks |
| --- | --- |
| Earlier control of electrolyte/metabolic derangement | Iatrogenic episodes of hemodynamic instability that may impede kidney repair and recovery |
| Earlier control of acid–base derangement | Insertion of dialysis catheter and risk of catheter-associated complication (i.e., bleeding, thrombosis, bloodstream infection, and pneumothorax) |
| Avoidance and earlier control of complications of uremia | Uncertain clearance of micronutrients, trace elements and sub-therapeutic levels of vital medications (i.e., antimicrobials, anti-epileptics) |
| Earlier management of fluid status and avoidance of excessive fluid accumulation and overload | Unnecessary exposure to RRT in those who will spontaneously recover kidney function with conservative management |
| Avoidance of unnecessary diuretic exposure | Need for immobilization |
| Potentially beneficial immunomodulation | Use of health resources and increased health care costs |

RRT may be considered as one of the core life sustaining technologies used to support patients with critical illness, multiple organ dysfunction and AKI [12]. In general, the main goals of RRT are to: (1) achieve and maintain fluid and electrolyte, acid–base, and uremic solute homeostasis; and (2) facilitate additional supportive measures (i.e., enable the delivery of antimicrobials or other vital medications, nutritional support, and blood transfusions without limitation or complications as indicated). In addition, RRT in critical illness should also serve: (3) to prevent additional or worsening non-renal organ dysfunction that may have been contributed to by AKI; (4) to help avoid further insults to the kidney; and importantly; (5) to facilitate renal recovery; and (6) to improve patient outcome [1].

The optimal time to initiate RRT in critically ill patients with AKI remains uncertain, which unfortunately results in practice variation for the prescription and delivery of acute RRT in this population [13]. Life-threatening complications of AKI such as cardiac toxicity attributable to hyperkalemia, profound acidemia, and fluid overload precipitating pulmonary edema can be readily corrected with RRT [12]. In these situations, the need to initiate RRT is unequivocal. However, for patients who have severe AKI in the absence of overt or impending life-threatening complications, the optimal time for starting RRT is unknown [14, 15].

Earlier initiation of RRT in critically ill patients with AKI, in the absence of overt life-threatening complications, will theoretically lead to better electrolyte, acid–base, and uremic homeostasis, better control of extracellular volume accumulation, and potentially modulate systemic inflammation (Table 12.1). Similarly, earlier RRT may prevent the development of life-threatening complications such as hyperkalemia or pulmonary edema. Accordingly, earlier RRT would appear at face value to confer a variety of benefits and is supported by data from observational studies [16–18].

On the other hand, there is no robust high quality evidence to support the practice that earlier initiation of RRT, in the absence of a life-threatening complication of AKI, impacts important patient centered outcomes such as renal recovery or survival. These perceived benefits of RRT have to naturally be balanced with the potential harm attributable to RRT, including risks associated with iatrogenic episodes of hemodynamic instability, central venous insertion of a dialysis catheter, exposure of blood to an extracorporeal circuit, need for anticoagulation of the extracorporeal circuit, uncertain medication clearance (i.e., antimicrobials) and unwanted depletion of micronutrients. In addition, there is a possibility that with a more conservative strategy of supportive management and watchful waiting, and initiation of RRT only when a life-threatening complication develops, some patients with severe AKI may indeed recover kidney function spontaneously [19]. As a result, early RRT in some patients may unnecessarily expose patients to the risks of RRT and result in less favorable outcomes, unnecessary bedside resources and incremental costs [20].

## 12.2 Triggers for Starting RRT

When considering whether to initiate RRT, most clinicians make this decision based on the following clinical, physiologic and laboratory factors and their trajectories: serum creatinine, and urea including the presence of uremic complications, serum potassium, acid–base status, urine output, fluid balance, overall course and prognosis of the patient's illness, and the patient's preferences for escalation of life-sustaining therapy with RRT [21]. Among these triggers, some are considered absolute indications to avert potentially life threatening complications and others are considered more relative (Table 12.2). Recently, the issue of fluid balance,

**Table 12.2** Summary of absolute and relative indications for starting RRT in critically ill patients with AKI

| Absolute indications | In the absence of contraindications or limitations of organ support, indications for urgent/emergency RRT include: |
| --- | --- |
| | Refractory, rapidly rising, or cardiac toxicity associated hyperkalemia (K > 6.5 mmol/L) |
| | Refractory metabolic acidosis (pH ≤7.2 despite normal or low arterial $pCO_2$) |
| | Refractory pulmonary or non-renal organ edema unresponsive to diuretic therapy |
| | Symptoms or complications attributable to uremia (i.e., pericarditis, enccphalopathy, and coagulopathy) |
| | Overdose/toxicity from a dialyzable drug/toxin |
| Relative indications | In the absence of life threatening complications of AKI, important factors that might influence the decision to start RRT include: |
| | Limited physiological reserve to tolerate the consequences of AKI (i.e., pre-morbid advanced CKD) |
| | Advanced non-renal organ dysfunction intolerant to excessive fluid accumulation (i.e., impaired cardiac function) |
| | Anticipated solute burden (i.e., tumor lysis syndrome; rhabdomyolysis; and intravascular hemolysis) |
| | Need for large fluid administration (i.e., nutritional support, medications, or blood products) |
| | Severity of the underlying disease (affecting the likelihood of recovery of kidney function) |
| | Concomitant accumulation of poisons or toxic drugs which can be removed by RRT (i.e., salicylates, ethylene glycol, methanol, and metformin) |

accumulation and/or overload has received focused attention as a potential modifiable factor associated with outcome and has emerged as a determinant for considering RRT [22–24]. To know whether there is a role for the application of routine RRT primarily for immunomodulation to remove inflammatory mediators such as in sepsis is the focus of ongoing investigations [25].

## 12.3   Literature Review

The optimal timing for RRT remains unclear [26, 27]. Very few randomized clinical trials and numerous observational studies of variable methodological rigor have evaluated the issue of timing of RRT initiation in critically ill patients with AKI [16–18]. These studies vary widely in their criteria for defining "early" and "late" RRT, often using arbitrary cut-offs for serum creatinine, serum urea or urine output, fluid balance, time from ICU admission or duration of AKI. This has created challenges for making clear inferences to inform clinical practice.

In a pilot trial, Bouman et al randomized 106 critically ill predominantly cardiac surgical patients with oliguric AKI despite fluid resuscitation, inotropic support and diuretic therapy, to a strategy of early versus late initiation of RRT [28]. The early group started RRT within 12 h of fulfilling eligibility, defined by oliguria (<30 ml/h for 6 h and no response to a diuretic challenge or hemodynamic optimization), or a creatinine clearance <20 ml/min. The late group started RRT when classic indications were fulfilled including a serum urea >40 mmol/L, potassium of >6.5 mmol/L or evidence of pulmonary edema. In this study, there were no differences in survival, recovery of kidney function or health resource utilization beyond RRT. However, this trial was not adequately designed to assess these outcomes; was not viewed as widely generalizable due to an unexpectedly high observed survival and a large number of patients who had cardiac surgery-associated AKI. Notably, six patients allocated to the late group did not start RRT (four due to renal recovery; and two due to death) and of those who started RRT, 50 % had developed fluid overload and pulmonary edema. In a small single-centre trial from India, 208 hospitalized patients with community-acquired AKI were randomized to either (1) early RRT, characterized by starting RRT after serum urea exceeded 23 mmol/L or serum creatinine exceeded 618 μmol/L irrespective of other AKI complications, or (2) standard of care where RRT was only initiated in the setting of medically-refractory hyperkalemia, acidosis or volume overload or in the setting of uremic symptoms [29]. In this study, there were no observed differences in mortality or recovery of kidney function. This trial also has limited generalizability due to the young demographics of enrolled patients (mean age 42 years), the predominant aetiology of AKI (>50 % tropical infections or obstetric complications), and due to most patients not being critically ill.

Several single-centre controlled trials in cardiac surgery patients have suggested that earlier RRT, most often defined as initiation within 8 h of surgery, can reduce morbidity, improve survival and reduce overall post-operative resource use [30–35]. The concluding inference from these small non-randomized trials is that early initiation of RRT for patients with AKI following cardiac surgery should be triggered by a worsening oliguria rather than actual serum creatinine results.

Several observational studies have also evaluated the optimal timing of RRT for critically ill patients with AKI, as summarized in recent systematic reviews [16–18]. While these studies have numerous methodological limitations, low quality, and high risk of bias, the majority have suggested that "earlier" initiation of RRT was associated with improved outcomes [36–41].

In a secondary analysis of the multinational Beginning and Ending Supportive Therapy (BEST) for the Kidney cohort study, the timing of initiation of RRT was evaluated in 1,238 critically ill patients with AKI [42]. Late RRT, defined relative to time from ICU admission ($\geq$5 days) was associated with higher adjusted-mortality (OR, 1.95; 95 % CI, 1.30–2.92; $p=0.001$). Furthermore, the duration of RRT and hospitalization, and the rate of RRT dependence at hospital discharge, were greater when the interval from ICU admission to RRT initiation was prolonged. Other studies have shown similar results [20, 36]. In a multi-centre prospective Canadian study, the characteristics of critically ill patients with AKI at the time RRT was initiated, were evaluated [43]. At RRT initiation, serum creatinine and urea were 331 (225–446) μmol/L and 22.9 (13.9–32.9) mmol/L, respectively. Oligo-anuria (<400 mL/24 h) was present in 32.9 %, and 92.2 % had a positive fluid balance. Notably, only 16.2 % had hyperkalemia (serum potassium $\geq$5.5 mmol/L) and 33.8 % had metabolic acidosis (serum bicarbonate $\leq$15 mmol/L) at RRT initiation. These data highlight that the decision to initiate RRT was often influenced by numerous patient-specific factors and that the majority (>80 %) had two or more recognized triggers; however, this study also found that the occurrence of life threatening urgent indications for RRT initiation was relatively infrequent in the ICU. In a secondary analysis of 239 critically ill patients with severe AKI treated with RRT in the FINNAKI study, the impact of the presence of classic indications for RRT on 90-day all-cause mortality were evaluated [44]. The primary exposure was the timing of starting RRT relative to evidence of developing one or more "conventional" indications for RRT which included hyperkalemia, severe acidemia, uremia, oligo-anuria and severe fluid overload with pulmonary edema. Timing was classified as "pre-emptive" if RRT was started in the absence of these criteria; "classic – urgent" if started within 12 h of developing one of these indications; and "classic – delayed" when started more than 12 h after developing one of these indications. In multivariable and propensity-adjusted analyses, pre-emptive RRT was associated with lower 90-day mortality compared with RRT after a classic indication developed (30 % vs. 49 %; odds ratio [OR] 2.1; 95 % CI 1.0–4.1). Ninety-day mortality was also markedly lower among patients having "classic – urgent" RRT compared with when RRT was delayed (39 % vs. 68 %; OR 3.9; 95 % CI 1.5–10.2). Moreover, mortality among patients with pre-emptive RRT was found lower compared to those with AKI not treated with RRT in an adjusted propensity-matched analysis.

## 12.4  Current Clinical Practice Guideline Recommendations

Since 2012, the *Kidney Disease Improving Global Outcomes* (KDIGO) consortium and the *National Institute for Health and Care Excellence* (NICE) in the United Kingdom have published official recommendations related to the timing of RRT [26, 27].

The KDIGO Clinical Practice Guideline (CPG) for AKI acknowledged that both the ideal indication and the optimal timing for initiation of RRT in patients with AKI were uncertain, [26] and accordingly, by consensus, KDIGO provided the following recommendations:

(i) *Initiate RRT emergently when life-threatening changes in fluid, electrolyte, and acid–base balance exist* (Sect. 5.1.1 – *Not Graded*).

(ii) *Consider the broader clinical context, the presence of conditions that can be modified with RRT, and trends of laboratory tests—rather than single BUN and creatinine thresholds alone—when making the decision to start RRT* (Sect. 5.1.2 – *Not Graded*)

The KDIGO CPG clearly recognizes that there is a paucity of a strong evidence base for these recommendations and suggests that clinicians assess not only the presence of life-threatening complications when considering RRT, but also the wider clinical status of the patient, including the underlying trajectory of illness severity, burden of non-renal organ dysfunction and the expectation of whether complications attributable to AKI will arise.

Similarly, the NICE CPG for AKI, based on the findings from two randomized trials and three prospective observational studies, made the following recommendations pertaining to initiation of RRT [27]:

(i) *Discuss any potential indications for renal replacement therapy with a nephrologist, pediatric nephrologist and/or critical care specialist immediately to ensure that the therapy is started as soon as needed.*

(ii) *Refer adults, children and young people immediately for RRT if any of the following are not responding to medical management:*
- *Hyperkalemia*
- *Metabolic acidosis*
- *Complications of uremia (i.e., pericarditis or encephalopathy)*
- *Fluid overload*
- *Pulmonary edema*

(iii) *Base the decision to start RRT on the condition of the adult, child or young person as a whole and not on an isolated urea, creatinine or potassium value.*

The NICE recommendations also highlight the lack of evidence to support when to optimally start RRT. Moreover, NICE emphasizes that better tools are needed to identify those patients with AKI who are less likely to recover renal function with a conservative strategy alone and need a period of renal support, and patients in whom

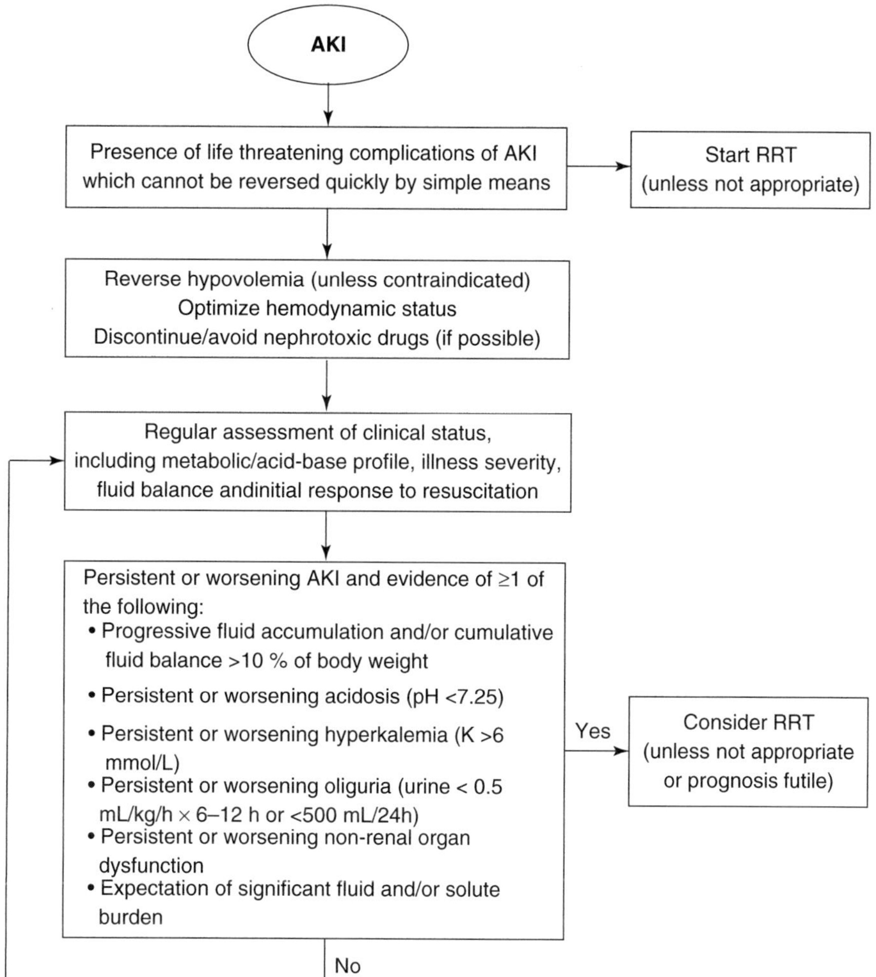



**Fig. 12.1** Proposed algorithm to aid in clinical decision making on when to initiate RRT in critically ill patients with AKI [21]

RRT can be safely avoided. It is possible that some of the newly discovered biomarkers for AKI will fulfil this role. Figure 12.1 gives some guidance for clinical management and decision making at the bedside [21].

## 12.5 Discontinuation of RRT in the ICU

There is a relative paucity of data about the optimal circumstance and time to wean and/or discontinue RRT in critically ill patients with AKI [45, 46]. In the BEST Kidney study, an increase in urine output was the most important determinant of recovery of kidney function and likelihood of successful weaning from RRT [45]. Those patients with a spontaneous urine output >400–450 mL/day without diuretics or >2,300 mL/day with exposure to diuretics had a >80 % probability of sustained weaning from RRT. In a similar retrospective study of 304 post-operative patients with severe AKI treated with RRT from the National Taiwan University Surgical, I. C. U. Acute Renal Failure Study Group, predictors of successful weaning from RRT were higher (and increasing) urine output on the day following cessation of RRT along with a shorter cumulative duration of renal support, younger age and lower non-renal organ dysfunction [46]. Accordingly, apart from increasing spontaneous urine output, there are few reliable clinical signs or tests to predict recovery sufficient to successfully wean RRT.

## 12.6 Future Clinical Trials

In addition to the limited high quality evidence on optimal timing of RRT for critically ill patients with AKI, there are a number of ongoing or recently completed randomized controlled trials (RCTs) addressing this issue. In Canada, the STARRT-AKI trial, a multi-centre pilot RCT has recently been completed [47].This trial enrolled critically ill patients with severe AKI to a strategy of early RRT (within 12 h of eligibility) or standard initiation of RRT (based on persistent AKI and/or development of more classic indications).The ongoing IDEAL-ICU trial is a multi-centre RCT in France with a target enrolment of 824 patients that seeks to randomize critically ill patients with septic shock and severe AKI (defined as a three-fold rise in serum creatinine and urine output <0.3 mL/kg/h for 12 h) [48]. The early strategy calls for starting RRT within 12 h of fulfilling AKI criteria whereas in the late arm RRT commences 48–60 h thereafter. Finally, the AKIKI trial, another multi-centre RCT in France, proposes to enrol 620 critically ill patients with AKI randomized to early RRT immediately upon fulfilling Risk-Injury-Failure-End-stage-Loss (RIFLE) category FAILURE or a conservative strategy whereby RRT is started only after fulfilling RIFLE FAILURE criteria and an additional classical indication for RRT [49]. The findings from these trials are eagerly awaited and should help to better inform practice on when to optimally initiate RRT and reduce unnecessary variation in practice.

## 12.7 Conclusions: Decision Making on Starting RRT at the Bedside

The accumulated evidence from clinical studies to date would imply that the optimal timing of starting RRT for critically ill patients with AKI is uncertain and that the decision should largely be individualized and informed by best practice whenever possible. Evidence from high quality RCTs addressing this issue are anticipated and will hopefully help to inform best clinical practice, reduce unnecessary variation in how RRT is prescribed, and provide critical data to update clinical practice guidelines. In the absence of life threatening complications of AKI, the patient's current and evolving illness severity, burden of non-renal organ dysfunction, fluid balance, and physiological reserve to the consequences of AKI and response to medical treatment should all be considered and continuously reassessed when deciding whether RRT should be initiated. These factors should naturally be weighted in the context of the perceived risks associated with starting RRT along with the patient's stated preferences for life-sustaining therapy.

## References


1. Bellomo R, Kellum JA, Ronco C. Acute kidney injury. Lancet. 2012;380:756–66.
2. Bagshaw SM, George C, Bellomo R. Changes in the incidence and outcome for early acute kidney injury in a cohort of Australian intensive care units. Crit Care. 2007;11:R68.
3. Hsu RK, McCulloch CE, Dudley RA, Lo LJ, Hsu CY. Temporal changes in incidence of dialysis-requiring AKI. J Am Soc Nephrol. 2013;24:37–42.
4. Vaara ST, Pettila V, Reinikainen M, Kaukonen KM. Population-based incidence, mortality and quality of life in critically ill patients treated with renal replacement therapy: a nationwide retrospective cohort study in Finnish intensive care units. Crit Care. 2012;16:R13.
5. Hoste EA, Clermont G, Kersten A, et al. RIFLE criteria for acute kidney injury are associated with hospital mortality in critically ill patients: a cohort analysis. Crit Care. 2006;10:R73.
6. Nisula S, Kaukonen KM, Vaara ST, et al. Incidence, risk factors and 90-day mortality of patients with acute kidney injury in Finnish intensive care units: the FINNAKI study. Intensive Care Med. 2013;39:420–8.
7. Uchino S, Kellum JA, Bellomo R, et al. Acute renal failure in critically ill patients: a multinational, multicenter study. JAMA. 2005;294:813–8.
8. Hamel MB, Phillips RS, Davis RB, et al. Outcomes and cost-effectiveness of initiating dialysis and continuing aggressive care in seriously ill hospitalized adults. SUPPORT Investigators. Study to Understand Prognoses and Preferences for Outcomes and Risks of Treatments. Ann Intern Med. 1997;127:195–202.
9. Korkeila M, Ruokonen E, Takala J. Costs of care, long-term prognosis and quality of life in patients requiring renal replacement therapy during intensive care. Intensive Care Med. 2000;26:1824–31.
10. Wald R, Quinn RR, Luo J, et al. Chronic dialysis and death among survivors of acute kidney injury requiring dialysis. JAMA. 2009;302:1179–85.
11. Bagshaw SM, Laupland KB, Doig CJ, et al. Prognosis for long-term survival and renal recovery in critically ill patients with severe acute renal failure: a population-based study. Crit Care. 2005;9:R700–9.
12. Joannidis M, Forni LG. Clinical review: timing of renal replacement therapy. Crit Care. 2011;15:223.
13. Ricci Z, Ronco C, D'Amico G, et al. Practice patterns in the management of acute renal failure in the critically ill patient: an international survey. Nephrol Dial Transplant. 2006;21:690–6.
14. Bagshaw SM, Uchino S, Kellum J, et al. Association between renal replacement therapy in critically ill patients with severe acute kidney injury and mortality. J Crit Care. 2013;28(6):1011–8.
15. Clec'h C, Gonzalez F, Lautrette A, et al. Multiple-center evaluation of mortality associated with acute kidney injury in critically ill patients: a competing risks analysis. Crit Care. 2011;15:R128.
16. Karvellas CJ, Farhat MR, Sajjad I, et al. A comparison of early versus late initiation of renal replacement therapy in critically ill patients with acute kidney injury: a systematic review and meta-analysis. Crit Care. 2011;15:R72.

17. Seabra VF, Balk EM, Liangos O, Sosa MA, Cendoroglo M, Jaber BL. Timing of renal replacement therapy initiation in acute renal failure: a meta-analysis. Am J Kidney Dis. 2008;52:272–84.
18. Wang X, Jie Yuan W. Timing of initiation of renal replacement therapy in acute kidney injury: a systematic review and meta-analysis. Ren Fail. 2012;34:396–402.
19. Clark EG, Bagshaw SM. Unnecessary renal replacement therapy for acute kidney injury is harmful for renal recovery. Semin Dial. 2015;28(1):6–11.
20. Shiao CC, Ko WJ, Wu VC, et al. U-curve association between timing of renal replacement therapy initiation and in-hospital mortality in postoperative acute kidney injury. PLoS One. 2012;7, e42952.
21. Ostermann M, Dickie H, Barrett NA. Renal replacement therapy in critically ill patients with acute kidney injury–when to start. Nephrol Dial Transplant. 2012;27(6):2242–8.
22. Bouchard J, Soroko SB, Chertow GM, et al. Fluid accumulation, survival and recovery of kidney function in critically ill patients with acute kidney injury. Kidney Int. 2009;76:422–7.
23. Prowle JR, Echeverri JE, Ligabo EV, Ronco C, Bellomo R. Fluid balance and acute kidney injury. Nat Rev Nephrol. 2010;6:107–15.
24. Sutherland SM, Zappitelli M, Alexander SR, et al. Fluid overload and mortality in children receiving continuous renal replacement therapy: the prospective pediatric continuous renal replacement therapy registry. Am J Kidney Dis. 2010;55(2):316–25.
25. Rimmele T, Kellum JA. Clinical review: blood purification for sepsis. Crit Care. 2011;15:205.
26. Kidney Disease: Improving Global Outcomes (KDIGO) Acute Kidney Injury Work Group. KDIGO clinical practice guideline for acute kidney injury. Kidney Int. 2012;2012:1–138.
27. National Institute for Health and Care Excellence Acute Kidney Injury Workgroup. Acute kidney injury: prevention, detection and management of acute kidney injury up to the point of renal replacement therapy. Clinical guidelines, CG169. (http://guidance.nice.org.uk/CG169).
28. Bouman CS, Oudemans-Van Straaten HM, Tijssen JG, Zandstra DF, Kesecioglu J. Effects of early high-volume continuous venovenous hemofiltration on survival and recovery of renal function in intensive care patients with acute renal failure: a prospective, randomized trial. Crit Care Med. 2002;30:2205–11.
29. Jamale TE, Hase NK, Kulkarni M, et al. Earlier-start versus usual-start dialysis in patients with community-acquired acute kidney injury: a randomized controlled trial. Am J Kidney Dis. 2013;62:1116–21.
30. Demirkilic U, Kuralay E, Yenicesu M, et al. Timing of replacement therapy for acute renal failure after cardiac surgery. J Card Surg. 2004;19:17–20.
31. Durmaz I, Yagdi T, Calkavur T, et al. Prophylactic dialysis in patients with renal dysfunction undergoing on-pump coronary artery bypass surgery. Ann Thorac Surg. 2003;75:859–64.
32. Elahi MM, Lim MY, Joseph RN, Dhannapuneni RR, Spyt TJ. Early hemofiltration improves survival in post-cardiotomy patients with acute renal failure. Eur J Cardiothorac Surg. 2004;26(5):1027–31.
33. Manche A, Casha A, Rychter J, Farrugia E, Debono M. Early dialysis in acute kidney injury after cardiac surgery. Interact Cardiovasc Thorac Surg. 2008;7:829–32.
34. Sugahara S, Suzuki H. Early start on continuous hemodialysis therapy improves survival rate in patients with acute renal failure following coronary bypass surgery. Hemodial Int. 2004;8: 320–5.
35. Iyem H, Tavli M, Akcicek F, Buket S. Importance of early dialysis for acute renal failure after an open-heart surgery. Hemodial Int. 2009;13:55–61.
36. Andrade L, Cleto S, Seguro AC. Door-to-dialysis time and daily hemodialysis in patients with leptospirosis: impact on mortality. Clin J Am Soc Nephrol. 2007;2:739–44.
37. Gettings LG, Reynolds HN, Scalea T. Outcome in post-traumatic acute renal failure when continuous renal replacement therapy is applied early vs. late. Intensive Care Med. 1999;25: 805–13.
38. Shiao CC, Wu VC, Li WY, et al. Late initiation of renal replacement therapy is associated with worse outcomes in acute kidney injury after major abdominal surgery. Crit Care. 2009;13: R171.

39. Wu VC, Ko WJ, Chang HW, et al. Early renal replacement therapy in patients with postoperative acute liver failure associated with acute renal failure: effect on postoperative outcomes. J Am Coll Surg. 2007;205:266–76.
40. Carl DE, Grossman C, Behnke M, Sessler CN, Gehr TW. Effect of timing of dialysis on mortality in critically ill, septic patients with acute renal failure. Hemodial Int. 2010;14:11–7.
41. Liu KD, Himmelfarb J, Paganini E, et al. Timing of initiation of dialysis in critically ill patients with acute kidney injury. Clin J Am Soc Nephrol. 2006;1:915–9.
42. Bagshaw SM, Uchino S, Bellomo R, et al. Timing of renal replacement therapy and clinical outcomes in critically ill patients with severe acute kidney injury. J Crit Care. 2009;24:129–40.
43. Bagshaw SM, Wald R, Barton J, et al. Clinical factors associated with initiation of renal replacement therapy in critically ill patients with acute kidney injury-a prospective multicenter observational study. J Crit Care. 2012;27:268–75.
44. Vaara ST, Reinikainen M, Wald R, Bagshaw SM, Pettila V, for the FINNAKI Study Group FS. Timing of RRT based on the presence of conventional indications. Clin J Am Soc Nephrol. 2014;9:1577–85.
45. Uchino S, Bellomo R, Morimatsu H, et al. Discontinuation of continuous renal replacement therapy: a post hoc analysis of a prospective multicenter observational study. Crit Care Med. 2009;37:2576–82.
46. Wu VC, Ko WJ, Chang HW, et al. Risk factors of early redialysis after weaning from postoperative acute renal replacement therapy. Intensive Care Med. 2008;34:101–8.
47. Smith OM, Wald R, Adhikari NK, et al. Standard versus accelerated initiation of renal replacement therapy in acute kidney injury (STARRT-AKI): study protocol for a randomized controlled trial. Trials. 2013;14:320.
48. Initiation of Dialysis Early Versus Late in Intensive Care Unit. ClinicalTrials.gov, 2013. Accessed 20 Dec 2014, at https://clinicaltrials.gov/ct2/show/NCT01682590.
49. Artificial Kidney Initiation in Kidney Injury, a Multicenter Randomised Trial. ClinicalTrials.gov, 2013. Accessed 20 Dec 2014, at https://clinicaltrials.gov/ct2/show/NCT01932190.

# Dose of Renal Replacement Therapy in AKI

**13**


Catherine S.C. Bouman, Marlies Ostermann,
Michael Joannidis, and Olivier Joannes-Boyau


## 13.1 Introduction

The intention to initiate renal replacement therapy (RRT) in patients with acute kidney injury (AKI) requires a prescription, outlining mode, target dose, type of anticoagulation, target fluid balance and measures of adequacy, similar to RRT in patients with end-stage renal disease (ESRD). However, acute RRT is often not formally prescribed, and effective delivery is not always measured [1]. One potential reason for this omission is lack of consensus on the best way of measuring intensity of RRT and conflicting data related to the optimal dose. In the chronic setting, Kt/V and/or urea reduction ratio (URR) are routinely used to measure adequacy of dialysis but these parameters are not appropriate in the acute setting and alternative methods are needed.

This chapter will provide guidance on how to prescribe RRT dose and monitor its efficacy in critically ill patients with AKI.


C.S.C. Bouman, MD, PhD (✉)
Department of Intensive Care, Academic Medical Center,
University of Amsterdam, PO Box 22660, 1100 DD Amsterdam, The Netherlands
e-mail: c.s.bouman@amc.uva.nl

M. Ostermann, MD, PhD
Department of Critical Care, King's College London,
Guy's and St Thomas' Foundation Trust, London SE1 7EH, UK
e-mail: Marlies.Ostermann@gstt.nhs.uk

M. Joannidis, MD, PhD
Division of Intensive Care and Emergency Medicine, Department of Internal Medicine,
Medical University Innsbruck, Innsbruck A-6020, Austria
e-mail: michael.joannidis@i-med.ac.at

O. Joannes-Boyau, MD
Service d'Anesthésie-Réanimation, Centre Hospitalier
Universitaire (CHU) de Bordeaux, Bordeaux 33000, France
e-mail: olivier.joannes-boyau@chu-bordeaux.fr



© Springer International Publishing 2015
H.M. Oudemans-van Straaten et al. (eds.), *Acute Nephrology for the Critical Care Physician*, DOI 10.1007/978-3-319-17389-4_13

## 13.2    Prescription of Dose of RRT

The dose of RRT is a measure of the quantity of a solute that is removed from the patient during extracorporeal treatment and is reasonably representative of other solutes which require removal [1, 2]. In patients on chronic hemodialysis, dose of treatment is expressed as URR or Kt/V ($K$ = dialyzer clearance of urea, $t$ = dialysis time and $V$ = volume of distribution of urea). Both parameters have important limitations in critically ill patients with AKI where neither urea generation rate nor volume of distribution can be clearly defined. In patients receiving continuous renal replacement therapy (CRRT), clearance of small uncharged molecules such as urea and creatinine is essentially equal to the delivered effluent rate. Therefore, the effluent rate roughly corresponds to the prescribed replacement or dialysis rate and is often used as a surrogate of urea clearance. Following the landmark study by Ronco et al. in 2000, it was suggested to index the flow rate to the patient's body weight [3]. As a result, the dose of CRRT is often expressed as the amount of dialysis/hemofiltration flow delivered to the patient in ml/kg per hour. Whether to use actual body weight or ideal body weight is unclear [3–8].

Degree of 'pre-dilution' and 'filter-down' time are important factors which reduce the effective dose. They need to be taken into account when prescribing and reviewing the dose of RRT. Infusion of replacement solution as pre-dilution will reduce effective effluent dose by the degree to which the plasma is diluted. The final dilution effect is dependent on circuit blood flow, replacement fluid rate, and haematocrit. Furthermore, discrepancies between prescribed doses and measured creatinine clearance increase with higher doses over time as demonstrated for predilution continuous veno-venous hemodiafiltration (CVVHD) [9]. Premature circuit clotting or need for investigations outside the ICU are common reasons for unintended interruptions in treatment which can lead to reduced clearance [10]. It is therefore necessary to review regularly whether the delivered dose of RRT matches the prescribed target and to adjust the prescription if necessary.

Of note, effluent rate only represents clearance of small solutes but not larger molecules or molecules with high protein binding. In addition, there are many other important aspects of RRT which need to be considered when prescribing a dose, like acid–base homeostasis, nutritional support and, perhaps most importantly, fluid balance.

## 13.3    Dose Intensity of RRT in AKI and Outcome

Since 2000, there have been eight randomized controlled trials (RCTs) on intensity of RRT in AKI [3–8, 11, 12]. Two studies evaluated RRT doses in patients receiving intermittent haemodialysis (IHD) [11, 12], five studies in patients on CRRT [3–5, 7, 8] and one study enrolled patients on IHD, slow extended dialysis (SLED) and CRRT [6]. Two single center studies showed better outcomes with increased intensity of small solute clearance [3, 7]. In contrast, the two largest multi-center RCTs, the ATN study ($n = 1,124$) and the RENAL study ($n = 1,464$), showed no benefit in survival or recovery of renal function with higher doses of RRT [4, 6]. A subsequent meta-analysis of all eight RCTs concluded that higher intensity RRT did not reduce mortality rates or improve renal recovery in patients with AKI [13]. Current international guidelines recommend delivering an effluent volume of 20–25 ml/kg/h for post dilution CRRT in AKI [14, 15]. Increasing the dose beyond 20–25 ml/kg/h has not been shown to be beneficial and may potentially result in losses of important solutes including phosphate and antibiotics, and heat. In patients receiving CRRT in pre-dilution mode, the target dose should be increased to 25–30 ml/kg/h in order to achieve a delivered dose of 20–25 ml/kg/h. For patients receiving intermittent RRT for AKI, international recommendations differ. While the guideline by the Kidney Disease Improving Global Outcome (KDIGO) expert group recommends a target Kt/V of 3.9 per week for intermittent or extended acute RRT [15], the European Renal Best Practice (ERBP) guideline recommends not to use Kt/V as a marker of adequacy and to adapt the duration of IHD to metabolic and volume status [14].

It is important to acknowledge that in the RCTs mentioned earlier, the RRT dose was not adjusted for severity of disease or degree of catabolism. Instead, patients were treated with a fixed dose indexed to the patient's body weight. Finally, the above mentioned RCTs evaluated different doses of RRT but did not study possible pleiotropic effects of RRT in patients with sepsis or the effect of fluid balance on outcome.

## 13.4   Fluid Overload and RRT

There is increasing evidence that fluid overload is detrimental to both renal outcome and survival in critically ill patients with AKI, including patients treated with RRT [16, 17]. In a retrospective analysis of the RENAL study the authors found that a negative daily fluid balance during the treatment period was independently associated with a shorter ICU and hospital stay and lower 90 day mortality [18]. The multicenter observational FINNAKI study demonstrated an association between fluid overload at RRT initiation and increased 90-day mortality, which remained significant after adjustment for common risk factors [18, 19].

The relationship between fluid accumulation, AKI and outcome is complex. Fluid overload may be a marker of the severity of AKI but may also be causing harm as a result of interstitial edema, visceromegaly and secondary organ dysfunction. Based on existing data, it would be advisable to target a negative fluid balance in patients on RRT, as soon as the patient is adequately resuscitated and hemodynamic status allows.

It is not possible to recommend a general net ultrafiltration rate. Instead, the ultrafiltration rate should be tailored to the patients' needs and haemodynamic and fluid status.

## 13.5  High-Volume Hemofiltration in Septic Shock

It is rather inopportune that studies in the literature have defined high-volume hemofiltration (HV-HF) by ultrafiltrate rates of 35–200 ml/kg/h. In RCTs in animals HV-HF was only beneficial when using very high ultrafiltrate rates (>100 mL/kg/h) and initiating hemofiltration early (i.e., before or very early after the septic challenge) [20, 21]. The number of RCTs in humans is limited and their size is small [22–26]. Important differences among animal and human studies include the later initiation of HV-HF, the lower ultrafiltrate rates and the use of antibiotics in humans [20]. The two largest recent RCTs were negative: a Chinese study in 280 patients comparing high volume (50 ml/kg/h) versus very high volume (80 ml/kg/h) [26] and the IVOIRE study in 140 patients comparing 35 ml/kg/h versus 70 ml/kg/h [25]. In a recent systematic review and meta-analysis HV-HF was defined as continuous high-volume treatment with an effluent rate of 50–70 ml/kg/h (for 24 h per day) or intermittent very high volume treatment with an effluent rate of 100–120 ml/kg/h for a 4–8 h period followed by conventional renal dose hemofiltration [27]. Four studies (470 participants) were included and the authors concluded that HVHF, compared with standard renal dose had no significant impact on short-term mortality, kidney recovery, improvement in hemodynamic profile, or reduction in ICU or hospital length-of-stay. Another more extensive systematic review and meta-analysis including 7 RCTs (558 patients) using the same cut-off of 50 ml/kg/h but additionally investigating pulse HV-HF with 85–100 ml/kg/h over 8 h confirmed the lack of effect on relevant endpoints such as renal recovery as well as vasopressor requirements or cytokine clearance [28]. The application of continuous HV-HF hemofiltration or pulse very HV-HF in severe sepsis and septic shock cannot be recommended based on the results of human studies.

## 13.6  Risks of "Too Little" and "Too Much" RRT

Insufficient metabolic clearance correlates with inadequate treatment and should be avoided. However, it is not clear what the lowest acceptable dose of acute RRT is. In the chronic setting, ESRD patients receiving thrice-weekly intermittent haemodialysis with URR <60 % had a higher mortality compared to patients with URR of 65–69 % (odds ratio for mortality 1.28 for URR of 55–59 % and 1.39 for URR <55 %) [29]. Thrice-weekly IHD with an estimated URR <60 % provides azotemic control similar to that of approximately 10–15 mL/kg/h of CRRT. Since it is unlikely that critically ill patients have a lower requirement for RRT in comparison with stable haemodialysis patients, it has been suggested that CRRT doses of <15 ml/kg/h are too low in critically ill patients, especially in the acute phases of illness.

High dose CRRT is associated with higher clearance of urea and creatinine but also increased losses of other substances. Some losses may be obvious (ie phosphate) but others may be hidden and not immediately recognized, for instance trace elements and micronutrients [25]. There is also increasing recognition that high dose CRRT increases drug clearance and may potentially lead to sub-therapeutic drug levels, including antibiotics, resulting in treatment failure [5, 30, 31]. The IVOIRE study clearly demonstrated reduced average elimination half-life of administered antibiotics when using high doses of 70 ml/kg/h [25].

Awareness about the potential dangers of increased clearance is necessary and close drug monitoring is essential when using RRT above the current recommended doses.

**Key Messages**
1. CRRT dose is expressed as the amount of dialysis/hemofiltration flow delivered to the patient in ml/kg per hour.
2. Current international guidelines recommend *delivering* an effluent volume of 20–25 ml/kg per hour for post-dilution CRRT in AKI, taking into account the degree of 'pre-dilution' and 'filter-down' time.
3. CRRT doses of <15 ml/kg per hour are believed to be too low in critically ill patient, especially in the acute phases of illness.
4. Increasing evidence suggests that fluid overload is detrimental to both renal outcome and survival in critically ill patients with AKI. It is not possible to recommend a general net ultrafiltration rate, instead the ultrafiltration rate should be tailored to the patients' needs and hemodynamic and fluid status.
5. The application of high-volume hemofiltration in severe sepsis and septic shock is not recommended based on the results of human studies.
6. Drug clearance, including antibiotics, is affected by (high dose) CRRT and may potentially lead to sub-therapeutic drug levels resulting in treatment failure.

# References


1. Ronco C, Ricci Z, Bellomo R. Current worldwide practice of dialysis dose prescription in acute renal failure. Curr Opin Crit Care. 2006;12(6):551–6.
2. Ricci Z, Ronco C, Bachetoni A, D'amico G, Rossi S, Alessandri E, et al. Solute removal during continuous renal replacement therapy in critically ill patients: convection versus diffusion. Crit Care. 2006;10(2):R67.
3. Ronco C, Bellomo R, Homel P, Brendolan A, Dan M, Piccinni P, et al. Effects of different doses in continuous veno-venous haemofiltration on outcomes of acute renal failure: a prospective randomised trial. Lancet. 2000;356(9223):26–30.
4. Bellomo R, Cass A, Cole L, Finfer S, Gallagher M, Lo S, et al. Intensity of continuous renal-replacement therapy in critically ill patients. N Engl J Med. 2009;361(17):1627–38.
5. Bouman CS, Oudemans-van Straaten HM, Tijssen JG, Zandstra DF, Kesecioglu J. Effects of early high-volume continuous venovenous hemofiltration on survival and recovery of renal function in intensive care patients with acute renal failure: a prospective, randomized trial. Crit Care Med. 2002;30(10):2205–11.
6. Palevsky PM, Zhang JH, O'Connor TZ, Chertow GM, Crowley ST, Choudhury D, et al. Intensity of renal support in critically ill patients with acute kidney injury. N Engl J Med. 2008;359(1):7–20.

7. Saudan P, Niederberger M, De SS, Romand J, Pugin J, Perneger T, et al. Adding a dialysis dose to continuous hemofiltration increases survival in patients with acute renal failure. Kidney Int. 2006;70(7):1312–7.

8. Tolwani AJ, Campbell RC, Stofan BS, Lai KR, Oster RA, Wille KM. Standard versus high-dose CVVHDF for ICU-related acute renal failure. J Am Soc Nephrol. 2008;19(6):1233–8.

9. Lyndon WD, Wille KM, Tolwani AJ. Solute clearance in CRRT: prescribed dose versus actual delivered dose. Nephrol Dial Transplant. 2012;27(3):952–6.

10. Uchino S, Fealy N, Baldwin I, Morimatsu H, Bellomo R. Continuous is not continuous: the incidence and impact of circuit "down-time" on uraemic control during continuous veno-venous haemofiltration. Intensive Care Med. 2003;29(4):575–8.

11. Faulhaber-Walter R, Hafer C, Jahr N, Vahlbruch J, Hoy L, Haller H, et al. The Hannover Dialysis Outcome study: comparison of standard versus intensified extended dialysis for treatment of patients with acute kidney injury in the intensive care unit. Nephrol Dial Transplant. 2009;24(7):2179–86.

12. Schiffl H, Lang SM, Fischer R. Daily hemodialysis and the outcome of acute renal failure. N Engl J Med. 2002;346(5):305–10.

13. Jun M, Heerspink HJ, Ninomiya T, Gallagher M, Bellomo R, Myburgh J, et al. Intensities of renal replacement therapy in acute kidney injury: a systematic review and meta-analysis. Clin J Am Soc Nephrol. 2010;5(6):956–63.

14. Jorres A, John S, Lewington A, ter Wee PM, Vanholder R, Van BW, et al. A European Renal Best Practice (ERBP) position statement on the Kidney Disease Improving Global Outcomes (KDIGO) Clinical Practice Guidelines on Acute Kidney Injury: part 2: renal replacement therapy. Nephrol Dial Transplant. 2013;28(12):2940–5.

15. Khwaja A. KDIGO clinical practice guidelines for acute kidney injury. Nephron Clin Pract. 2012;120(4):179–84.

16. Bouchard J, Soroko SB, Chertow GM, Himmelfarb J, Ikizler TA, Paganini EP, et al. Fluid accumulation, survival and recovery of kidney function in critically ill patients with acute kidney injury. Kidney Int. 2009;76(4):422–7.

17. Payen D, de Pont AC, Sakr Y, Spies C, Reinhart K, Vincent JL. A positive fluid balance is associated with a worse outcome in patients with acute renal failure. Crit Care. 2008;12(3):R74.

18. Bellomo R, Cass A, Cole L, Finfer S, Gallagher M, Lee J, et al. An observational study fluid balance and patient outcomes in the Randomized Evaluation of Normal vs. Augmented Level of Replacement Therapy trial. Crit Care Med. 2012;40(6):1753–60.

19. Vaara ST, Korhonen AM, Kaukonen KM, Nisula S, Inkinen O, Hoppu S, et al. Fluid overload is associated with an increased risk for 90-day mortality in critically ill patients with renal replacement therapy: data from the prospective FINNAKI study. Crit Care. 2012;16(5):R197.

20. Bouman CS, Oudemans-van Straaten HM, Schultz MJ, Vroom MB. Hemofiltration in sepsis and systemic inflammatory response syndrome: the role of dosing and timing. J Crit Care. 2007;22(1):1–12.

21. Grootendorst AF, van Bommel EF, van der Hoven B, van Leengoed LA, van Osta AL. High volume hemofiltration improves right ventricular function in endotoxin-induced shock in the pig. Intensive Care Med. 1992;18(4):235–40.

22. Boussekey N, Chiche A, Faure K, Devos P, Guery B, d'Escrivan T, et al. A pilot randomized study comparing high and low volume hemofiltration on vasopressor use in septic shock. Intensive Care Med. 2008;34(9):1646–53.

23. Cole L, Bellomo R, Journois D, Davenport P, Baldwin I, Tipping P. High-volume haemofiltration in human septic shock. Intensive Care Med. 2001;27(6):978–86.

24. Ghani RA, Zainudin S, Ctkong N, Rahman AF, Wafa SR, Mohamad M, et al. Serum IL-6 and IL-1-ra with sequential organ failure assessment scores in septic patients receiving high-volume haemofiltration and continuous venovenous haemofiltration. Nephrology (Carlton). 2006;11(5):386–93.

25. Joannes-Boyau O, Honore PM, Perez P, Bagshaw SM, Grand H, Canivet JL, et al. High-volume versus standard-volume haemofiltration for septic shock patients with acute kidney injury (IVOIRE study): a multicentre randomized controlled trial. Intensive Care Med. 2013;39(9):1535–46.
26. Zhang P, Yang Y, Lv R, Zhang Y, Xie W, Chen J. Effect of the intensity of continuous renal replacement therapy in patients with sepsis and acute kidney injury: a single-center randomized clinical trial. Nephrol Dial Transplant. 2012;27(3):967–73.
27. Clark E, Molnar AO, Joannes-Boyau O, Honore PM, Sikora L, Bagshaw SM. High-volume hemofiltration for septic acute kidney injury: a systematic review and meta-analysis. Crit Care. 2014;18(1):R7.
28. Lehner G, Wiedermann C, Joannidis M. High volume hemofiltration in critically ill patients – a systematic review and meta-analysis. Minerva Anestesiol. 2014;80(5):595–609.
29. Owen Jr WF, Lew NL, Liu Y, Lowrie EG, Lazarus JM. The urea reduction ratio and serum albumin concentration as predictors of mortality in patients undergoing hemodialysis. N Engl J Med. 1993;329(14):1001–6.
30. Jamal JA, Economou CJ, Lipman J, Roberts JA. Improving antibiotic dosing in special situations in the ICU: burns, renal replacement therapy and extracorporeal membrane oxygenation. Curr Opin Crit Care. 2012;18(5):460–71.
31. Roberts DM, Roberts JA, Roberts MS, Liu X, Nair P, Cole L, et al. Variability of antibiotic concentrations in critically ill patients receiving continuous renal replacement therapy: a multicentre pharmacokinetic study. Crit Care Med. 2012;40(5):1523–8.

# Type of Renal Replacement Therapy

**14**

Michael Joannidis and Lui G. Forni

## 14.1 Principles of Diffusion and Convection

Simplistically, the two predominant techniques employed in terms of renal support for patients with acute kidney injury may be viewed as either diffusion based (dialysis) or convective (filtration) in nature. Hybrids of these techniques are also available and may offer theoretical advantages, but in order to understand any potential benefits of one technique over another, the fundamental processes involved must be understood. Both convection and diffusion are intimately related in that both processes are required for the separation of molecular species and although haemodialysis, for example, is viewed as a diffusive therapy, it also relies on convection. Similarly, techniques such as haemofiltration relies, in part, on diffusion as well as convection [1].

Convection describes the movement of any given molecular species within the medium in which it is embedded. The movement of any given molecule is at a speed identical to that of the components of the medium itself and thus all molecular components consequently move at the same rate (Fig. 14.1a). It follows, therefore, that convection per se is of little use in terms of separation of molecular species. However, convection is an essential process in that it allows transport of molecular species to a boundary where they *can* be separated: this may be via a semipermeable

M. Joannidis
Medical Intensive Care Unit, Department of General Internal Medicine,
Medical University, Innsbruck, Austria

L.G. Forni (✉)
Department of Intensive Care Medicine, Royal Surrey County Hospital NHS
Foundation Trust, Surrey Perioperative Anaesthesia Critical Care Collaborative
Research Group (SPACeR) and Faculty of Health Care Sciences,
University of Surrey, Guildford, UK
e-mail: luiforni@nhs.net

© Springer International Publishing 2015
H.M. Oudemans-van Straaten et al. (eds.), *Acute Nephrology for the Critical Care Physician*, DOI 10.1007/978-3-319-17389-4_14

"""

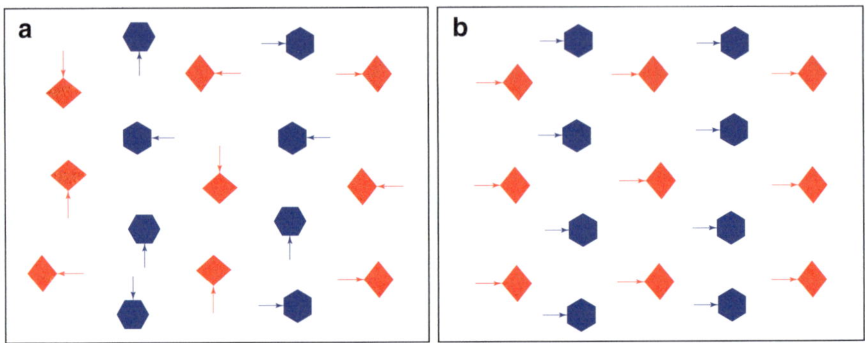

**Fig. 14.1** (**a**) Representation of unhindered ordinary diffusion demonstrating a non-uniform distribution and movement throughout the solvent. (**b**) Representation of convection without diffusion moves all molecular species equally and does not result in separation

membrane, for example. Therefore, without convection, diffusive therapies could not occur efficiently. Convection is often thought of as the process which drives ultrafiltration, the removal of water from a solution. However, water removal in dialysis is actually accomplished through forced diffusion through pressure across a semi-permeable membrane. Where highly permeable membranes are used such as in haemofiltration, the predominant driving force is hydrostatic promoting convection through the filter. Given that convection implies that all molecular components move at the same rate then all molecular components will travel with the water (so-called solvent drag) but molecular separation will also depend on the characteristics of the membrane or filter employed (Fig. 14.1b) [2].

Diffusive therapies rely on several phenomena including ordinary diffusion and forced diffusion. Ordinary (or Fickian) diffusion describes the molecular movement induced by random movements coupled to the non-uniform distribution in space of the species. This is shown in Fig. 14.1b, where eventual uniform distribution of molecular species will be seen within a solution. The rate of this process is defined by the diffusive flux. The flux is defined as the number of molecules that pass through a unit area in a unit time. Clearly the flux is also dependent on any concentration gradient involving the diffusing substance and this process, for any given molecular species *A*, is described by Fick's law [3]:

$$N_A = -D_A \nabla C_A$$

where $\nabla_C$ is the gradient and D is the Fickian diffusivity. Ordinary diffusion effectively scatters molecular species throughout the medium and is dependent on numerous factors including molecular size and properties of the solution. Separation, however, is determined by the introduction of a further element such as a membrane or gel. These will affect diffusion coefficients significantly, allowing molecular separation to occur, which in turn is limited by the available concentration gradients. Forced diffusion describes the application of an external force which acts differently on the molecular species present facilitating separation. Thus in a dialysis machine separation is enhanced not only by the membrane but by concentration gradients (ordinary diffusion) but also by pressure changes through the application of blood pumps (forced diffusion). In practice this results in the passage of a molecular species along a concentration gradient, and this solute transport can be expressed as:

$$Jd = DTA \left( \frac{\partial c}{\partial x} \right)$$

where DTA are the diffusion coefficient (which varies with the cubed root of the molecular weight), temperature and the surface area of the membrane and $\partial c$ is the concentration gradient across the membrane with $\partial d$ being the membrane thickness. This differs from convective based treatments (Fig. 14.2) where clearance of a molecular species is, as indicated, driven by hydrostatic pressures and convection. The hydrostatic pressure driving convection is that pressure generated across the membrane (TMP). This transmembrane pressure is defined as:

$$TMP = Pb - Pd - \pi$$

where Pb is the hydrostatic pressure in the blood compartment and Pd is the hydrostatic pressure on the ultrafiltrate side of the membrane. The oncotic pressure is given by $\pi$. It follows from this equation that convective flux (Jf) of any given molecular species will be given by:

$$Jf = Kf \times TMP$$

with Kf being the membrane permeability coefficient. The rate at which molecular species cross the membrane depends on the membrane rejection coefficient ($\sigma$) which is effectively zero for small species such as urea but approaches 1 for larger molecules such as albumin. The sieving coefficient (Sc) is given by:

$$Sc = 1 - \sigma$$

This can be determined by measuring the concentration of a given solute in the plasma water and the ultrafiltrate. Thus a simple view of solute clearance ($K$) in convective treatments is the product of:

$$K = Qf.Sc$$

where Qf is the ultrafiltration rate. It follows that where Sc = 1, the clearance is equal to Qf. Solute clearance using diffusion-based systems may be calculated from:

$$K = (Qdo \times Cdo) / Cbi$$

with Qdo and Cdo being the dialysate effluent flow and solute concentration in the effluent dialysate (that leaving the dialyser). Cbi is the concentration of the solute of interest entering the dialyser [4]. In summary, diffusion provides the main basis for the separation of molecular species in dialysis aided by convection, whereas in filtration convection is aided by diffusion, and as such the two processes often act simultaneously with any division being somewhat artificial.

| Typical Settings | Type of Renal Replacement Therapy | | | |
|---|---|---|---|---|
| | Inermittent Haemodialysis (IHD) | Continuous Haemodialysis (CVVHD) | Continuous Venovenous Haemofiltration (CVHD) | Continuous Venovenous Haemodialfiltration (CVVHDF) |
| | 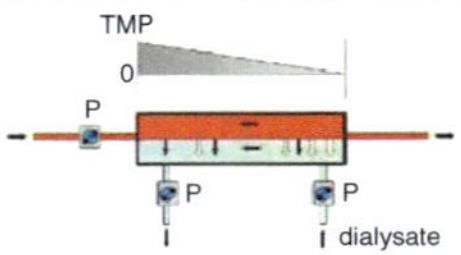  | 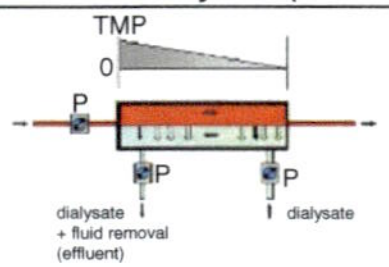  | 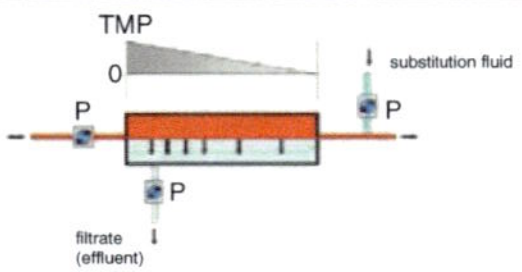  | 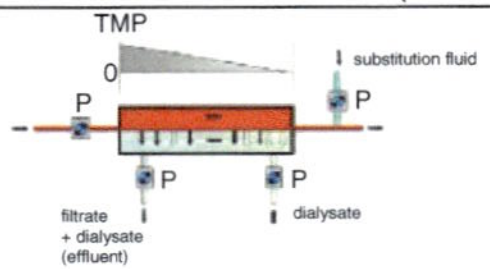  |
| Blood Flow ($Q_B$) | 200–400 ml/min | 80–150 ml/min | 150–250 ml/min | 100–250 ml/min |
| Dialystae Flow ($Q_D$) | 500–800 ml/min | 10–35 ml/min | | 10–35 ml/min |
| Filtrate Rate ($Q_F$) | | | 25–50 ml/min | 10–50 ml/min |
| Convection | + | + | +++ | +++ |
| Diffusion | +++ | +++ | − | +++ |
| Adsorption | + | + | + | + |

Schematics show an outline of the techniques described. P = Pump and TMP = Trans Membrane Pressure. Typical settings are outlined as are the predominant physiochemical processes involved.

**Fig. 14.2** Schematics show an outline of the techniques described. *P* Pump and *TMP* Transmembrane Pressure. Typical settings are outlined, as are the predominant physiochemical processes involved

> **Key Messages**
> - Convection and diffusion are essential processes needed to drive molecular separation.
> - Convective therapies transport solutes and solvent across a semipermeable membrane through the application of a transmembrane pressure gradient.
> - Diffusive therapies rely on solute transport across a semipermeable membrane driven by a concentration gradient such that the solute concentration will tend to reach equilibrium in the available distribution space on both sides of the membrane.
> - Convection and diffusion often occur simultaneously and as such any distinction is somewhat artificial.

## 14.2 Types of Renal Replacement Therapy for AKI: Intermittent versus Continuous

RRT for AKI may be applied in several guises. In essence these can be simplistically thought of as being continuous therapies, intermittent therapies and more recently hybrid technologies. Although each technique may have its proponents, there are advantages (and disadvantages!) of each mode. All extracorporeal techniques share many features including access to the circulation as well as an extracorporeal circuit offering molecular separation the nature of which is technique dependent. There are many acronyms used when describing the various techniques to provide renal support. The consensus recommends the use of the term renal replacement therapy (RRT) which may be intermittent or continuous and described as IRRT or CRRT, respectively. The extracorporeal circuit type is then described, for example, pumped venovenous—VV. This is followed by the method of blood purification, for example, haemofiltration—H, haemodiafiltration—HDF and haemodialysis—HD. Therefore, continuous venovenous haemodiafiltration would be represented by CVVHDF [5, 6].

### 14.2.1 Intermittent Techniques

Intermittent techniques, specifically intermittent haemodialysis, are the standard treatment modality for renal replacement in patients with end stage renal disease. In intermittent haemodialysis, blood is pumped into a dialyser containing two fluid compartments with blood in the first compartment being pumped along one side of a semipermeable membrane while a crystalloid solution (dialysate) is pumped along the other side in a contraflow fashion. As described, the concentration gradients of solute between blood and dialysate lead to the desired biochemical changes. In order to prevent filtration of the dialysate back into the bloodstream, this compartment is under negative pressure relative to the blood compartment.

Compared to continuous techniques, relatively high blood flows are used (200–400 mL/min) coupled with dialysate flow rates of 500–800 mL/min (see Fig. 14.2). Such flows enable high solute clearance rates over a relatively short period of time which may be associated with complications in the critically ill patient. For example, rapid removal of urea during dialysis may be associated with the dialysis disequilibrium syndrome. This is a clinical phenomenon of acute central nervous system dysfunction attributed to cerebral oedema occurring during or just after renal replacement therapy. Although generally accepted that cerebral oedema plays a major role in the development of the dialysis disequilibrium syndrome, the definitive pathophysiology is incompletely described [7, 8]. Of the mechanisms proposed, the increased urea removal from the plasma over that of the cerebrospinal fluid resulting in movement of water into the brain—the so-called reverse urea effect hypothesis—is probably the most universally accepted. Features of the dialysis disequilibrium syndrome include nausea, headache, vomiting, tremors and seizures [9]. There is no treatment as such for the dialysis disequilibrium syndrome, and despite a lack of evidence base, preventive measures include shorter session length, lower blood flow rates and use of smaller surface area filters. Low-dose continuous therapies could also be applied.

Perhaps, in critically ill patients, intermittent therapies result in higher rates of hypotension, which is significantly influenced by the amount of fluid removal required during each dialysis session and often prevents achievement of desired fluid balance (Table 14.1). To minimize the adverse haemodynamic effects of intermittent therapies, several groups have described techniques whereby modifications are made to avoid the dialysis disequilibrium syndrome as well as haemodynamic intolerance [10]. These include:

- Limiting maximal blood flow at 150 mL/min with a minimal session duration of 4 h
- Simultaneously connection of the circuit with a catheter primed with 0.9 % saline
- Setting dialysate sodium concentration >145 mmol/L
- Setting dialysate temperature <37°C with cooling to 35°C in haemodynamically unstable patients
- Commencing session with dialysis for a short period followed by ultrafiltration

Intermittent therapies do have some potential advantages which include facilitated patient mobilization as well lower costs principally due to a lack of expense of replacement fluids with online dialysate production. However, this presumes that

**Table 14.1** Outline of techniques viewed suitable for RRT in AKI

| Therapeutic aim | Patient characteristics | Suitable techniques |
| --- | --- | --- |
| Solute removal | Stable | Intermittent |
| | Unstable | Continuous/Hybrid |
| Fluid removal | Stable | Ultrafiltration |
| | Unstable | Ultrafiltration/SCUF |
| Solute & fluid removal | Stable | Intermittent |
| | Unstable | Continuous/Hybrid |

the therapy is delivered by dedicated ICU staff and not additional specified renal nurses. Often choice of treatment is a matter of preference and local practice, although many intensive care doctors would regard haemodynamic instability as a major concern and hence influence treatment choice for acute kidney injury in the ICU. Treatment of acute kidney injury in the renal unit, however, when present as single organ failure is almost exclusively delivered as intermittent therapies [11].

However, there continues to be a growing body of evidence which points to worse renal outcomes when intermittent therapies are employed in the critical care unit. Although this evidence is retrospective, it is impelling and implies that initial treatment choice may well influence the outcomes of survivors of acute kidney injury [12, 13].

## 14.2.2 Continuous Therapies

Although renal replacement therapy implies the total replacement of kidney function, practically this is not the case. Although no current technology can mimic the function of the kidney, continuous therapies may be viewed as providing good clinical tolerance coupled with the recovery of metabolic homeostasis. Historically, continuous therapies developed from ultrafiltration systems dependent on arterial flow rates to provide the hydrostatic pressures driving the filtration process. In the critically ill, there is often relative hypotension which precludes adequate perfusion of an extracorporeal circuit, which in turn is reflected in inefficient molecular clearance and inadequate dosing of treatment when driven by the systemic arterial pressure. The development of non-occlusive venous pumping systems allowed the development of venovenous circuitry, which overcame this problem. Such blood pumps assure a fast and stable blood flow that can be set at rates tolerated by the patient [14]. Occasionally, catabolic patients with an increased urea load may require higher flow rates but continuous techniques do allow more predictable blood flow rate and thus the ability to achieve a higher filtration rate.

Several techniques and modality types are currently available to deliver renal support continuously on the intensive care unit. Continuous venovenous haemofiltration (CVVH: Fig. 14.2) has found favour as the mainstay of renal replacement techniques in the critically ill, certainly within Europe and Australasia [15]. Solute transport is achieved predominantly by convection utilizing a high-flux membrane. This produces an ultrafiltrate which is replaced by a substitution fluid with volume balance being achieved by the degree of replacement. The replacement fluid may be infused before or after the filter (see below). Continuous venovenous haemodialysis (CVVHD) again is a process driven by a venovenous pump through an extracorporeal circuit and, through a haemodialyser containing a semipermeable membrane. This allows adequate exchange of small molecular weight solutes into the dialysate and hence their removal from the body. In general, haemodialysis is effective for the removal of small molecular weight solutes and becomes increasingly less efficient as molecular weight rises above a thousand daltons. Continuous venovenous haemodialfiltration (CVVHDF) is adapted from that technique originally introduced to increase the limited clearance of urea and other small molecular weight solutes in arterial-driven haemofiltration systems. CVVHDF does combine the two processes of diffusion and convection by introducing a countercurrent flow of dialysate into the non-blood-containing compartment of the haemodiafilter. This theoretically increases the efficiency of clearance of small molecular weight solutes over that of haemofiltration without dialysis.

### 14.2.3 Continuous versus Intermittent Therapies

To date there is a paucity of evidence to support one approach over another with current data suggesting that the two principal outcomes measured, namely survival and renal recovery, are similar whatever technique is used [6]. As such they are viewed as complementary therapies in patients with acute kidney injury. Conclusions from the limited number of randomized prospective studies are also somewhat contradictory. For example, one of the earliest studies randomized 166 patients with acute kidney injury to either continuous or intermittent techniques and demonstrated a higher all-cause mortality with continuous therapies. However, on adjustment for severity of illness no such association was observed [16]. A larger, prospective study on some 360 patients also failed to demonstrate any survival benefit, as defined by 60-day mortality, when comparing IHD to CVVHDF [17]. With regard to renal recovery, often defined as the need for long-term renal replacement therapy, again no definitive conclusions can be driven, although several meta-analyses point to a benefit with continuous treatments although when just randomized trials are included no difference is seen [12, 18].

> **Key Messages**
> - Continuous treatment is often an aspirational treatment goal and there are often many reasons why treatment may be interrupted.
> - Intermittent therapies are the mainstay of treatment for chronic kidney disease.
> - Continuous therapies may be associated with less treatment associated hypotension or disequilibrium syndromes.
> - There is a paucity of definitive, high-quality data supporting one technique over another, although meta-analyses tend to support a potential survival and renal recovery benefit with continuous treatments.

### 14.3 'Hybrid' Technologies: Prolonged Intermittent Renal Replacement Therapy for AKI

As discussed, the therapeutic aims of continuous RRT are correction and maintenance of volume and acid–base homeostasis in the critically ill without undue haemodynamic disturbance. This originally led to the introduction of continuous therapies but more recently several newer technologies have sought to achieve this aim without necessarily being continuous in nature. The aim, therefore, is to optimize the potential advantages offered by both approaches thus solute clearances achieved, for example, may not be as efficient as intermittent dialysis but the techniques are maintained for longer periods of time. Numerous regimens/techniques have evolved which can be collectively referred to by the umbrella term 'hybrid therapies'. An alternative description is 'prolonged (daily) intermittent renal replacement therapy' (PIRRT). These techniques have various approaches which differ slightly and include techniques such as:

- Sustained low efficiency (daily) dialysis (SLEDD)
- Sustained low efficiency (daily) diafiltration (SLEDD-f)
- Extended daily dialysis (EDD)
- Extended daily dialysis with filtration (EDDf)

Advocates of these technologies claim that such techniques combine the logistic and cost advantages of intermittent haemodialysis with the theoretical therapeutic advantages of continuous replacement therapies. Potential benefits include efficient solute removal with reduced ultrafiltration rate, thereby minimizing haemodynamic instability. Furthermore, there may be lower anticoagulant needs as well as reduced costs and perhaps most importantly improved patient mobility particularly in the rehabilitative phase of critical illness. Indeed, a randomized controlled trial of PIRRT versus CRRT demonstrated cardiovascular stability during treatment [19]. Patients were randomly assigned to either PIRRT or CRRT, achieving a total ultrafiltration of 3 L over 12 h and 3.3 L over 24 h during the hybrid treatment and CRRT, respectively. No significant difference in inotrope dose or number was observed. Although a trend to lower blood pressure and cardiac output was observed, this did not reach significance and no difference in outcomes were observed. Although at present these techniques account for less than 10 % of treatments offered to critically ill patients with acute kidney injury, the potential benefits including that of cost may mean that they become more prevalent.

> **Key Messages**
> - Hybrid therapies may deliver desired solute clearance without haemodynamic compromise.
> - Hybrid therapies have a considerable cost advantage and as such may increasingly be seen as a favourable approach.
> - No data as yet has suggested that hybrid therapies confer any survival or renal recovery differences compared to conventional intermittent or continuous treatments.

## 14.4 Postdilution versus Predilution

As discussed above, continuous convective therapies such as continuous venovenous haemofiltration (CVVH) require the replacement of fluids to achieve net solute removal and to achieve prescribed volume balance. The replacement fluid may be returned to the circuit either before (predilution) or after the haemofilter (postdilution).

### 14.4.1 Postdilution

Where replacement fluid is reinfused through the venous line of the circuit (postdilution), the effect on solute clearance and ultrafiltration rate is relatively straightforward. Solute clearance will be, in the main, determined by the sieving coefficient and the ultrafiltration rate. Although postdilution haemofiltration provides higher solute clearance, it is limited by the attainable blood flow rate. Specifically, this is governed by the filtration fraction. The filtration fraction in continuous therapies (only relevant for CVVH and CVVHDF) can be simply calculated by dividing the ultrafiltration rate by the plasma flow rate (Blood pump speed × 1-Haematocrit = equivalent to renal blood flow). Therefore,

$$(1\text{-Hct}) \times \text{Blood flow rate} = \text{plasma flow (PF) rate}$$

and

$$\text{ultrafiltration rate (UFR)/plasma flow (PF)} = \text{filtration fraction (FF)}.$$

In CRRT, a filtration fraction above 25 % significantly increases clotting risk through haemoconcentration. Thus, if a blood pump speed of 250 mL/min is used with a haematocrit of 0.3, then Plasma Flow = 175 mL/min. In order to maintain the filtration fraction at <25 %, the UFR must be set no higher than 45 mL/min. At filtration fractions that are greater than 25 %, secondary membrane effects and concentration polarization both impair filter performance.

### 14.4.2 Predilution

Predilution reinfusion does have a few theoretical advantages with regard to solute removal but these must be tempered by the effect of dilution on plasma solute concentration. In turn, this affects the amount of solute removed by convection as well as increasing the replacement fluid utilization. However, filter viability is improved by predilution as it reduces the risk of clotting in the filter by reducing the haematocrit.

**Key Messages**
- Replacement fluids can be delivered to the extracorporeal circuit before the filter (predilution) or after the filter (postdilution).
- The blood flow rate within the filter determines replacement fluid requirements as this influences the filtration fraction.
- The filtration fraction should be maintained at <25 % in order to minimize deleterious effects on filter performance and filter life.

## References


1. EF Leonard. The bases of mass seperation processes. In: Ronco C, Bellomo R, Kellum JA, editor. Critical care nephrology. Philadelphia: Saunders Elsevier; 2009. p. 1131–5.
2. Bird RB, Stewart WE, Lightfoot EN. Transport phenomena. New York: J Wiley; 2002.
3. Lightfoot EN. Transport phenomena and living systems: biomedical aspects of momentum and mass transport. New York: Wiley; 1974.
4. Ricci Z, Bellomo R, Ronco C. Renal replacement techniques: descriptions, mechanisms, choices and controversies. In: Bellomo R, Ronco C, Kellum JA, editors. Critical care nephrology. Philadelphia: Saunders Elsevier; 2009. p. 1136–41.
5. Kellum JA, Mehta RL, Angus DC, Palevsky P, Ronco C, ADQI Workgroup. The first international consensus conference on continuous renal replacement therapy. Kidney Int. 2002;62(5): 1855–63.
6. Group, K.D.I.G.O.K.A.K.I.W. KDIGO clinical practice guideline for acute kidney injury. Kidney Int. 2012;2((S 1)):1–138.
7. Bunchman TE, et al. Prevention of dialysis disequilibrium by use of CVVH. Int J Artif Organs. 2007;30(5):441–4.
8. Ronco C, Bellomo R, Brendolan A, Pinna V, La Greca G. Brain density changes during renal replacement in critically ill patients with acute renal failure: continuous hemofiltration versus intermittent hemodialysis. J Nephrol. 1999;12(3):173–8.
9. Patel N, Dalal P, Panesar M. Dialysis disequilibrium syndrome: a narrative review. Semin Dial. 2008;21(5):493–8.
10. Schortgen F, Soubrier N, Delclaux C, Thuong M, Girou E, Brun-Buisson C, Lemaire F, Brochard L. Hemodynamic tolerance of intermittent hemodialysis in critically ill patients usefulness of practice guidelines. Am J Respir Crit Care Med. 2000;162:197–202.
11. Fieghen H, Wald R, Jaber BL. Renal replacement therapy for acute kidney injury. Nephron Clin Pract. 2009;112(4):c222–9.
12. Bagshaw SM, et al. Continuous versus intermittent renal replacement therapy for critically ill patients with acute kidney injury: a meta-analysis. Crit Care Med. 2008;36(2):610–7.
13. Schneider AG, et al. Choice of renal replacement therapy modality and dialysis dependence after acute kidney injury: a systematic review and meta-analysis. Intensive Care Med. 2013;39(6):987–97.
14. Forni LG, Hilton PJ. Continuous hemofiltration in the treatment of acute renal failure. N Engl J Med. 1997;336:1303–9.
15. Uchino S, Kellum JA, Bellomo R, Doig GS, Morimatsu H, Morgera S, Schetz M, Tan I, Bouman C, Macedo E, Gibney N, Tolwani A, Ronco C for the Beginning and Ending Supportive Therapy for the Kidney (BEST Kidney) Investigators. Acute renal failure in critically ill patients a multinational, multicenter study. JAMA. 2005;294(7):813–8.
16. Mehta RL, McDonald B, Gabbai FB, Pahl M, Pascual MT, Farkas A, Kaplan RM, Collaborative Group for Treatment of ARF in the ICU. A randomized clinical trial of continuous versus intermittent dialysis for acute renal failure. Kidney Int. 2001;60(3):1154–63.
17. Vinsonneau C, Camus C, Combes A, de Beauregard MA C, Klouche K, Boulain T, Pallot JL, Chiche JD, Taupin P, Landais P, Dhainaut JF, Hemodiafe Study Group. Continuous venovenous haemodiafiltration versus intermittent haemodialysis for acute renal failure in patients with multiple-organ dysfunction syndrome- a multicentre randomised trial. Lancet. 2006;368: 379–85.
18. Ronco C, Bellomo R. Dialysis in intensive care unit patients with acute kidney injury: continuous therapy is superior. Clin J Am Soc Nephrol. 2007;2(3):597–600.
19. Kielstein JT, Kretschmer U, Ernst T, Hafer C, Bahr MJ, Haller H, Fliser D. Efficacy and cardiovascular tolerability of extended dialysis in critically ill patients: a randomized controlled study. Am J Kidney Dis. 2004;43(2):342–9.

# Anticoagulation for Continuous Renal Replacement Therapy

# 15


Heleen M. Oudemans-van Straaten, Anne-Cornelie J.M. de Pont, Andrew Davenport, and Noel Gibney


## 15.1 Heparin Anticoagulation for Continuous Venovenous Hemofiltration (CRRT)


Anne-Cornelie J.M. de Pont


Unfractionated heparin (UFH) is the anticoagulant most frequently used to prevent thrombosis in the extracorporeal circuit [1]. Its anticoagulant effect is mediated by the binding to antithrombin through a high affinity pentasaccharide sequence, thereby inactivating factors IIa, Xa, IXa, XIa and XIIa. By inactivating thrombin (IIa), UFH also inhibits thrombin-induced activation of platelets and factors V, VIII and XI [2]. After intravenous injection, UFH binds to endothelial cells, macrophages and plasma proteins such as the acute phase proteins factor VIII and fibrinogen, often elevated in critically ill patients. This explains why the response to UFH among critically ill patients is often reduced, a phenomenon known as heparin


H.M. Oudemans-van Straaten (✉)
Department of Intensive Care, VU University Medical Center, Amsterdam, The Netherlands
e-mail: hmoudemans@gmail.com

A.C.J.M. de Pont
Department of Intensive Care, Academic Medical Center, Amsterdam, The Netherlands
e-mail: a.c.depont@amc.uva.nl

A. Davenport
UCL Centre for Nephrology, Royal Free Hospital, University College London Medical School, London, UK
e-mail: andrewdavenport@nhs.net

N. Gibney
Division of Critical Care Medicine, 3C1.16 University of Alberta Hospital, Edmonton, AB, Canada
e-mail: ngibney@ualberta.ca



© Springer International Publishing 2015
H.M. Oudemans-van Straaten et al. (eds.), *Acute Nephrology for the Critical Care Physician*, DOI 10.1007/978-3-319-17389-4_15

resistance. UFH is cleared from the circulation by cellular binding and renal elimination. Binding to endothelial cells and macrophages leads to rapid internalization and depolymerization, whereas renal elimination is a much slower process. Two small studies demonstrated that UFH is not cleared by continuous venovenous hemofiltration [3, 4].

The anticoagulant effect of UFH is generally monitored by means of the activated partial thromboplastin time (APTT) or the activated clotting time (ACT). The APTT tests the intrinsic and common pathways of the coagulation cascade, requiring the presence of coagulation factors I, II, V, VIII, IX, X, XI and XII to yield a normal result. The ACT is a point of care test, measuring the time to clotting of whole blood added to a surface activator such as celite, glass or kaolin. The ACT is less accurate than the APTT and is not recommended for the monitoring of treatment with heparin in the intensive care setting [5].

UFH can be used both for priming the circuit and keeping it open during the treatment. Priming the circuit with UFH has not been extensively studied. A small prospective randomized crossover study showed less thrombogenicity after priming the circuit with UFH, but differences in circuit survival were not mentioned [6]. To prevent thrombosis in the extracorporeal circuit during the treatment, UFH can be used systemically or regionally. No dose finding studies have been performed to establish the systemically administered UFH dose needed to prevent thrombosis in this setting. A maximum loading dose of 5,000 IU, followed by a maintenance dose of 5–10 IU/kg/h, aiming at an APTT up to 1.4 times the upper limit of normal has been recommended [7, 8]. Two small studies investigated the efficacy of regional anticoagulation with UFH, infusing UFH before the filter and reversing its action with protamine after the filter to prevent systemic anticoagulation. In the first study, circuit survival times during systemic and regional anticoagulation with UFH were similar, whereas in the second study, circuit survival was shorter during regional anticoagulation with UFH than during systemic anticoagulation with nadroparin [9, 10]. A prospective controlled study among 110 intensive care patients demonstrated that regional anticoagulation with UFH and protamine combined with intravenous prostacyclin increased circuit survival when compared with systemically administered UFH only [11]. Given the many safe citrate protocols (see below), regional anticoagulation with heparin–protamin is nowadays not recommended anymore.

Treatment with UFH carries the risks of both drug resistance and bleeding. Drug resistance is associated with antithrombin deficiency, increased heparin clearance and elevation in heparin binding proteins such as the acute phase proteins factor VIII and fibrinogen [12]. In critically ill patients, elevated levels of factor VIII may shorten the APTT without diminishing the antithrombotic effect of UFH. In this case, monitoring through an anti-Xa assay is recommended, since the result of this assay more closely mirrors the antithrombotic effect of UFH. The risk of heparin-associated bleeding increases with the dose. When doses exceeding 35,000 IU/24 h are used, monitoring by means of the anti-Xa assay is recommended [2].

The use of UFH has several advantages: Its half-life is relatively short (0.5–3 h), it is easily reversible with protamine, the experience with it is large and it is cheap. However, both drug resistance and bleeding are common and UFH carries a 1–5 % risk of heparin induced thrombocytopenia (HIT).

Low molecular weight heparins (LMWHs) are also being used to prevent thrombosis in the extracorporeal circuit, although less often than UFH [1]. The mechanism of action of LMWHs is similar to that of UFH, but because of reduced binding to plasma proteins, their pharmacokinetics are more predictable. They exhibit linear pharmacokinetics with stationary distribution volume and clearance processes, obviating the need of anti-Xa monitoring during continuous dosing. However, a small study reported resistance to LMWH in critically ill patients as well [13]. LMWHs are partially metabolized by desulfatation and depolymerization, and 5–10 % of the injected dose is eliminated by urinary excretion. Clearance by hemofiltration is insignificant [13]. The half-life is longer than that of UFH (2–4 h) and the anticoagulant action is not fully reversible with protamine. However, the incidence of HIT is much lower (0.5–1 %). Several studies have investigated the use of LMWHs during hemofiltration. The drugs most frequently investigated are dalteparin, enoxaparin and nadroparin. LMWHs differ in their ratio of anti-Xa versus anti-IIa inhibition, enoxaparin having the greatest ratio (3.8) and tinzaparin the smallest (1.9) [14]. The use of dalteparin as an anticoagulant during hemofiltration was investigated in three studies, with loading doses of 15–20 IU/kg and maintenance doses of 4–10 IU/kg/h reaching circuit survival times from 15 to 47 h [15, 16]. Enoxaparin was investigated in two studies: A dose of 0.05 – 0.06 mg/kg/h was recommended, reaching circuit survival times of 22–31 h [17]. Nadroparin has been investigated in three studies with doses of 328–475 IU/h reaching circuit survival times of 15–40 h [10, 16, 18].

In summary, when carefully dosed and monitored, both UFH and LMWHs can be used for the prevention of thrombosis in the extracorporeal circuit.

**Key Messages Heparin**
- Both UFH and LMWH can be used to prevent coagulation in the extracorporeal circuit if carefully dosed and monitored.
- Both heparin and LMWH increase the risk of bleeding.
- Half-life of UFH is 0.5–3 h; UFH is easily reversible with protamine.
- Half-life of LMWH is 2–4 h; anticoagulant action is only partially reversible with protamine.
- Critically ill patients can exhibit heparin resistance due to antithrombin deficiency and increased heparin binding to acute phase proteins and cells.
- The risk of heparin-induced thrombocytopenia (HIT) is lower with use of LMWH than with heparin.

## 15.2    Heparin Induced Thrombocytopenia

Andrew Davenport

Heparins, both unfractionated heparins and low molecular weight heparins can bind to platelet factor 4 on the surface of platelets, causing activation and a reduction in the peripheral platelet count [19]. This is termed heparin induced thrombocytopenia type 1, and the fall in peripheral platelet count is typically modest, and the platelet count recovers spontaneously. On the other hand heparin induced thrombocytopenia type 2 leads to marked thrombocytopenia (typically >50 % fall in peripheral platelet count) due to autoantibody mediated platelet activation which can be life-threatening, and necessitates heparin withdrawal to aid recovery [20].

Heparins are large negatively charged proteoglycans which can nonspecifically bind to proteins. As such heparins bind to platelet factor 4 (PF4), but when heparin is in excess (heparin:PF4 27 IU:1 mg) this leads to unfolding of the PF4 molecule, exposing new epitopes to which autoantibodies form. These antibodies then bind to platelet surface FcγIIa receptors activating platelets, and also to endothelial cells increasing tissue factor expression. The ratio of heparin to PF4 is critical, and as such heparin induced thrombocytopenia type 2 is most commonly observed when patients are exposed to larger doses of heparins, for example following cardiac, major vascular and orthopaedic surgery [21]. Similarly the amount of negative charge on the heparin molecule is also important in causing changes in the shape of the PF4 molecule, so the incidence is greater with unfractionated than low molecular weight heparins, and bovine compared to porcine derived heparins. Similarly the incidence of HIT is increased in patients with solid organ malignancies and critically ill patients. Although IgA, IgG and IgM autoantibodies may be formed to the heparin-PF4 complex, it is thought that only IgG are pathological [22].

The diagnosis of heparin induced thrombocytopenia type 2 (HIT) remains a clinical diagnosis. In the critically ill patient there are often many other potential causes of peripheral thrombocytopenia, ranging from reduced platelet production to increased consumption [23]. To aid the clinician in estimating the probability of HIT, Warkentin proposed the 4 Ts scoring system (Table 15.1) [24]. Even so if the diagnosis of HIT is clinically suspected then heparin should be withdrawn, including catheter locks and line flushes whilst awaiting laboratory testing. Most laboratories now have access to ELISA assays designed to detect antibodies to heparin-PF4, but most assays are not specific for the IgGisotype, and report positive results with IgA and IgM antibodies [21, 22]. Only a few laboratories worldwide are able to perform the gold standard 5HT platelet release test for diagnosing HIT. Comparative studies between these assays have suggested that although most ELISA assays report a positive result with an optical density (OD) of >0.6, to have clinically significant disease, the OD is >1.0. As such platelet agglutination assays should also be performed to confirm the ELISA assay result. The reason that HIT remains a clinical diagnosis is that antibodies can also form from other proteins released by activated platelets.

**Table 15.1** The "4 Ts" scoring system to estimate probability for heparin induced thrombocytopenia, prior to laboratory testing for HIT antibodies

| score | 2 points | 1 point | zero |
|---|---|---|---|
| Thrombocytopenia ×10 9 1 | 20–100 or Fall > 50 % | 10 – 19 or Fall 30–50 % | <10 or Fall <30 % |
| Timing of onset in fall platelets[a] | 5–10 days heparin Rx | >10 days or timing not evident | <1 day heparin exposure |
| Thrombosis or Acute systemic symptoms | Proven thrombosis Skin necrosis or Acute systemic reaction | Progressive, recurrent, silent thrombosis or erythematous skin lesions | none |
| Other aetiology for thrombocytopenia | None evident | possible | probable |

Adapted from Ref. [6]

Low probability ≤3, intermediate probability 4–6, high probability ≥6

[a]This assumes the patient has not been previously exposed to heparins. In cases of prior heparin exposure, then HIT can develop within 24 h if preformed antibodies are already present

The lower the peripheral platelet count reflects greater platelet activation and platelet adhesion to the endothelium, with greater risk of thrombosis. HIT can lead to both major venous and arterial thrombosis and platelet activation in the lung can lead to acute lung injury, so-called "pseudo-pulmonary" embolus. The management of HIT centers on both withdrawal of all heparins (including heparin flushes, catheter locks and subcutaneous administration) and also systemic anticoagulation to prevent thrombosis. The lower the platelets count the greater the risk of thrombosis and need for systemic anticoagulation. Typically thrombocytopenia starts to recover within 72 h following heparin withdrawal, and if there is no response to heparin withdrawal, then an alternative explanation for thrombocytopenia should be considered. Currently systemic anticoagulation options include the direct thrombin inhibitor argatroban, and the heparinoids, danaparoid and fondaparinux [25, 26]. Although danaparoid may cause cross reactivity with ELISA assays for HIT, this has not been reported to have adverse clinical consequences. Argatroban is a reversible thrombin inhibitor and requires a continuous infusion, with the infusion adjusted to maintain an activated partial thromboplastin ratio (aPPTr) of 2.0–2.5, and as it is hepatically metabolised then much lower dosages are required for patients with liver disease. Both danaparoid and fondaparinux are renally excreted and accumulate in patients with acute kidney injury and chronic kidney disease. As they have minimal effect on the aPPTr, monitoring requires measurement of anti-Xa activity, aiming for a therapeutic window of 0.4–0.6 IU/ml. Given the procoagulant nature of HIT, regional anticoagulants such as citrate for CRRT do not provide the systemic anticoagulation required to prevent systemic thrombosis, and as such additional systemic anticoagulation should be considered.

Once the platelet count has recovered to >150,000 × $10^6$/l, then warfarin therapy can be considered, as there is a risk of precipitating skin gangrene if warfarin therapy is started before the platelet count has recovered. Argatroban prolongs the prothrombin time, and therefore caution is required when converting patients from intravenous argatroban to oral warfarin therapy. For the majority of patients HIT antibodies are a temporary phenomenon and disappear over time. However before considering rechallenging patients with heparin, then both ELISA and platelet agglutination assays should be negative on at least two occasions (Table 15.1).

> **Key Messages Heparin Induced Thrombocytopenia**
> - Consider heparin induced thrombocytopenia in any patient with a 50 % fall in peripheral platelet count after starting heparin within the previous 10 days.
> - Heparin induced thrombocytopenia remains a clinical diagnosis. Use the "4 Ts" scoring system to estimate probability.
> - With a score $\geq 6$, withdraw all heparins immediately whilst awaiting confirmation with ELISA and platelet agglutination assays, and start alternative systemic anticoagulation with argatroban as first choice and consider additional citrate anticoagulation for the circuit.
> - With a score between 3 and 6, order ELISA testing, while continuation of heparins awaiting results seems to be justified.
> - The lower the platelet count the greater the risk of thrombosis and systemic anticoagulation is required.
> - For a definite diagnosis of HIT, positive ELISA testing should be confirmed with a platelet agglutination assay.

## 15.3 Prostacyclin

Noel Gibney

Prostacyclin is an anti-hemostatic prostaglandin that inhibits platelet function, activation and adhesion by diminishing the expression of platelet fibrinogen receptors and P-selectin and reduces heterotypic platelet-leukocyte aggregation. At higher infusion doses it is also a potent smooth muscle relaxant and vasodilator. It is available for clinical therapy as a synthetic analogue, epoprostenol. It is produced primarily in the endothelial and smooth muscle cells of blood vessels. Prostacyclin has a short half-life of 2–3 min with a clinical effect on end-organs and platelets of approximately 30 min [27, 28]. It has been used in combination with low dose heparin infusions and on its own as an adjunct to prolong hemofilter life during intermittent dialysis and CRRT [29–31].

### 15.3.1 Indication

Prostacyclin has primarily been used as an anti-hemostatic to enhance hemofilter life in patients with acute kidney injury and acute liver failure and concern to avoid hemorrhage. Although many such patients have severe coagulopathy, some continually thrombosehemofilters during CRRT, even while suffering from ongoing hemorrhage, usually gastrointestinal. This is likely due to deficiencies in the synthesis of anti-thrombotic substances such as anti-thrombin III, protein C and protein S [32]. Since prostacyclin exerts its effect on platelet function, it unlikely to be of significant value in patients with severe thrombocytopenia.

Although regional citrate anticoagulation has been shown to be more effective in maintaining hemofilter patency, its use is often not possible as these patients are at risk of citrate accumulation as citrate is primarily metabolized in the liver [33]. In this difficult clinical situation, the use of prostacyclin may be valuable in prolonging hemofilter life without adding extra risk of bleeding [34].

## 15.3.2 Practical Considerations

Prostacyclin is available clinically as epoprostenol in a freeze dried powder which must be reconstituted as directed, only using the supplied diluent containing a glycine buffer to maintain a pH of 10–11. It must be infused via a separate infusion line to avoid inactivation by acidic drugs such as catecholamine vasopressor agents. It is important that only syringe infusion pumps with noncompliant intravenous tubing external to the pumps on the CRRT machine are used for infusion when using prostacyclin with CRRT. The infusion pumps on some CRRT machines, although ostensibly syringe pumps, operate by using "micro boluses" of drug rather than a smooth continuous infusion and may be associated with the development of intermittent episodes of hypotension. A similar issue may be seen using other infusion pumps that use peristaltic mechanisms. Since prostacyclin does not interfere with the coagulation systems, there is no simple clinical means of readily monitoring and titrating the infusion dose although thromboelastography could be used for this purpose [27].

## 15.3.3 Alone or Incombination with Heparin

Prostacyclin has been used both as a sole anti-hemostatic agent and in combination with unfractionated heparin. It has been shown to extend hemofilter survival, particularly when used in combination with low dose heparin [22–24].

The use of prostacyclin combined with regional anticoagulation with prefilter heparin and postfilter protamine has been studied in a prospective randomized trial and provided excellent filter survival and minimal bleeding when compared with conventional heparin [11].

## 15.3.4 Dose and Side Effects

Because of its vasodilator properties, prostacyclin can cause hypotension, although, the typical infusion doses used to enhance hemofilter life by antagonism of platelet activation and aggregation is in the range of 3–5 ng/kg/min and, generally does not impact on blood pressure significantly in most patients, although occasionally the dose of vasopressor infusions needs to be increased. (The typical dose required to achieve pulmonary vasodilatation is up to 35 ng/kg/min).

The main side effect of prostacyclin is hypotension caused by vasodilatation which may be managed by ensuring adequate fluid volume status, by reducing the rate of infusion or by titrating a vasopressor infusion. Theoretically, the risk of bleeding increases with platelet inhibition. However, in an observational study of 51 critically ill patients undergoing CRRT with prostacyclin as sole anti-hemostatic agent there was minimal bleeding (one episode per 1,000 h treatment) although 15 % required either fluids or vasopressor therapy either for the first time or an increase in dose following initiation of prostacyclin [34]. Prostacyclin is relatively expensive, but at the low doses used for CRRT the cost is similar to citrate regional anticoagulation.

## 15.4 Citrate Anticoagulation for Continuous Renal Replacement Therapy

Heleen M. Oudemans-van Straaten

### 15.4.1 Summary

Citrate acts as anticoagulant by chelating ionized calcium (iCa) and thereby causing hypocalcemia in the filter. At an iCa concentration of 0.25 mmol/L, anticoagulation is maximal. Part of the citrate is removed by dialysis or filtration, the remains enter the systemic circulation. Citrate is rapidly metabolized in the mitochondria, the chelated calcium is released and the lost calcium is replaced. Citrate therefore provides regional anticoagulation and does not increase the risk of bleeding.

Sodium citrate is a buffer as well provided that citrate is metabolized. The buffer strength is equivalent to 3 mmol bicarbonate per mmol citrate if all cations are sodium (trisodium citrate) and less so if part of the cations are hydrogen (citric acid).

Citrate anticoagulation is better tolerated than heparin, and is associated with less bleeding and generally longer circuit survival. Its main risk is accumulation due to decreased metabolism as a result of liver failure or systemic hypoperfusion. Accumulation is characterized by a decrease in iCa, a rise in total Ca and metabolic acidosis. It is monitored by measuring systemic iCa (to adjust calcium replacement) and acid–base balance. A rise in total/iCa is the most sensitive marker of accumulation.

### 15.4.2 Introduction

Sodium citrate has become the first choice anticoagulant for continuous renal replacement therapy (CRRT). It provides regional anticoagulation of the circuit, without increasing the patient's risk of bleeding. Its anticoagulant properties are due to the chelation of ionized calcium (iCa) thereby causing hypocalcemia in the circuit. Calcium is a necessary cofactor in the formation of thrombin. Coagulation is inhibited as soon as ionCa falls below 0.50 mmol/L, and is maximal at an iCa concentration of 0.25 mmol/l [35].

### 15.4.3 Regional Anticoagulation

Within the CRRT circuit, sodium citrate is administered before the filter. Citrate dose is titrated to blood flow. Postfilter iCa can be monitored to fine-tune anticagulation by adjusting citrate dose to iCa targets (0.25–0.35 mmol/L),but many protocols use a fixed citrate to blood flow proportion. Part of the calcium citrate complexes are removed by dialysis or filtration. The remains enter the patient's circulation to be metabolized in the Krebs cycle of liver, kidney and muscle. The chelated calcium is released, while the calcium lost by dialysis or filtration is replaced. Regional anticoagulation is the result, and this is the main benefit of citrate [8, 36].

### 15.4.4 Citrate Is a Buffer

Sodium citrate is a buffer base as well. According to the classical concept, each mole of trisodium citrate provides a buffer equivalent of three moles of bicarbonate, if and when citrate is metabolized. According to the Stewart concept of acid–base [30], sodium citrate increases the strong ion difference $(SID = (Na^+ + K^+ + Ca^{2+} + Mg^{2+}) - (Cl^- + lactate^-))$ provided that citrate is metabolized. This concept explains why the buffer strength of the citrate solution depends on the accompanying cation [31]. The buffer strength is higher when using a trisodium citrate solution and lower when part of the cations are hydrogen, as is the case in the acid dextrose citrate (ACD-A) solution, as used in some protocols, in which 30 % of the cations consist of hydrogen [37–39].

### 15.4.5 Principles of the Citrate Circuit

Citrate is administered before the filter, either as a separate more or less concentrated trisodium citrate solution [18, 40–43] or as part of an isotonic balanced calcium-free predilution hemofiltration solution. In the latter, the bicarbonate is replaced by citrate and the solution is calcium-free [44–46]. When a separate sodium citrate solution is used, the associated dialysate or postdilution hemofiltration solution contains no or less bicarbonate and less sodium to compensate for the citrate buffer and the sodium content of the citrate solution. In most protocols, calcium is replaced separately. It should be noted that citrate additionally chelates magnesium and that citrate CRRT can lead to a negative magnesium balance because the magnesium content of most CRRT solutions is too low [47].

### 15.4.6 Modalities

Different modalities for citrate are in use: Hemodialysis [41],predilution hemofiltration [44–46], postdilution hemofiltration [18, 43] or hemodiafiltration [42]. Modern CRRT devices have a strict citrate protocol incorporated in the software, allowing for choices to determine the desired citrate concentration in the filter (2.5–4.5 mmol/L blood flow), to adjust acid–base derangements (more or less buffer supply) and to adjust calcium infusion rate to compensate for calcium loss (zero calcium balance). Each protocol has strict rules for citrate dosing, acid base compensation and calcium replacement. These rules depend on the composition of the fluids in use and cannot be generalized. The use of a strict protocol, adherence to the protocol and training are crucial for safety of the method.

### 15.4.7 Monitoring of Citrate Anticoagulation

Citrate anticoagulation is monitored by measuring ion- and total calcium concentration and blood gas analysis (for acid–base) in systemic blood at 6–8 h interval. Chloride and lactate can be measured to monitor anion gap and tissue perfusion, but this is not obligatory. Postfilter iCa can be measured to fine-tune anticoagulation.

### 15.4.8 Citrate Accumulation

Metabolism of citrate is conditional for its safe use. Citrate is metabolized in the mitochondria of liver, kidney and muscle and is decreased in patients with liver cirrhosis [43] and systemic hypoperfusion. Although a high lactate concentration at the start of CRRT should raise awareness of the risk of citrate accumulation, septic patients with a high lactate level and other shock patients generally tolerate citrate remarkably well if circulation improves. Citrate anticoagulation is even feasible in patients severe lactate acidosis due to metformine intoxication (personal experience). Citrate is likely to accumulate in patients with persistent severe cardiogenic shock, ischemic hepatitis and poor muscle perfusion [44], because the Krebs cycle only operates under aerobic conditions. However, most critically ill patients tolerate citrate better than heparin [18, 48]. Even in patients with liver failure, the use of citrate is feasible with intensified monitoring [49].

When citrate accumulates, iCa concentration in the patient's blood falls, while total calcium rises due to chelation with citrate and replacement of calcium according to the protocol. A rise of total/iCa ratio is the most sensitive sign of citrate accumulation [50]. A rise above 2.25–2.5 indicates citrate accumulation. Second, if citrate is not metabolized, acidosis will ensue and anion gap will rise, because the alkalizing effect of citrate depends on its metabolism. Due to liver failure or severe hypoperfusion, citrate accumulation is associated with a rise in lactate as well. Citrate accumulation is seen in the most severely ill patients and seems a predictor of mortality [51].

Thus iCa, total calcium, total/iCa ratio, blood gas analysis (for acid base) and lactate are used to monitor citrate accumulation. In patients at risk, intensified monitoring is recommended, initially at 2-h interval. If the total/iCa ratio rises, the risks of continuing citrate should be weighed against the use of alternative anticoagulation (heparin) with risk of bleeding or CRRT without anticoagulation (early circuit clotting). In general, citrate is not toxic. If acid–base is in balance and ionized calcium can be controlled with additional calcium supplementation, the continuation of citrate seem safer than the alternatives [49]. If calcium ratio plateaus, monitoring interval can be prolonged.

## 15.4.9 Benefits of Citrate Anticoagulation

Clinical benefits of citrate are primarily related to less bleeding, a better circuit survival and lower requirement for blood products. The use of citrate does not increase the patient's risk of bleeding. In addition, anticoagulation with citrate seems more effective than with heparin, especially when higher doses are used, and the calcium is replaced outside the CRRT circuit. Three meta-analyses, one including up to six randomized controlled trials (comparing citrate to unfractionated heparin) [52, 53], to low molecular weight heparin [18] or to heparin/protamine [54] with a total of 417 patients and one including four studies (comparing citrate to unfractionated heparin) found less bleeding and a longer circuit survival time with citrate [55–57]. After this meta-analysis, a large multicenter trial has appeared, showing that citrate was superior in terms of safety, efficacy and costs [58]. The largest randomized controlled trial (200 patients) found an unexpected survival benefit for citrate. This benefit could not be fully explained by less bleeding and not to less circuit clotting. It was especially seen in younger patient, surgical patients, and patients with sepsis or those with a high degree of organ failure, suggesting a role of citrate limiting inflammation or oxidative stress [18]. Compared to heparin, citrate confers less complement activation and neutrophil degranulation in the filter and less endothelial activation [58]. Up to now, this survival benefit had not been confirmed by other studies.

> **Key Messages Citrate**
> - Citrate anticoagulation is first choice anticoagulant for CRRT.
> - The main benefit of citrate anticoagulation for CRRT is that it does not increase the patient's risk of bleeding.
> - Citrate anticoagulation is associated with a less bleeding, less transfusion and longer circuit life than heparin in patients without an increased risk of bleeding.
> - The main limitation of citrate anticoagulation is accumulation, developing in case of hypoperfusion or severe liver dysfunction.
> - Citrate accumulation is associated with a decrease in iCa, a rise in total Ca and increase in total/iCa ratio, metabolic acidosis and an increase in lactate.
> - If the total/iCa ratio is higher than 2.5, continuation of citrate is only safe when acid base balance and ionized calcium concentration are under control. If not, citrate should be reduced or discontinued.

## 15.5	CRRT Without Anticoagulation

Most authors and guidelines recommend the use of some form of anticoagulation to maintain circuit patency during CRRT. This is to minimize blood loss in clotted hemofilters, maximize delivered dose of therapy and reduce nursing workload and complexity of care [55]. It has been shown that frequent hemofilter clotting is associated with more blood transfusions due to blood loss in the discarded hemofilters [59].

One of the major concerns with the use of CRRT is that, in order to maintain the extracorporeal circuit continuously, it usually requires some form of anticoagulation to prevent frequent circuit clotting. Although heparin is the most commonly used anticoagulant, it has been shown to be associated with bleeding complications, especially in high-risk patients receiving CRRT [60].

Because of this, using no anticoagulation is an option to be considered during CRRT in critically ill patients with severe coagulopathy and thrombocytopenia. Interestingly, using CRRT without anticoagulation has been reported more commonly than the use of anticoagulation in some large randomized trials of CRRT. In the NIH ATN trial, 55 % of patients treated with CVVHDF received no anticoagulation while 20 % were anticoagulated with heparin, 20 % received citrate regional anticoagulation and 5 % received other forms of anticoagulation [61]. Over 1,500 patients were treated with CVVHDF in the RENAL study. In that study, 46 % received no anticoagulation while the others received some form of anticoagulation with heparin [62]. This suggests that, despite guidelines suggesting that anticoagulation should be provided, using CRRT without anticoagulation is a default strategy for some prescribing physicians and in some critical care units.

Some studies have shown little difference in CRRT hemofilter survival between circuits with no anticoagulation compared to low dose heparin [1, 63, 64]. In general, hemofilter life is longer with more intensive heparin anticoagulation. It is noteworthy, however, that platelet levels were significantly lower in the group without anticoagulation suggesting consumption in the extracorporeal circuit. While some studies have shown a mean hemofilter life of up to 20 h without anticoagulation, this appears to be population dependent with other studies demonstrating more typical hemofilter survival times of 11–16 h. A study comparing circuit survival with citrate regional anticoagulation or no anticoagulation showed significantly longer CRRT circuit survival with citrate with a mean circuit survival time of 41 h using citrate versus 12 h with no anticoagulation [45]. Despite this, many critical care units find the relative complexity of citrate regional anticoagulation intimidating and prefer to perform CRRT without anticoagulation despite the shorter hemofilter survival.

## 15.6	Non-anticoagulant Measures to Maximize Hemofilter Survival

It is important to consider non-anticoagulant aspects of CRRT circuit management to optimize hemofilter survival, especially if no anticoagulation or low heparin doses are used [29]. The most important of these is to ensure the placement of a large bore

**Table 15.2** Recommended doses of anticoagulants for CRRT

|  | Loading dose | Maintenance dose | Target |
|---|---|---|---|
| Unfractionated heparin | 2,000–5,000 IU | 5–10 IU/kg/h | APTT 1–1.4 times normal |
| Nadroparin, dalteparin | 15–25 IU/kg | 5 IU/kg/h | Anti-Xa 0.25–0.35 IU/ml |
| Enoxaparin | 0.15 mg/kg | 0.05 mg/kg/h | Anti-Xa 0.25–0.35 IU/ml |
| Prostacyclin | None | 3–5 ng/kg/min | |
| Citrate | None | 3–4 mmol/L blood flow | Circuit iCa 0.25 mmol/L |

double lumen central venous hemodialysis catheter in the right jugular or femoral position (straight course) to minimize blood flow interruptions, which promote clotting [64]. It is also important to ensure that the filtration fraction (the proportion of blood flow per minute that is removed as plasma filtrate) is maintained at 25 % or less to avoid hemoconcentration and red blood cell sludging in the hemofilter.

It has been suggested by some authors that delivering replacement fluid in a predilution mode may improve hemofilter life [1, 10, 63], while others show no significant difference [45].

Some CRRT machines incorporate deaeration chambers with a blood/air interface. This tends to encourage clotting but can be prevented by the infusion of at least some or all of the replacement fluid postfilter so that there is an air/replacement fluid/blood interface (Table 15.2).

# References


1. Uchino S, Bellomo R, Morimatsu H, Morgera S, Schetz M, Tan I, et al. Continuous renal replacement therapy: a worldwide practice survey. The beginning and ending supportive therapy for the kidney (B.E.S.T. kidney) investigators. Intensive Care Med. 2007;33(9):1563–70.
2. Garcia DA, Baglin TP, Weitz JI, Samama MM. Parenteral anticoagulants: antithrombotic therapy and prevention of thrombosis, 9th ed: American College of Chest Physicians evidence-based clinical practice guidelines. Chest. 2012;141(2 Suppl):e24S–43S.
3. Singer M, McNally T, Screaton G, Mackie I, Machin S, Cohen SL. Heparin clearance during continuous veno-venous haemofiltration. Intensive Care Med. 1994;20(3):212–5.
4. Despotis GJ, Levine V, Filos KS, Joiner-Maier D, Joist JH. Hemofiltration during cardiopulmonary bypass: the effect on anti-Xa and anti-IIa heparin activity. Anesth Analg. 1997;84(3):479–83.
5. De Waele JJ, Van Cauwenberghe S, Hoste E, Benoit D, Colardyn F. The use of the activated clotting time for monitoring heparin therapy in critically ill patients. Intensive Care Med. 2003;29(2):325–8.
6. Richtrova P, Opatrny Jr K, Vit L, Sefrna F, Perlik R. The AN69 ST haemodialysis membrane under conditions of two different extracorporeal circuit rinse protocols a comparison of thrombogenicity parameters. Nephrol Dial Transplant. 2007;22(10):2978–84.
7. De Pont AC, On behalf of the NVIC Committee Nephrology and Intensive Care. Guidelines for anticoagulation with unfractionated heparin and low molecular weight heparins during continuous venovenous hemofiltration in the intensive care. Neth J Crit Care. 2005;9:308–12.

8. Oudemans-Van Straaten HM, Wester JP, de Pont AC, Schetz MR. Anticoagulation strategies in continuous renal replacement therapy: can the choice be evidence based? Intensive Care Med. 2006;32(2):188–202.

9. Biancofiore G, Esposito M, Bindi L, Stefanini A, Bisa M, Boldrini A, et al. Regional filter heparinization for continuous veno-venous hemofiltration in liver transplant recipients. Minerva Anestesiol. 2003;69(6):527–34; 34–8.

10. van der Voort PH, Gerritsen RT, Kuiper MA, Egbers PH, Kingma WP, Boerma EC. Filter run time in CVVH: pre- versus post-dilution and nadroparin versus regional heparin-protamine anticoagulation. Blood Purif. 2005;23(3):175–80.

11. Fabbri LP, Nucera M, Al Malyan M, Becchi C. Regional anticoagulation and antiaggregation for CVVH in critically ill patients: a prospective, randomized, controlled pilot study. Acta Anaesthesiol Scand. 2010;54(1):92–7.

12. Young E, Podor TJ, Venner T, Hirsh J. Induction of the acute-phase reaction increases heparin-binding proteins in plasma. Arterioscler Thromb Vasc Biol. 1997;17(8):1568–74.

13. Oudemans-Van Straaten HM, van Schilfgaarde M, Molenaar PJ, Wester JP, Leyte A. Hemostasis during low molecular weight heparin anticoagulation for continuous venovenous hemofiltration: a randomized cross-over trial comparing two hemofiltration rates. Crit Care. 2009;13(6):R193.

14. Davenport A. Review article: low-molecular-weight heparin as an alternative anticoagulant to unfractionated heparin for routine outpatient haemodialysis treatments. Nephrology (Carlton). 2009;14(5):455–61.

15. Reeves JH, Cumming AR, Gallagher L, O'Brien JL, Santamaria JD. A controlled trial of low-molecular-weight heparin (dalteparin) versus unfractionated heparin as anticoagulant during continuous venovenous hemodialysis with filtration. Crit Care Med. 1999;27(10):2224–8.

16. de Pont AC, Oudemans-Van Straaten HM, Roozendaal KJ, Zandstra DF. Nadroparin versus dalteparin anticoagulation in high-volume, continuous venovenous hemofiltration: a double-blind, randomized, crossover study. Crit Care Med. 2000;28(2):421–5.

17. Tsang DJ, Tuckfield A, Macisaac CM. Audit of safety and quality of the use of enoxaparin for anticoagulation in continuous renal replacement therapy. Crit Care Resusc. 2011;13(1):24–7.

18. Oudemans-Van Straaten HM, Bosman RJ, Koopmans M, van der Voort PH, Wester JP, van der Spoel JI, et al. Citrate anticoagulation for continuous venovenous hemofiltration. Crit Care Med. 2009;37(2):545–52.

19. Davenport A. Antibodies to heparin-platelet factor 4 complex: pathogenesis, epidemiology, and management of heparin-induced thrombocytopenia in hemodialysis. Am J Kidney Dis. 2009;54(2):361–74.

20. Lee GM, Arepally GM. Diagnosis and management of heparin-induced thrombocytopenia. Hematol Oncol Clin North Am. 2013;27(3):541–63.

21. Keeling D, Davidson S, Watson H. The management of heparin-induced thrombocytopenia. Br J Haematol. 2006;133(3):259–69.

22. Arnold DM, Kukaswadia S, Nazi I, Esmail A, Dewar L, Smith JW, et al. A systematic evaluation of laboratory testing for drug-induced immune thrombocytopenia. J Thromb Haemost. 2013;11(1):169–76.

23. Warkentin TE, Cook DJ. Heparin, low molecular weight heparin, and heparin-induced thrombocytopenia in the ICU. Crit Care Clin. 2005;21(3):513–29.

24. Cuker A, Gimotty PA, Crowther MA, Warkentin TE. Predictive value of the 4Ts scoring system for heparin-induced thrombocytopenia: a systematic review and meta-analysis. Blood. 2012;120(20):4160–7.

25. Kelton JG, Arnold DM, Bates SM. Nonheparin anticoagulants for heparin-induced thrombocytopenia. N Engl J Med. 2013;368(8):737–44.

26. Eichler P, Friesen HJ, Lubenow N, Jaeger B, Greinacher A. Antihirudin antibodies in patients with heparin-induced thrombocytopenia treated with lepirudin: incidence, effects on aPTT, and clinical relevance. Blood. 2000;96(7):2373–8.

27. Scheeren T, Radermacher P. Prostacyclin (PGI2): new aspects of an old substance in the treatment of critically ill patients. Intensive Care Med. 1997;23(2):146–58.

28. Langenecker SA, Felfernig M, Werba A, Mueller CM, Chiari A, Zimpfer M. Anticoagulation with prostacyclin and heparin during continuous venovenous hemofiltration. Crit Care Med. 1994;22(11):1774–81.
29. Camici M, Evangelisti L. Prostacyclin and heparin during haemodialysis: comparative effects. Life Support Syst. 1986;4(3):205–9.
30. Zusman RM, Rubin RH, Cato AE, Cocchetto DM, Crow JW, Tolkoff-Rubin N. Hemodialysis using prostacyclin instead of heparin as the sole antithrombotic agent. N Engl J Med. 1981;304(16):934–9.
31. Davenport A, Will EJ, Davison AM. Comparison of the use of standard heparin and prostacyclin anticoagulation in spontaneous and pump-driven extracorporeal circuits in patients with combined acute renal and hepatic failure. Nephron. 1994;66(4):431–7.
32. Agarwal B, Gatt A, Riddell A, Wright G, Chowdary P, Jalan R, et al. Hemostasis in patients with acute kidney injury secondary to acute liver failure. Kidney Int. 2013;84(1):158–63.
33. Balik M, Waldauf P, Plasil P, Pachl J. Prostacyclin versus citrate in continuous haemodiafiltration: an observational study in patients with high risk of bleeding. Blood Purif. 2005;23(4):325–9.
34. Fiaccadori E, Maggiore U, Rotelli C, Minari M, Melfa L, Cappe G, et al. Continuous haemofiltration in acute renal failure with prostacyclin as the sole anti-haemostatic agent. Intensive Care Med. 2002;28(5):586–93.
35. Calatzis A, Toepfer M, Schramm W, Spannagl M, Schiffl H. Citrate anticoagulation for extracorporeal circuits: effects on whole blood coagulation activation and clot formation. Nephron. 2001;89(2):233–6.
36. Joannidis M, Oudemans-Van Straaten HM. Clinical review: patency of the circuit in continuous renal replacement therapy. Crit Care. 2007;11(4):218.
37. Swartz R, Pasko D, O'Toole J, Starmann B. Improving the delivery of continuous renal replacement therapy using regional citrate anticoagulation. Clin Nephrol. 2004;61(2):134–43.
38. Gupta M, Wadhwa NK, Bukovsky R. Regional citrate anticoagulation for continuous venovenous hemodiafiltration using calcium-containing dialysate. Am J Kidney Dis. 2004;43(1):67–73.
39. Mariano F, Tedeschi L, Morselli M, Stella M, Triolo G. Normal citratemia and metabolic tolerance of citrate anticoagulation for hemodiafiltration in severe septic shock burn patients. Intensive Care Med. 2010;36(10):1735–43.
40. Mehta RL, McDonald BR, Aguilar MM, Ward DM. Regional citrate anticoagulation for continuous arteriovenous hemodialysis in critically ill patients. Kidney Int. 1990;38(5):976–81.
41. Morgera S, Scholle C, Melzer C, Slowinski T, Liefeld L, Baumann G, et al. A simple, safe and effective citrate anticoagulation protocol for the genius dialysis system in acute renal failure. Nephron Clin Pract. 2004;98(1):c35–40.
42. Tolwani AJ, Prendergast MB, Speer RR, Stofan BS, Wille KM. A practical citrate anticoagulation continuous venovenous hemodiafiltration protocol for metabolic control and high solute clearance. Clin J Am Soc Nephrol. 2006;1(1):79–87.
43. Monchi M, Berghmans D, Ledoux D, Canivet JL, Dubois B, Damas P. Citrate vs. heparin for anticoagulation in continuous venovenous hemofiltration: a prospective randomized study. Intensive Care Med. 2004;30(2):260–5.
44. Palsson R, Niles JL. Regional citrate anticoagulation in continuous venovenous hemofiltration in critically ill patients with a high risk of bleeding. Kidney Int. 1999;55(5):1991–7.
45. Nurmohamed SA, Vervloet MG, Girbes AR, Ter Wee PM, Groeneveld AB. Continuous venovenous hemofiltration with or without predilution regional citrate anticoagulation: a prospective study. Blood Purif. 2007;25(4):316–23.
46. Egi M, Naka T, Bellomo R, Cole L, French C, Trethewy C, et al. A comparison of two citrate anticoagulation regimens for continuous veno-venous hemofiltration. Int J Artif Organs. 2005;28(12):1211–8.
47. Brain M, Anderson M, Parkes S, Fowler P. Magnesium flux during continuous venovenous haemodiafiltration with heparin and citrate anticoagulation. Crit Care Resusc. 2012; 14(4):274–82.

48. Schilder L, Azam Nurmohamed SA, Bosch FH, Purmer IM, den Boer SS, Kleppe CG, et al. Citrate anticoagulation versus systemic heparinisation in continuous venovenous hemofiltration in critically ill patients with acute kidney injury: a multi-center randomized clinical trial. Crit Care. 2014;18(4):472.
49. Faybik P, Hetz H, Mitterer G, Krenn CG, Schiefer J, Funk GC, et al. Regional citrate anticoagulation in patients with liver failure supported by a molecular adsorbent recirculating system. Crit Care Med. 2011;39(2):273–9.
50. Bakker AJ, Boerma EC, Keidel H, Kingma P, van der Voort PH. Detection of citrate overdose in critically ill patients on citrate-anticoagulated venovenous haemofiltration: use of ionised and total/ionised calcium. Clin Chem Lab Med. 2006;44(8):962–6.
51. Link A, Klingele M, Speer T, Rbah R, Poss J, Lerner-Graber A, et al. Total-to-ionized calcium ratio predicts mortality in continuous renal replacement therapy with citrate anticoagulation in critically ill patients. Crit Care. 2012;16(3):R97.
52. Hetzel GR, Schmitz M, Wissing H, Ries W, Schott G, Heering PJ, et al. Regional citrate versus systemic heparin for anticoagulation in critically ill patients on continuous venovenous haemofiltration: a prospective randomized multicentre trial. Nephrol Dial Transplant. 2011; 26(1):232–9.
53. Betjes MG, van Oosterom D, van Agteren M, van de Wetering J. Regional citrate versus heparin anticoagulation during venovenous hemofiltration in patients at low risk for bleeding: similar hemofilter survival but significantly less bleeding. J Nephrol. 2007;20(5):602–8.
54. Fealy N, Baldwin I, Johnstone M, Egi M, Bellomo R. A pilot randomized controlled crossover study comparing regional heparinization to regional citrate anticoagulation for continuous venovenous hemofiltration. Int J Artif Organs. 2007;30(4):301–7.
55. Zhang Z, Hongying N. Efficacy and safety of regional citrate anticoagulation in critically ill patients undergoing continuous renal replacement therapy. Intensive Care Med. 2012;38(1):20–8.
56. Liao YJ, Zhang L, Zeng XX, Fu P. Citrate versus unfractionated heparin for anticoagulation in continuous renal replacement therapy. Chin Med J (Engl). 2013;126(7):1344–9.
57. Wu MY, Hsu YH, Bai CH, Lin YF, Wu CH, Tam KW. Regional citrate versus heparin anticoagulation for continuous renal replacement therapy: a meta-analysis of randomized controlled trials. Am J Kidney Dis. 2012;59(6):810–8.
58. Schilder L, Nurmohamed SA, Ter Wee PM, Paauw NJ, Girbes AR, Beishuizen A, et al. Citrate confers less filter-induced complement activation and neutrophil degranulation than heparin when used for anticoagulation during continuous venovenous haemofiltration in critically ill patients. BMC Nephrol. 2014;15(1):19.
59. Cutts MW, Thomas AN, Kishen R. Transfusion requirements during continuous veno-venous haemofiltration: the importance of filter life. Intensive Care Med. 2000;26(11):1694–7.
60. van de Wetering J, Westendorp RG, van der Hoeven JG, Stolk B, Feuth JD, Chang PC. Heparin use in continuous renal replacement procedures: the struggle between filter coagulation and patient hemorrhage. J Am Soc Nephrol. 1996;7(1):145–50.
61. Palevsky PM, Zhang JH, O'Connor TZ, Chertow GM, Crowley ST, Choudhury D, et al. Intensity of renal support in critically ill patients with acute kidney injury. N Engl J Med. 2008;359(1):7–20.
62. Bellomo R, Cass A, Cole L, Finfer S, Gallagher M, Lo S, et al. Intensity of continuous renal-replacement therapy in critically ill patients. N Engl J Med. 2009;361(17):1627–38.
63. Tan HK, Baldwin I, Bellomo R. Continuous veno-venous hemofiltration without anticoagulation in high-risk patients. Intensive Care Med. 2000;26(11):1652–7.
64. Baldwin I, Bellomo R, Koch B. Blood flow reductions during continuous renal replacement therapy and circuit life. Intensive Care Med. 2004;30(11):2074–9.

# Metabolic Aspects of CRRT

# 16

Heleen M. Oudemans-van Straaten, Horng-Ruey Chua, Olivier Joannes-Boyau, and Rinaldo Bellomo

## 16.1 Acidosis

Horng-Ruey Chua and Rinaldo Bellomo

### 16.1.1 Summary

Acidosis is common in patients with AKI in the ICU and often associated with acidemia. It is typically secondary to the accumulation of lactate, chloride and unmeasured anions. Its correction appears desirable and can be more reliably and safely achieved with CRRT. Use of bicarbonate-based fluids is safest as the initial approach. However, lactate- and citrate-buffered fluids can also correct acidosis if appropriately metabolized by the liver and other key organs. CRRT can also be used to correct extreme acidosis in the absence of a major degree of renal impairment. As

H.M. Oudemans-van Straaten (✉)
Department of Intensive Care, VU University Medical Center, Amsterdam, The Netherlands
e-mail: hmoudemans@gmail.com

H.-R. Chua
Division of Nephrology, Department of Medicine, National University Hospital,
Singapore, Singapore

O. Joannes-Boyau
Service d'Anesthésie-Réanimation 2, Centre Hospitalier Universitaire de Bordeaux,
Bordeaux, France
e-mail: Olivier.joannes-boyau@chu-bordeaux.fr

R. Bellomo
Department of Intensive Care, Austin Hospital,
145 Studley Road, Level 2 Austin Tower, Heidelberg, VIC 3084, Australia
e-mail: rinaldo.bellomo@austin.org.au

© Springer International Publishing 2015
H.M. Oudemans-van Straaten et al. (eds.), *Acute Nephrology for the Critical Care Physician*, DOI 10.1007/978-3-319-17389-4_16

CRRT controls volume status easily, it would additionally enable bicarbonate infusion to occur for more rapid correction of acidemia.

In patients with acute kidney injury (AKI), metabolic acidosis is especially common [1]. Although the exact mechanisms of metabolic acidosis in AKI are complex, excess of retained metabolic acids is likely to contribute, together with other general acid–base disorders of critical illness (hyperlactatemia and/or hyperchloremia) [2]. Depending on its severity, correction may require different levels on intervention including renal replacement therapy (RRT) [3].

Both intermittent hemodialysis (IHD) and continuous RRT (CRRT) correct metabolic acidosis. However, the rate and degree of correction differ significantly. CRRT normalizes metabolic acidosis more rapidly and more effectively in the first 24 h. Moreover, IHD is associated with a higher incidence of metabolic acidosis than CRRT during the subsequent treatment period. Accordingly, CRRT is physiologically superior in terms of correction of metabolic acidosis [4]. The plasma concentration of solutes available for ultrafiltration, the composition of the dialysis or replacement fluid, and the rate of ultrafiltration all appear to determine the effect of RRT on acid–base status.

Once CRRT is commenced, even acidemia is typically corrected within 24 h. CRRT appears to correct metabolic acidosis in acute renal failure through its effect on unmeasured anions, phosphate and chloride. Once CRRT is established, it becomes the dominant force in controlling metabolic acid–base status and, in stable patients, it typically results in a degree of metabolic alkalosis [5].

During CRRT, according to conventional acid–base thinking, there is a substantial loss of "buffers." Lactate and bicarbonate have been used as "buffers" during RRT [6, 7]. Citrate has been used as "buffer" and anticoagulation. These "buffers" affect acid–base balance. Bicarbonate has the major advantage of being the physiological buffer and is now the dominant or sole buffer used in CRRT in developed countries. Moreover, lactate, if not metabolized and still present in blood, acts as a strong anion, which would have the same acidifying effect of chloride. Accordingly, iatrogenic hyperlactatemia can cause a metabolic acidosis. The administration of lactate-buffered fluids can induce significant hyperlactatemia and acidosis in patients with liver failure because the metabolic rate is insufficient to meet the additional lactate load.

Citrate has been used for regional anticoagulation. During this procedure, citrate is administered to the circuit before the filter and chelates calcium, thus impeding coagulation. Once citrate enters the circulation, it is metabolized to $CO_2$ and then bicarbonate on a 1:3 basis; thus, 1 mmol of citrate yields 3 mmol of $CO_2$ and then bicarbonate. Under these circumstances, citrate acts as the "buffer" as well as the anticoagulant [8, 9]. Its administration can lead to metabolic alkalosis (up to 25 % of cases). Attention must be paid in patients with liver disease who may not be able to metabolize citrate. In these patients, citrate may accumulate and result in severe ionized hypocalcemia and metabolic acidosis because the citrate anion acts as an unmeasured anion and increases the SIG, which has acidifying effects.

When oxidizable anions are used in the replacement fluids, the anion must be completely oxidized to $CO_2$ and $H_2O$ in order to generate bicarbonate. If the metabolic conversion of non-bicarbonate anions proceeds without accumulation, their buffering capacity is equal to that of bicarbonate. Thus, under most circumstances, the effect on acid–base status depends on the "buffer" concentration rather than on the kind of "buffer" used. The nature and extent of acid–base changes during CRRT is therefore governed by the intensity of plasma water exchange/dialysis, by the "buffer" content of the replacement fluid/dialysate and by the metabolic rate for these anions.

CRRT can be also used to correct severe metabolic acidosis even in the absence of severe acute kidney injury. If the dose of treatment is titrated to achieve such a goal, essentially even the most dramatic metabolic acidosis can be corrected. In addition, because volume can be controlled, if deemed necessary, a bicarbonate infusion can be started at 100–200 mmol/h and the volume removed simultaneously by CRRT. Such an approach can expedite the correction of even the most severe level of acidemia.

**Key Messages**
- Acidosis and/or acidemia are common in critically ill patients with AKI.
- The acidosis of AKI in ICU is complex and involves the accumulation of lactate, chloride and unmeasured anions.
- Correction of acidosis appears desirable and can be achieved with renal replacement therapy.
- CRRT is superior to IHD in correcting metabolic acidosis in critically ill patients with AKI.
- Bicarbonate is the safest buffer to achieve correction of acidosis, but citrate- and lactate-based fluids can also achieve such correction, provided they are correctly and rapidly metabolized.

## 16.2 Electrolyte Management During CRRT

Olivier Joannes-Boyau and Heleen M. Oudemans-van Straaten

### 16.2.1 Summary

Electrolyte balance of CRRT depends on baseline plasma concentrations, the composition of the dialysate or replacement fluids, CRRT dose and type of anticoagulation. Hypokalemia and hypophosphatemia are the most faced electrolyte disturbances during RRT. During citrate CRRT, calcium balance depends on the target plasma ionized calcium concentration of the protocol, but is often negative. Some algorithms provide a zero calcium balance option. During heparin CRRT, calcium balance is generally slightly positive. Magnesium balance is generally negative, more so during citrate than during other anticoagulation, due to the low magnesium concentration of commercial fluids. During CRRT, plasma concentrations of potassium, phosphate, calcium and magnesium should be monitored. Choose replacement fluids with concentrations close to target plasma concentrations or supplement these electrolytes separately.

### 16.2.2 Introduction

Continuous renal replacement therapy (CRRT) is used to support renal function but also to recover homeostasis; electrolyte management is actually a challenge in that case. The electrolyte balance of CRRT depends on baseline plasma concentrations, the composition of the dialysate or replacement fluids, CRRT dose and type of anticoagulation.

### 16.2.3 Potassium and Phosphate

The most common electrolyte disorders observed during CRRT are hypokalemia and hypophosphatemia [10–12]. Due to frequent hyperkalemia in patients with acute kidney injury before start of CRRT, solutions with a low potassium concentration (0–2 mmol/L) are developed. Then, hyperkalemia is rapidly normalized by CRRT. However, after some hours of treatment, hypokalemia occurs. This is more so for phosphate, because most replacement fluids are phosphate-free. Hypophosphatemia can occur early during hemofiltration treatment, especially with higher CRRT dose. Although few disturbances are registered in some studies (in particular with pediatrics patients [11, 13], other electrolytes are correctly regulated, because concentrations in the substitution fluids are close to normal [14, 15].

### 16.2.4 Role of Effluent Volume

There are clearly some differences between the different modalities of RRT treatment in terms of electrolytes removal and acid–base equilibrium. The diffusion principle used in the dialysis mode is more effective for small molecule removal (as electrolytes) than hemofiltration at standard dose (25 ml/kg/h). However, the convection principle used in the hemofiltration mode can remove much more electrolytes when used at high volume (more than 35 ml/kg/h) [16]. However, the most important parameter for electrolyte removal remains the dose of renal replacement (effluent volume). Electrolyte deficiencies are more frequent when high effluent volumes are used [17]. In two large randomized controlled trials comparing low- and high-intensity RRT, more electrolyte imbalances were found in the high-intensity group [2, 3].

## 16.2.5 Intermittent Versus Continuous

Furthermore, continuous techniques are more able to normalize hyperkalemia or hyperphosphatemia than intermittent hemodialysis, but are also more likely to induce electrolyte deficits like hypophosphatemia [9]. Accordingly, CVVH achieves better acid–base balance and electrolyte removal than extended daily dialysis, but can also induce severe hypophosphatemia [18].

The big challenge for the industry is to provide fluids as close as possible to the plasma composition [15, 17].

## 16.2.6 Calcium

The typical calcium concentration of the bicarbonate- and lactate-buffered fluids is about 1.75 mmol/L, substantially higher than the plasma ionized calcium concentration, which is the amount accessible for filtration or dialysis. Thus, calcium balance during conventional CRRT is generally slightly positive (about 5–12 mmol/day) [19, 20]. However, during citrate CRRT, calcium handling is different and calcium balance of many protocols is negative [19, 20]. Most fluids used for citrate CRRT are calcium-free and calcium is generally replaced by separate infusion. For calcium replacement, each protocol has its own ionized plasma calcium target, ranging between 1.0 and 1.35 mmol/L. Especially with lower plasma calcium targets, calcium balance is negative, 12–96 mmol/day is reported [19, 20]. Of note, a negative calcium balance does not necessarily cause systemic hypocalcemia, due to a rapid parathormone response, which leads to unwanted calcium release from bone [21]. Targeting a higher plasma calcium concentration seems to suppress PTH release, which may limit calcium mobilization from bone. However, PTH measurements in critically ill patients should be interpreted with caution, because the normal assay measures oxidized PTH as well, which is biologically inactive [22]. Some modern CRRT devices incorporate an algorithm with a 100 % calcium compensation option, which seems attractive. Up to now, optimal calcium targets are not known. Hypocalcemia is common in patients with sepsis, and it is not known whether correction is beneficial [23]. However, a prolonged negative calcium balance for days should likely be avoided.

## 16.2.7 Magnesium

Magnesium balance during CRRT has gained little attention. The typical magnesium concentration of commercial CRRT fluids is about 0.5 mmol/L, while high normal or increased magnesium concentrations are targeted in ICU patients to prevent arrhythmias, promote vasodilatation and anti-inflammatory and anti-oxidant defense [24]. When using these fluids, mean magnesium balance during CVVHDF was −17 mmol/day in heparin circuits and −26 mmol/day in circuits anticoagulated with citrate [25]. Apart from calcium, citrate chelates magnesium, explaining the higher magnesium loss during citrate CRRT in this study. Hypomagnesemia is reported by others as well [26] and is even associated with non-recovery of renal function [27]. Given the important role of magnesium during critical illness, additional magnesium should be supplemented, the amount depending on the fluids in use, the local CRRT protocol and the plasma magnesium concentration.

### 16.2.8 Monitoring of Electrolytes During CRRT

Standard electrolyte monitoring should include potassium (two to four times daily), phosphate and magnesium (twice daily), total calcium (once daily) and ionized calcium (four times daily during citrate anticoagulation). See also the chapter on citrate anticoagulation.

> **Key Messages**
> - Electrolyte balance of CRRT depends on baseline plasma concentrations, the composition of the dialysate or replacement fluids, CRRT dose and type of anticoagulation.
> - Hypokalemia and hypophosphatemia are the most faced electrolyte disturbances during RRT.
> - During citrate CRRT, calcium balance depends on the target plasma ionized calcium concentration of the protocol, but is often negative. Some algorithms provide a zero calcium balance option.
> - During heparin CRRT, calcium balance is generally slightly positive.
> - Magnesium balance is generally negative, more so during citrate than during other anticoagulation, due to the low magnesium concentration of commercial fluids.
> - Choose replacement fluids with concentrations close to target plasma concentrations or supplement these electrolytes separately.

## 16.3    Nutrition and Micronutrients

Horng-Ruey Chua and Rinaldo Bellomo

### 16.3.1 Summary

In patients receiving renal replacement therapy, enteral nutrition is preferred. Specific so-called renal feeding preparations are not needed. The dose of protein should be between 1 and 1.5 g/kg/day. Energy provision should likely be between 20 and 25 kcal/kg/day. Amino acid loss through the filter accounts for 10–20 % of administered protein. Water soluble vitamins are lost and should be replaced. Lipid soluble vitamins are not lost and do not require regular replacement. Some trace elements are lost and regular trace element administration seems prudent. However, all recommendations regarding nutrition in these patients are based on weak evidence.

## 16.3.2 General Recommendations

The preferred mode of nutritional support in critical illness is early enteral nutrition (EN) [28, 29]. In the absence of more definite evidence, CRRT patients should receive EN within 24–48 h following admission titrated to gut tolerance. EN is preferred to parenteral nutrition (PN) because of its safety, low cost, and its physiological route and hormonal signalling. The role of supplemental PN in CRRT patients is unknown.

The target goal of nutrition remains ill defined. Providing 20–35 kcal/kg/day of calories with 1.5–1.8 g/kg/day of protein in patients with AKI on CRRT appears to allow a reasonable balance between protein catabolism and nitrogen balance [30]. This empirical caloric amount seems consistent with calculated requirements [31]. Due to water soluble vitamin losses, it seems prudent to administer water soluble vitamins daily or second daily. As some trace elements are also lost, it seems prudent to administer trace elements daily or second daily.

These recommendations for CRRT patients are based on clinical observational studies, small studies with physiological outcomes and physiological reasoning. They are low-level recommendations (level C) and open to challenge. Such lack of evidence suggests the need for level 1 studies in this field.

## 16.3.3 Protein

The optimal protein intake is unclear, and the flexibility of adjusting intake is limited by the composition in standard enteral formulas. For example, Isosource® 1.5 cal (Nestle) contains 1.5 kcal/ml of calories and 67.6 g of protein per litre. Intake of 30 kcal/kg/day only delivers 1.4 g/kg/day of protein. Higher protein intake of 2.5 g/kg/day results in a near positive or positive nitrogen balance and offers the only active measure to reduce the negative nitrogen balance so commonly seen in these patients [32, 33]. A positive nitrogen balance is associated with improved patient survival in critical illness, but improved survival is not a direct effect of increased protein intake [31]. However, there may be a dose-related association between increased protein intake and clinically significant improvement in renal function in critically ill patients [34]. Supplemental PN does not lead to improved clinical outcomes [35] and, if given early, may lead to clinical problems [36]. There is no evidence that specific administration of essential AA in preference to general AA preparations leads to any improved clinical outcomes.

## 16.3.4 Amino Acids (AA)

The molecular weights of proteins range from 55 to 220 kDa, well above the cut-off of standard CRRT membranes, while that of AA is only 110 Da (75–204 Da). AA loss during CRRT has been studied mostly in the context of total parenteral nutrition (PN).

Most AA have a high sieving coefficient (easily filtered) of near 1.0, such as cysteine, arginine, alanine and glutamine, except for glutamic acid (0.25–0.5) [37–39]. AA clearances range from 20 to 45 ml/min in patients on CRRT [40], as compared to about 200 ml/min in patients with AKI on intermittent hemodialysis [41]. In general AA loss represents about 11–12 % of total (parenteral) protein intake. The amount of AA lost in each patient depends on the intensity of CRRT but also in great part on AA blood levels, which in turn depend on the amount administered and route of administration.

Protein intake of more than 1.5 g/kg/day is associated with AA loss of about 12 g/day [39], and AA loss seems less with lower protein intake [41]. AA losses can account for 5 % to a substantial 20 % of daily AA intake [37–39, 41]. Individual blood AA levels correlate well to corresponding losses in CRRT [41], and overall AA loss is higher with higher intensity of treatment [37]. In addition, there is selectivity in individual AA losses, with glutamine and alanine being lost in greater absolute amounts [39, 41], and tyrosine having the highest fractional loss per intake [37]. All three are non-essential AA under normal physiological states.

Total nitrogen loss in CRRT is about 25 g/day [38, 39]—the vast majority of which is due to urea nitrogen with 10–20 % (2–5 g/day) contributed by AA nitrogen loss [37–39]—while the rest is likely from protein catabolism; this results in a negative nitrogen balance. Intermittent hemodialysis has been reported to lead to losses of 6–8 g/session [17].

## 16.3.5 Lipids

Effluent samples in CRRT are lipid free, with trace amounts of cholesterol and triglycerides detectable, and there is no arteriovenous gradient for lipids across the hemodiafilter to suggest membrane adsorption. Lipid homeostasis is not significantly affected by CRRT and lipid soluble vitamins are not lost.

## 16.3.6 Vitamins and Trace Elements

These micronutrients have important wound healing, immunomodulatory and antioxidant effects in critical illness [42]. There is observational evidence that during CRRT, water soluble vitamins are lost, especially vitamin C and folic acid [43].

In patients on CRRT, blood levels of vitamins C and E, zinc and selenium are lower, while that of chromium is higher, than healthy controls and normal reference ranges. Low vitamin levels might be associated with increased oxidative utilization in critical illness, and higher chromium might reflect its dependence on renal excretion [42]. Hours to days of CRRT can reduce blood levels of folate, pyridoxine-5′-phosphate (P-5′-P, an important moiety of vitamin B6), zinc and selenium significantly [44].

Losses of micronutrients enough to cause significant decrease in blood levels or large fractional losses of usual intake include vitamins C, B1, B6 (P-5′-P), folate, chromium and selenium. Specifically, about 68 mg/day of vitamin C, 0.3 mg/day of folate and 4 mg/day of vitamin B1 (thiamine) are lost [42, 44, 45]. More than twice the daily supplementation of vitamin B1 and selenium can be lost. Zinc, however, is present in some citrate preparations and replacement fluids, which may instead result in a net gain [42, 44, 45]. The effect of intensity and mode of CRRT on these losses are unclear.

> **Key Messages**
> - It is unclear whether patients receiving renal replacement therapy should receive a nutritional regimen different from that of other critically ill patients.
> - However, due to amino acid losses of 10–20 % of administered dose and due to water soluble and trace element losses, appropriate adjustments (protein intake of 1–1.5 g/kg/day and regular vitamin and trace element supplementation) seem prudent.

## 16.4 Energy Balance of CRRT

Heleen M. Oudemans-van Straaten

### 16.4.1 Summary

Potential sources of energy gain by CRRT consist of glucose and lactate, and less so of citrate, while energy can be lost by the removal of glucose and amino acids. Net energetic gain is equivalent to the net amount infused or diffused (which depends on the composition of the fluids) minus the amount removed by CRRT. Sieving coefficients are close to one and caloric equivalents per mmol are 0.73 kcal (3.06 kJ) for glucose, 0.33 kcal (1.37 kJ) for lactate, 0.59 kcal (2.48 kJ) for citrate and about 4.5 kcal/g for amino acids. Energy delivery by lactate can mount to 600 kcal/day and by glucose to 950 kcal/day. The clinical consequences remain unknown; however, clinicians should be aware of the energy balance of their CRRT modality and adjust nutritional intake and insulin dose when necessary.

### 16.4.2 Introduction

Potential sources of energy gain by CRRT consist of glucose, lactate and citrate, while energy can be lost by the removal of glucose and amino acids. Net energetic gain is equivalent to the net amount infused or diffused (which depends on the composition of the fluids) minus the amount removed by CRRT [46–48]. Sieving coefficients are close to one [48–50] and caloric equivalents per mmol are 0.73 kcal

(3.06 kJ) for glucose, 0.33 kcal (1.37 kJ) for lactate and 0.59 kcal (2.48 kJ) for citrate. The caloric equivalent of amino acids largely varies among individual amino acids and their metabolic pathway, but is about 4.5 kcal/g on average [51].

### 16.4.3 Glucose

CRRT can confer either a net loss or net gain of glucose. Glucose balance depends on glucose concentration in plasma, replacement fluid and/or dialysate. Glucose concentration in most modern solutions is 5.5 mmol/L (100 mg/dl). With tight glucose control, glucose balance will be about zero. However, if plasma glucose concentration are higher, 7.7–10 mmol/L (140–180 mg/dl), the net caloric loss per day will be about 70–160 kcal (290–669 kJ) for a CRRT dose of 2 L/h. Of note, some older lactate solutions contain 11–14 mmol glucose per litre, increasing the caloric load of lactate replacement. Finally, the use of acid citrate dextrose (ACD-A) as citrate source, which contains 139 mmol glucose per litre, can convey about 550 kcal (2,400 kJ) glucose per day during 2 L/h CVVHD and 950 kcal glucose/day (4,200 kJ) during 2 L/h postdilution CVVH to the patient [46–48].

### 16.4.4 Lactate

When lactate is used as buffer, a considerable amount of energy is delivered to the patient [47, 52]. Assuming a lactate concentration in the replacement fluid of 40 mmol/L, a plasma lactate of 2 mmol/L and a CRRT dose of 2,000 ml/h, the patient receives about 602 kcal/day (2,518 kJ/day) from the lactate replacement. Furthermore, additional glucose is delivered with use of lactate solutions containing high glucose concentrations (see above).

### 16.4.5 Citrate

The dose of citrate infused depends on blood flow and target citrate concentration in the filter. Because hemodialysis is feasible at a lower blood flow for a similar CRRT dose, citrate infusion rate is lower and fractional citrate removal greater. Thus, less citrate enters the patient during hemodialysis compared to hemofiltration [53]. Total daily energy delivered by citrate during 24 h of CRRT at an assumed dose of 2 L/h varies between 200 and 350 kcal [46, 47]. However, when using a citrate dextrose solution (ACD-A) as citrate source [50, 54, 55], a substantial glucose load is delivered as well (see above).

### 16.4.6 Amino Acids

The energetic equivalent of an estimated daily loss of amino acids of 12 g/day [39] is small (54 kcal/226 kJ/day) (see also the paragraph on amino acids).

## 16.4.7 Consequences of the Caloric Balance

Depending on the modality, the caloric balance of CRRT may be positive or negative. When using citrate anticoagulation or lactate replacement, the balance is positive. Both citrate and lactate are easy fuel under stress [56–60]. Neither rely on insulin to enter the cell. Citrate enters cells directly, whereas lactate enters after oxidation to pyruvate, maintaining mitochondrial redox state under condition of hypoxia or limited substrate availability for the Krebs cycle and providing intermediates for amino acid and lipid synthesis [61, 62]. Lactate additionally enters the gluconeogenesis pathway to be metabolized to glucose and thereby increasing insulin requirements [52]. Of note, lactate delivery during CCRT may surpass the patient's metabolic capacity if metabolism is compromised in case of hypoperfusion or liver dysfunction. If lactate replacement is changed into bicarbonate, then energetic delivery abruptly falls and hypoglycaemia may ensue when insulin dose is not adjusted.

Glucose balance can be positive or negative, depending on the glucose concentration of the replacement/dialysate fluids (5.6–14 mmol/L), the use of ACD-A as citrate source (139 mmol/L) and actual glucose concentration in plasma [48]. Use of ACD-A as citrate source poses an unnecessary strain on carbohydrate metabolism, especially when used in combination with lactate-buffered replacement fluids [47].

The clinical consequences of all these bioenergetics remain unknown. Clinicians should be aware of the energy balance of their CRRT modality and adjust nutritional intake and insulin dose when necessary.

> **Key Messages**
> - Depending on the modality, the caloric balance of CRRT may positive or negative.
> - Potential sources of energy gain consist of glucose, lactate and citrate, while energy can be lost by the net removal of glucose and amino acids.
> - Glucose balance depends on the difference between the glucose concentration in plasma and replacement fluid and/or dialysate.
> - When using ACD-A as citrate source, an unintended glucose load is delivered as well (550–950 kcal/day).
> - The use of lactate-buffered solutions can provide an energy delivery of about 600 kcal/day.

## References


1. Naka T, Bellomo R. Bench-to-bedside review: treating acid-base abnormalities in the intensive care unit–the role of renal replacement therapy. Crit Care. 2004;8(2):108–14.
2. Rocktaschel J, Morimatsu H, Uchino S, Ronco C, Bellomo R. Impact of continuous venovenous hemofiltration on acid-base balance. Int J Artif Organs. 2003;26(1):19–25.
3. Hilton PJ, Taylor J, Forni LG, Treacher DF. Bicarbonate-based haemofiltration in the management of acute renal failure with lactic acidosis. QJM. 1998;91(4):279–83.

4. Uchino S, Bellomo R, Ronco C. Intermittent versus continuous renal replacement therapy in the ICU: impact on electrolyte and acid-base balance. Intensive Care Med. 2001;27(6):1037–43.
5. Demirjian S, Teo BW, Paganini EP. Alkalemia during continuous renal replacement therapy and mortality in critically ill patients. Crit Care Med. 2008;36(5):1513–7.
6. Tan HK, Uchino S, Bellomo R. The acid-base effects of continuous hemofiltration with lactate or bicarbonate buffered replacement fluids. Int J Artif Organs. 2003;26(6):477–83.
7. Morgera S, Heering P, Szentandrasi T, Manassa E, Heintzen M, Willers R, et al. Comparison of a lactate-versus acetate-based hemofiltration replacement fluid in patients with acute renal failure. Ren Fail. 1997;19(1):155–64.
8. Mehta RL, McDonald BR, Aguilar MM, Ward DM. Regional citrate anticoagulation for continuous arteriovenous hemodialysis in critically ill patients. Kidney Int. 1990;38(5): 976–81.
9. Oudemans-Van Straaten HM, Kellum JA, Bellomo R. Clinical review: anticoagulation for continuous renal replacement therapy–heparin or citrate? Crit Care. 2011;15(1):202.
10. Bellomo R, Cass A, Cole L, Finfer S, Gallagher M, Lo S, et al. Intensity of continuous renal-replacement therapy in critically ill patients. N Engl J Med. 2009;361(17):1627–38.
11. Santiago MJ, Lopez-Herce J, Urbano J, Solana MJ, del Castillo J, Ballestero Y, et al. Complications of continuous renal replacement therapy in critically ill children: a prospective observational evaluation study. Crit Care. 2009;13(6):R184.
12. Palevsky PM, Zhang JH, O'Connor TZ, Chertow GM, Crowley ST, Choudhury D, et al. Intensity of renal support in critically ill patients with acute kidney injury. N Engl J Med. 2008;359(1):7–20.
13. Tan HK, Uchino S, Bellomo R. Electrolyte mass balance during CVVH: lactate vs. bicarbonate-buffered replacement fluids. Ren Fail. 2004;26(2):149–53.
14. Honore PM, Joannes-Boyau O. High volume hemofiltration (HVHF) in sepsis: a comprehensive review of rationale, clinical applicability, potential indications and recommendations for future research. Int J Artif Organs. 2004;27(12):1077–82.
15. Aucella F, Di PS, Gesualdo L. Dialysate and replacement fluid composition for CRRT. Contrib Nephrol. 2007;156:287–96.
16. Joannes-Boyau O, Honore PM, Perez P, Bagshaw SM, Grand H, Canivet JL, et al. High-volume versus standard-volume haemofiltration for septic shock patients with acute kidney injury (IVOIRE study): a multicentre randomized controlled trial. Intensive Care Med. 2013;39(9):1535–46.
17. Davenport A. Potential adverse effects of replacing high volume hemofiltration exchanges on electrolyte balance and acid-base status using the current commercially available replacement solutions in patients with acute renal failure. Int J Artif Organs. 2008;31(1):3–5.
18. Baldwin I, Naka T, Koch B, Fealy N, Bellomo R. A pilot randomised controlled comparison of continuous veno-venous haemofiltration and extended daily dialysis with filtration: effect on small solutes and acid-base balance. Intensive Care Med. 2007;33(5):830–5.
19. van der Voort PH, Postma SR, Kingma WP, Boerma EC, de Heide LJ, Bakker AJ. An observational study on the effects of nadroparin-based and citrate-based continuous venovenous hemofiltration on calcium metabolism. Blood Purif. 2007;25(3):267–73.
20. Brain M, Parkes S, Fowler P, Robertson I, Brown A. Calcium flux in continuous venovenous haemodiafiltration with heparin and citrate anticoagulation. Crit Care Resusc. 2011;13(2):72–81.
21. Wang PL, Meyer MM, Orloff SL, Anderson S. Bone resorption and "relative" immobilization hypercalcemia with prolonged continuous renal replacement therapy and citrate anticoagulation. Am J Kidney Dis. 2004;44(6):1110–4.
22. Raimundo M, Crichton S, Lei K, Sanderson B, Smith J, Brooks J, et al. Maintaining normal levels of ionized calcium during citrate-based renal replacement therapy is associated with stable parathyroid hormone levels. Nephron Clin Pract. 2013;124(1–2):124–31.
23. Lind L, Carlstedt F, Rastad J, Stiernstrom H, Stridsberg M, Ljunggren O, et al. Hypocalcemia and parathyroid hormone secretion in critically ill patients. Crit Care Med. 2000;28(1):93–9.

24. Weglicki WB. Hypomagnesemia and inflammation: clinical and basic aspects. Annu Rev Nutr. 2012;32:55–71.
25. Brain M, Anderson M, Parkes S, Fowler P. Magnesium flux during continuous venovenous haemodiafiltration with heparin and citrate anticoagulation. Crit Care Resusc. 2012;14(4):274–82.
26. Morimatsu H, Uchino S, Bellomo R, Ronco C. Continuous veno-venous hemodiafiltration or hemofiltration: impact on calcium, phosphate and magnesium concentrations. Int J Artif Organs. 2002;25(6):512–9.
27. Alves SC, Tomasi CD, Constantino L, Giombelli V, Candal R, Bristot MD, et al. Hypomagnesemia as a risk factor for the non-recovery of the renal function in critically ill patients with acute kidney injury. Nephrol Dial Transplant. 2013;28:910–6.
28. McClave SA, Martindale RG, Vanek VW, McCarthy M, Roberts P, Taylor B, et al. Guidelines for the provision and assessment of nutrition support therapy in the adult critically ill patient: Society of Critical Care Medicine (SCCM) and American Society for Parenteral and Enteral Nutrition (A.S.P.E.N.). JPEN J Parenter Enteral Nutr. 2009;33(3):277–316.
29. Kreymann KG, Berger MM, Deutz NE, Hiesmayr M, Jolliet P, Kazandjiev G, et al. ESPEN guidelines on enteral nutrition: intensive care. Clin Nutr. 2006;25(2):210–23.
30. Macias WL, Alaka KJ, Murphy MH, Miller ME, Clark WR, Mueller BA. Impact of the nutritional regimen on protein catabolism and nitrogen balance in patients with acute renal failure. JPEN J Parenter Enteral Nutr. 1996;20(1):56–62.
31. Scheinkestel CD, Kar L, Marshall K, Bailey M, Davies A, Nyulasi I, et al. Prospective randomized trial to assess caloric and protein needs of critically Ill, anuric, ventilated patients requiring continuous renal replacement therapy. Nutrition. 2003;19(11–12):909–16.
32. Bellomo R, Tan HK, Bhonagiri S, Gopal I, Seacombe J, Daskalakis M, et al. High protein intake during continuous hemodiafiltration: impact on amino acids and nitrogen balance. Int J Artif Organs. 2002;25(4):261–8.
33. Scheinkestel CD, Adams F, Mahony L, Bailey M, Davies AR, Nyulasi I, et al. Impact of increasing parenteral protein loads on amino acid levels and balance in critically ill anuric patients on continuous renal replacement therapy. Nutrition. 2003;19(9):733–40.
34. Doig GS, Simpson F, Finfer S, Delaney A, Davies AR, Mitchell I, et al. Effect of evidence-based feeding guidelines on mortality of critically ill adults: a cluster randomized controlled trial. JAMA. 2008;300(23):2731–41.
35. Kutsogiannis J, Alberda C, Gramlich L, Cahill NE, Wang M, Day AG, et al. Early use of supplemental parenteral nutrition in critically ill patients: results of an international multicenter observational study. Crit Care Med. 2011;39(12):2691–9.
36. Casaer MP, Mesotten D, Hermans G, Wouters PJ, Schetz M, Meyfroidt G, et al. Early versus late parenteral nutrition in critically ill adults. N Engl J Med. 2011;365(6):506–17.
37. Davies SP, Reaveley DA, Brown EA, Kox WJ. Amino acid clearances and daily losses in patients with acute renal failure treated by continuous arteriovenous hemodialysis. Crit Care Med. 1991;19(12):1510–5.
38. Novak I, Sramek V, Pittrova H, Rusavy P, Lacigova S, Eiselt M, et al. Glutamine and other amino acid losses during continuous venovenous hemodiafiltration. Artif Organs. 1997;21(5):359–63.
39. Maxvold NJ, Smoyer WE, Custer JR, Bunchman TE. Amino acid loss and nitrogen balance in critically ill children with acute renal failure: a prospective comparison between classic hemofiltration and hemofiltration with dialysis. Crit Care Med. 2000;28(4):1161–5.
40. Kihara M, Ikeda Y, Fujita H, Miura M, Masumori S, Tamura K, et al. Amino acid losses and nitrogen balance during slow diurnal hemodialysis in critically ill patients with renal failure. Intensive Care Med. 1997;23(1):110–3.
41. Chua HR, Baldwin I, Fealy N, Naka T, Bellomo R. Amino acid balance with extended daily diafiltration in acute kidney injury. Blood Purif. 2012;33(4):292–9.
42. Berger MM, Shenkin A, Revelly JP, Roberts E, Cayeux MC, Baines M, et al. Copper, selenium, zinc, and thiamine balances during continuous venovenous hemodiafiltration in critically ill patients. Am J Clin Nutr. 2004;80(2):410–6.

43. Story DA, Ronco C, Bellomo R. Trace element and vitamin concentrations and losses in critically ill patients treated with continuous venovenous hemofiltration. Crit Care Med. 1999;27(1):220–3.
44. Fortin MC, Amyot SL, Geadah D, Leblanc M. Serum concentrations and clearances of folic acid and pyridoxal-5-phosphate during venovenous continuous renal replacement therapy. Intensive Care Med. 1999;25(6):594–8.
45. Klein CJ, Moser-Veillon PB, Schweitzer A, Douglass LW, Reynolds HN, Patterson KY, et al. Magnesium, calcium, zinc, and nitrogen loss in trauma patients during continuous renal replacement therapy. JPEN J Parenter Enteral Nutr. 2002;26(2):77–92.
46. Oudemans-Van Straaten HM, Ostermann M. Bench-to-bedside review: Citrate for continuous renal replacement therapy, from science to practice. Crit Care. 2012;16(6):249.
47. Balik M, Zakharchenko M, Leden P, Otahal M, Hruby J, Polak F, et al. Bioenergetic gain of citrate anticoagulated continuous hemodiafiltration-a comparison between 2 citrate modalities and unfractionated heparin. J Crit Care. 2013;28(1):87–95.
48. Stevenson JM, Heung M, Vilay AM, Eyler RF, Patel C, Mueller BA. In vitro glucose kinetics during continuous renal replacement therapy: implications for caloric balance in critically ill patients. Int J Artif Organs. 2013;36(12):861–8.
49. Chadha V, Garg U, Warady BA, Alon US. Citrate clearance in children receiving continuous venovenous renal replacement therapy. Pediatr Nephrol. 2002;17(10):819–24.
50. Mariano F, Morselli M, Bergamo D, Hollo Z, Scella S, Maio M, et al. Blood and ultrafiltrate dosage of citrate as a useful and routine tool during continuous venovenous haemodiafiltration in septic shock patients. Nephrol Dial Transplant. 2011;26(12):3882–8.
51. May ME, Hill JO. Energy content of diets of variable amino acid composition. Am J Clin Nutr. 1990;52(5):770–6.
52. Bollmann MD, Revelly JP, Tappy L, Berger MM, Schaller MD, Cayeux MC, et al. Effect of bicarbonate and lactate buffer on glucose and lactate metabolism during hemodiafiltration in patients with multiple organ failure. Intensive Care Med. 2004;30(6):1103–10.
53. Mariano F, Tedeschi L, Morselli M, Stella M, Triolo G. Normal citratemia and metabolic tolerance of citrate anticoagulation for hemodiafiltration in severe septic shock burn patients. Intensive Care Med. 2010;36(10):1735–43.
54. Swartz R, Pasko D, O'Toole J, Starmann B. Improving the delivery of continuous renal replacement therapy using regional citrate anticoagulation. Clin Nephrol. 2004;61(2):134–43.
55. Gupta M, Wadhwa NK, Bukovsky R. Regional citrate anticoagulation for continuous venovenous hemodiafiltration using calcium-containing dialysate. Am J Kidney Dis. 2004;43(1):67–73.
56. Chatham JC, Des RC, Forder JR. Evidence of separate pathways for lactate uptake and release by the perfused rat heart. Am J Physiol Endocrinol Metab. 2001;281(4):E794–802.
57. Mazer CD, Stanley WC, Hickey RF, Neese RA, Cason BA, Demas KA, et al. Myocardial metabolism during hypoxia: maintained lactate oxidation during increased glycolysis. Metabolism. 1990;39(9):913–8.
58. Kline JA, Thornton LR, Lopaschuk GD, Barbee RW, Watts JA. Lactate improves cardiac efficiency after hemorrhagic shock. Shock. 2000;14(2):215–21.
59. Levy B, Mansart A, Montemont C, Gibot S, Mallie JP, Regnault V, et al. Myocardial lactate deprivation is associated with decreased cardiovascular performance, decreased myocardial energetics, and early death in endotoxic shock. Intensive Care Med. 2007;33(3):495–502.
60. Leverve XM, Boon C, Hakim T, Anwar M, Siregar E, Mustafa I. Half-molar sodium-lactate solution has a beneficial effect in patients after coronary artery bypass grafting. Intensive Care Med. 2008;34(10):1796–803.
61. Vary TC, Hazen S. Sepsis alters pyruvate dehydrogenase kinase activity in skeletal muscle. Mol Cell Biochem. 1999;198(1–2):113–8.
62. Owen OE, Kalhan SC, Hanson RW. The key role of anaplerosis and cataplerosis for citric acid cycle function. J Biol Chem. 2002;277(34):30409–12.

# Continuous Renal Replacement Therapy in Sepsis: Should We Use High Volume or Specific Membranes?

17

Patrick M. Honore, Rita Jacobs, and Herbert D. Spapen

## 17.1 Introduction

Until recently, research on continuous renal replacement therapy (CRRT) in sepsis and systemic inflammatory response syndrome (SIRS) essentially focused on CRRT dose. However, some unconvincing and equivocal study results [1, 2] showing no benefit of a higher dose, tempered enthusiasm and incited to explore other treatment modalities to increase inflammatory mediator removal. Among those, the type of dialysis membrane used for CRRT gained considerable interest.

Many different dialysis membranes have indeed been marketed. Moreover, high cut-off membranes [3], highly adsorptive membranes, either non-selective [4] or semi-selective, enabling for instance to capture endotoxin [5], were specifically designed for the treatment of patients with sepsis and SIRS. A major advantage of these membranes is that they combine classic blood purging and anti-inflammatory capacities. Some membranes have been coated with antibiotics (e.g. polymyxin (PMX) B) [6]. Such membrane allows almost selective endotoxin adsorption but can only run in hemoperfusion mode.

Under specific manufacturing conditions, heparin is adsorbed passively or actively on the membrane surface [7]. Such heparin-soaked membranes can adequately capture mediators but are essentially developed for use in conditions that preclude systemic anticoagulation. Finally, sorbents will be discussed which are novel membranes structured in a cartridge exhibiting unselective or selective adsorption potential [7].

P.M. Honore, MD, PhD, FCCM (✉)
ICU Department, Universitair Ziekenhuis Brussel, Vrije Universitieit Brussel (VUB), 101, Laarbeeklaan, Jette, Brussels 1090, Belgium
e-mail: Patrick.Honore@uzbrussel.be

R. Jacobs, MD • H.D. Spapen, MD, PhD, FCCM
ICU Department, Universitair Ziekenhuis Brussel, Vrije Universitieit Brussel (VUB), Brussels, Belgium

## 17.2 High-Volume Hemofiltration

Until recently, high-volume hemofiltration (HVHF) was positioned as adjunctive treatment for septic shock complicated by acute kidney injury (AKI). Evidence for its use came from prospective interventional [8, 9] and small randomized studies [10], which showed an early significant hemodynamic benefit and faster weaning from inotropic support [11]. HVHF also reduced organ failure and ICU length of stay in some but not in all studies [8–11]. Finally, a survival benefit was suggested in cohort studies comparing observed with expected mortality [8, 9] but never confirmed in prospective randomized controlled studies [10, 12, 13].

The rationale behind the HVHF-related clinical effects in sepsis is not fully understood and has never been shouldered by mechanistic trials [14, 15]. Initially, "blood purification" was thought to help restoring immune homeostasis by attenuating the overwhelming systemic expression of pro- and anti-inflammatory mediators. Multiple mediators take part in this inflammatory response, often acting through complex and intertwined pathways [16]. Through the years, all attempts to modulate the inflammatory cascade by targeting one single component have failed [17]. Thus, non-specific removal of a wide array of inflammatory substances and microbial toxins seemed to be a logical step. Recently, new concepts to underpin the beneficial effects of blood purifying techniques have been proposed. First, Ronco and colleagues [18] hypothesized that preventing the cytokine burst during the early phase of sepsis might interrupt the inflammatory cascade and cause less endothelial, tissue, and organ damage. Second, Honoré and Matson [19] proposed the "threshold immunomodulation hypothesis." They postulated that removal of cytokines from the blood compartment would diminish tissue cytokine content due to an equilibration of cytokine concentrations between the two compartments. This theory explains why blood purifying techniques might improve outcome while leaving cytokine blood concentrations unmodified. Third, Di Carlo and Alexander [20] proposed the "mediator delivery hypothesis." Here, HVHF is thought to increase lymphatic flow because of the high amount of crystalloids used as replacement fluid. Inflammatory mediators are continuously dragged toward the blood compartment and subsequently removed [21]. Finally, Peng and colleagues [22] recently suggested that hemoadsorption or HVHF may directly act at cellular level and restore immune function through regulation or "reprogramming" of monocytes, neutrophils, and lymphocytes. However, the mechanism by which hemoadsorption interacts with HLA-DR expression remains unknown. Also, if this "cellular" theory is confirmed, blood purification would not be confined solely to the early phase of septic shock. Removal of mediators from plasma will restore their concentration gradient between plasma and infected tissues [22]. Because this gradient determines leukocyte tracking and bacterial clearance [22], a "cytokinetic concept" better explains the association between high cytokine levels and mortality than a cytotoxic model [22].

An important drawback of HVHF is that dose and duration are not unequivocally defined. Indeed, doses range from pulsed [8, 9, 23] to very high (up to 120 ml/kg/h) quantities and duration from very short [8] to extended (up to 8 h) periods. Moreover, performing continuous HVHF is recommended at doses of 50–70 ml/kg/h for at least 4 consecutive days [12, 13]. Actually, the most convenient definition was provided at the 2007 consensus conference in Pardubice [24–26]. Honoré and colleagues agreed that continuous HVHF should imply a 24-h high-volume (50–70 ml/kg/h) treatment and intermittent HVHF a 4- to 8-h very-high-volume (100–120 ml/kg/h) treatment, followed by conventional continuous veno-venous hemofiltration. In accordance with this definition, two large randomized HVHF trials were conducted [12, 13]. In the IVOIRE trial [12], 140 septic shock patients with AKI requiring CRRT were randomized toward receiving a dose of either 35 or 70 ml/kg/h for 4 consecutive days. The filter was systematically changed after 48 h. Delivered dose exceeded 95 % of the prescribed dose. Mortality at 28 and 90 days was comparable between groups. Hemodynamic parameters, duration of mechanical ventilation, and ICU length of stay were not different between groups. Renal recovery at 90 days was high with less than 5 % of patients remaining dialysis-dependent at 3 months. Compared with patients from other studies stratified by cardiovascular SOFA score, IVOIRE mortality rates at 28, 60, and 90 days were significantly lower [27–29]. This could be explained by a more early start of HVHF (at RIFLE injury level). In a recent meta-analysis on the use of HVHF according to the Pardubice definition, Bagshaw and Honoré found no effect of HVHF use on sepsis mortality [30]. Another trial by Zhang and colleagues [13] randomized 280 patients with severe sepsis (50 % septic shock) and AKI to receive a dose of 50 or 85 ml/kg/h. Mortality at 28, 60, and 90 days was also similar between groups. Interestingly, 90-day mortality was significantly higher than in the IVOIRE study (on average 61 % vs. 51 %) despite the lower proportion (50 % vs. 100 % in IVOIRE) of septic shock patients included. However, patients in the Zhang study received HVHF treatment at RIFLE failure level and considerably later (on average 5.5 days vs. 24 h from ICU admission!). Again, this underscores the importance of timing which has been completely neglected in some major dose-studying CRRT trials [31, 32]. Of note, starting HVHF in septic patients before the occurrence of AKI is not evidence-based and may even worsen organ failure [33]. Obviously, uncertainty about optimal timing to initiate HVHF may become fostered by the recent emergence of various biomarkers that detect AKI in the absence of oliguria and/or increased creatinine [34]. Finally, one single randomized study using HVHF (and one prospective interventional) could reproduce the high (above 27 %) filtration fraction obtained by Ronco et al. in the septic subgroup of patients receiving a dialysis dose of 45 ml/kg/h in his seminal study (2000) but all the other studies on HVHF failed to reach this high filtration fraction so far [35]. The study of Ronco et al. was not designed to look specifically at septic patients but a post-hoc analysis was looking than more closely to the septic subgroup [35]. Both the Oudemans (1999) [36] and the Bouman (2002) [37] studies used a high filtration fraction (33 %) and post-dilution as well (blood flow 200 ml/min, postdilution flow 4 l/h). These two trials were not specific sepsis studies but had a proportion of septic patients. Using this high filtration fraction (33 %), the Oudemans study has a positive impact in terms of mortality (observed mortality significantly lower than expected) whereas the Bouman study could not show in a prospective randomized study, the superiority of high volume (around 50 ml/kg/h) as compared to standard volume (around 20 ml/kg/h) in terms of 28 days mortality reduction. However, when compared to the seminal Ronco study, filters were not changed systematically every 24 h in the Bouman study which might have affect the elimination rate by convection of middle size molecules. In the Oudemans study, HVHF was done intermittently and not in a continuous mode and therefore limiting potential removal of middle size molecules. Indeed, in the pivotal study of Ronco, convection was performed in full post-dilution continuously with filters changed every 24 h to preclude early clotting and early clogging. Acknowledging the significant effect of a very high filtration fraction and the effect of frequent filter change on elimination rate of mediators and cytokines, a new trial using a filtration fraction around 30 % in post-dilution could be envisaged. This study may be performed more efficiently using citrate as regional anticoagulant [38] as this would allow attaining a high filtration fraction without needing frequent membrane changes in order to reproduce more exactly and better mimicking the convection elimination rate realized in the septic subgroup of the Ronco study. Awaiting this "ultimate" trial, HVHF can actually not be recommended in routine clinical practice.

## 17.3  CRRT Membranes for Non-septic Acute Kidney Injury

A membrane surface area of 1 m$^2$ is largely sufficient to provide optimal convection and diffusion [39]. However, adsorption requires a larger surface area and ideally approximates 1.5 m$^2$. Biocompatible, and not cuprophane, membranes should be used [39]. Even if regional citrate anticoagulation (RCA) is used, the membrane should be impregnated with heparin (10,000 U of unfractionated heparin in 2 l saline) as this improves adsorptive capacity [40]. To date, the utility of heparin soaking for preventing early filter clotting remains a matter of debate [40]. RCA permits to prolong membrane filter life span beyond 72 h if the hemopermeability index is preserved (i.e. preventing of filter clogging) [41].

### 17.3.1  Current Status and Recent Advances in Blood–Membrane Interactions

Evaluating biocompatibility in blood purification therapy is complex. Indeed, biocompatibility is not only associated with materials but may also be related to the method of sterilization, the eluted substance, the type of anticoagulation and even specific contaminating factors. It has impact on blood cells (leukocytes and platelets), humoral pathways (complement, coagulation and fibrinolysis, kallikrein-bradykinin system), and cytokines [42]. Bio-incompatibility observed during intermittent hemodialysis not only has prognostic significance but may also contribute to long-term complications such as immunodeficiency, cardiovascular disease, and dialysis-related amyloidosis [42, 43]. In critically ill patients, the impact is less clear. Still, in coronary artery bypass surgery it was found to be associated with the "post-pump syndrome" (i.e. remote organ damage with acute respiratory distress syndrome and AKI) [44].

Dialysis membrane material either is of cellulose origin such as cellulose triacetate or of synthetic nature including polyethersulfones (PES), polyacrylonitrile (PAN/AN69), PMMA, or ethylene vinyl alcohol. The use of highly biocompatible membranes (PES, PMMA, and PAN) has significantly diminished the risk of membrane-induced cellular lysis and humoral pathway activation. In contrast to the older AN69 membrane, the novel AN69 ST and Oxiris membranes do not induce a bradykinin syndrome in patients treated with ACE-inhibitors [45]. Awaiting definitive studies on the behavior of PES, PMMA, and PAN membranes in the critically ill, their use can be recommended.

## 17.3.2  CRRT Membranes for Sepsis and SIRS

### 17.3.2.1  High Cut-Off Membranes

Morgera et al. were the first to clinically evaluate the performance of high cut-off (HCO) membranes in septic patients with AKI [3]. Thirty patients were randomized to receive treatment with either an HCO membrane (60 kilodalton (kDa)/P2SH Gambro) or a classic cut-off membrane (35 kDa/Polyflux 11S). A significant reduction in noradrenaline dose ($p = 0.0002$) and a tenfold increase in IL-6 and IL-Ra clearance ($p = 0.0001$) was observed in the HCO group as compared with the classic membrane group.

Preliminary results of the High Cut-Off Sepsis study (HICOSS) were encouraging in terms of safety but not efficacy [46, 47]. In this study, patients with septic shock and AKI were randomized to treatment with either a conventional or a 60 kDa HCO membrane. Patients were treated for 5 consecutive days in continuous veno-venous hemodialysis (CVVHD) mode. The study was discontinued prematurely after enrolment of only 81 patients due to a lack of difference in 28-day mortality (31 % HCO vs. 33 % conventional). No difference was observed in vasopressor need, duration of mechanical ventilation, or length of ICU stay. Albumin levels were not different between the two groups, suggesting that the HCO membrane was safe for clinical use. Importantly, the use of CVVHD in this study precluded to observe the previously documented synergy between high-volume hemofiltration (HVHF) and high-permeability hemofiltration (HPHF) [13]. Blood from healthy volunteers, ex vivo spiked with endotoxin, was exposed to a 100 kDa HCO membrane at a filtering rate of either 16.6 or 80 ml/kg/h. Cytokine clearance was nearly tenfold higher in the HCO/HVHF group [46]. HCO membranes also permitted more effective clearance of myoglobin and other muscle degradation products in non-traumatic and traumatic rhabdomyolysis [47–50]. However, a cut-off of 60,000 Da enhances albumin loss. Instead, medium cut-off membranes (e.g. cut-off at 50,000 Da) which cause negligible albumin loss should be preferred [51].

Taken together, HCO membranes are still in experimental phase, yet hold an enormous potential for treatment of septic shock and rhabdomyolysis, in particular when used in combination with CVVH at a minimal dose of 35 ml/kg/h, although strong evidence for this dose is not available. Most experience has been accumulated with the septeX membrane which has a cut-off of approximately 60,000 Da preventing albumin loss [46, 47]. Future studies should concentrate on combinations of techniques, or so-called "hybrid" therapies [48].

### 17.3.3 Non-selective Highly Adsorptive Membranes

#### 17.3.3.1 Polyacrylonitrile and AN69 Surface Treated

Adsorption is a physicochemical process that allows to "catch" specific molecules on a given surface. Adsorption has been used in chronic dialysis patients for elimination of beta-2 microglobulin [52]. Later, it was found to be very efficient for removal of mediators, cytokines, antibiotics, and proteins in CRRT conditions. Based on polarity and ionic charges, CRRT membranes exhibit variable adsorption properties. Strong adsorbent membranes may also remove molecules with a molecular weight (MW) above cut-off value [53–56] and thus are able to eliminate pro- and anti-inflammatory mediators which have MWs ranging between 0.5 and 60 kDa. In a canine model of acute endotoxic shock, Rogiers et al. showed that hemoperfusion using a polyacrylonitrile membrane produced better, albeit transient, hemodynamic effects than when a polysulfone filter was applied, suggesting more effective adsorption of inflammatory mediators [54].

#### 17.3.3.2 AN69 ST Membrane

Recently, the polyacrylonitrile AN69 ST (Surface Treated) membrane was introduced [5]. Surface treatment consisted of grafting a second layer with polyethylenimine and a third layer with heparin on the membrane. The AN69 ST membrane differs from its AN69 Oxiris counterpart because it contains a threefold lower polyethylenimine concentration (precluding endotoxin adsorption) and a tenfold lower (and thus not biologically active) concentration of heparin. The AN69 ST membrane also has a greater bulk adsorption capacity as compared with former polyacrylonitrile membranes [5]. Adsorption properties of the AN 69 ST membrane have been enhanced by modifying membrane surface polarity. This permits leads to adsorption of various antibiotics (aminoglycosides, colistin, vancomycin, etc.) [55] and lactate. Additionally, AN 69 ST very effectively adsorbs the High Mobility Group Box 1 protein (HMGB-1), an upstream mediator in the inflammatory cascade secreted by endotoxin-stimulated macrophages which activates a wide variety of cytokines. Its MW of approximately 30 kDa precludes elimination by any form of filtration [4]. The AN 69 ST membrane markedly clears HMGB-1 from the circulation ($60.8 \pm 5.0$ ml/min at 15 min) with nearly 100 µg eliminated within the first hour of treatment "in vitro" [4]. A relationship between removal of HMGB-1 and improvement of clinical sepsis has recently been demonstrated [40, 46] but is not yet confirmed by larger randomized trials.

Slower adsorption due to membrane saturation can limit the time interval for cytokine clearance. Saturation occurs faster with smaller membrane size. Thus, a larger membrane surface area ($1.5 \ m^2$ at the least) is required [57–60] which might impair convection. Nevertheless, as adsorption not only occurs at the surface but also in the bulk of the membrane, saturation will occur more slowly for some mediators. Rapid saturation can also required regular membrane change. Although such procedure inherently increases CRRT costs and nursing workload [61], it permits to counteract de-adsorption processes which occurs with continuous use. Also, frequent membrane changes should be limited to the early phase of septic shock, when plasma endotoxin and cytokine levels are most increased. The best cost-benefit ratio for timing of membrane change remains to be determined.

The heparin-coated membrane AN69 ST that was conceived to run without anticoagulation are not superior to comparable membranes that lack heparin coating regarding circuit survival [62]. In fact, heparin coating may only safely and effectively supplant systemic anticoagulation in high-flow systems (e.g. extracorporeal membrane oxygenation).

AN69 ST membranes are promising albeit still experimental for use in sepsis or SIRS. When applied for CRRT, clinicians should be aware that antimicrobial agents and potentially other beneficial substances may be significantly removed as well.

### 17.3.3.3 PolyMethylMethAcrylate (PMMA) and Related Membranes

PMMA can adsorb mediators with MWs up to 65,000 Da [63] but has only half the AN69ST membrane adsorption capacity for HMGB-1 [4]. CVVH with a PMMA membrane removed more cytokines than when a hemofilter of different material was used [63]. This was principally due to a more adequate cytokine adsorption on the membrane [61]. CVVH with PMMA also caused a significant reduction of blood lactate levels [60].

Wrapping up, CRRT using non-selective highly adsorptive membranes could potentially revolutionize the current approach of septic shock by reducing the load of inflammatory mediators up- and downstream in the inflammatory cascade. Membrane saturation is a limiting factor but its impact may be lowered by the use of large surface membranes, more bulk adsorption, and frequent membrane changes. Large, prospective, randomized, interventional studies evaluating these membranes are awaited.

## 17.3.4 Endotoxin Selective Highly Adsorptive Membranes

### 17.3.4.1 Polyacrylonitrile and AN69 Oxiris Membranes

A new generation of membranes aiming at endotoxin adsorption [(Toraymyxin (Toray™) and Oxiris (Gambro™)] or specific immuno-adsorption [Prosorba (Fresenius™)] has emerged. Preliminary results are promising [61], and large randomized controlled trials are in preparation [63]. Prosorba, a sorbent used in apheresis, will be discussed separately [64].

### 17.3.4.2 AN69 Oxiris

As compared to the AN69ST, the AN69 Oxiris membrane has high polyethylenimine and heparin concentrations grafted in its three-layer structure. Membrane surface polarity was modified by adding a positively charged polycation that adhered to the negatively charged endotoxin. Compared with older polyacrylonitrile membranes, this ensured highly selective endotoxin adsorption at its membrane surface [15, 65, 66]. In addition, the AN69 Oxiris membrane has greater bulk adsorption capacity that permits unselective adsorption of a wide array of inflammatory mediators.

In a porcine model of septic shock, Rimmelé et al. compared the AN69 Oxiris with a standard AN69 membrane during a 6-h HVHF session. Hemodynamic parameters were better preserved and fluid requirements, lactic acidosis and pulmonary arterial hypertension less pronounced in the AN69 Oxiris-treated animals [67]. So far, this membrane has not been evaluated in human septic shock.

### 17.3.4.3 PolyMethylMethAcrylate (PMMA) and Related Membranes

Although not promoted by Toray™ for commercial reasons, the PMMA membrane adsorbs endotoxin almost as effectively as the AN69 Oxiris [68]. The adsorption of endotoxin is selective although the other components are not selectively adsorbed. Several unintended bonus effects were also observed. Patients dialyzed with this membrane had less beta-2 microglobulin activity and a lower incidence of carpal tunnel syndrome [69]. PMMA membranes with the largest pore size also effectively removed potentially noxious substances such as furancarboxylic acid, homocysteine, pentosidine, and soluble CD40 [67]. Membranes with an anionic component were found to clear substantial amounts of free immunoglobulin light chains [69]. Thus, PMMA membranes can "tackle" the sepsis cascade upstream (endotoxin) and downstream (soluble CD 40, cytokines). This apparent immunomodulating effect might be useful as an adjunctive treatment in severe sepsis [68, 69]. The clinical use of PMMA membranes is well documented. Early initiation of CRRT with a PMMA membrane in patients with septic shock resulted in a significant decrease of TNF-alpha, IL-6 and IL-8 and an increase in IL-10 levels. This was associated with improved hemodynamics, better oxygen transport, and reduced organ failure [63, 70].

### 17.3.4.4 Polymyxin-Coated Membrane

PMX B hemoperfusion employs a large selective membrane surface that specifically binds endotoxin. This membrane is not a CRRT membrane but a sorbent-like membrane that can run in a hemoperfusion device without delivering CRRT. The adsorption of endoxin is performed through a selective mechanism whereas the adsorption of other components is unselective. Since the publication of a meta-analysis on PMX B treatment during the course of septic shock [71], many studies have confirmed its beneficial hemodynamic effects. Cantaluppi et al. randomized 16 patients with gram-negative sepsis to receive standard treatment with or without PMX B therapy [72]. Plasma samples of both patient groups were incubated with renal tubular cells and glomerular podocytes [72]. PMX B therapy reduced the proapoptotic activity of septic plasma on these cells, mainly by modulating FAS upregulation and caspase activation [72]. The results of the EUPHAS (Early Use of Polymyxin B Hemoperfusion in Abdominal Sepsis) trial were recently published. This study targeted a population prone to high circulating endotoxin levels in which the source control was obtained surgically [6]. Sixty-four patients were randomly assigned to receive either standard treatment or standard treatment plus two sessions of PMX B therapy. The PMX B group had improved hemodynamic parameters, faster resolving of organ failure as assessed with the sequential organ failure assessment (SOFA) score and a lower 28-day mortality adjusted to initial SOFA score [6, 73]. PMX B treatment was also studied in solid organ transplant patients with severe sepsis and septic shock. Despite three PMX sessions, no hemodynamic improvement was noticed [74]. Mortality was not assessed in this population.

One could argue that PMX B treatment might completely supplant supportive CRRT in sepsis. Being a blood purification technique, it indeed eliminates endotoxin and could therefore prevent the occurrence of AKI. Nevertheless, CRRT will remain necessary in those patients who still develop AKI or do not recover metabolically and/or hemodynamically. More studies are definitely needed to determine the value of adjuvant PMX B in the critically ill.

## 17.3.5 New Sorbents Designed for Sepsis and SIRS

### 17.3.5.1 Cytokine Adsorbing and Related Columns

CytoSorb, CYT-860-DHP, Lixelle, CTR-001, and MPCF-X columns, though structurally different, have excellent adsorption rates for the most important inflammatory cytokines [73–75]. Cytokine-adsorbing columns have an enormous surface (up to 8,500 $m^2$) as compared with classic CRRT membranes [75]. The Cytosorb cartridge, for instance, contains 10 g of polystyrene divinylbenzene copolymer beads with a biocompatible polyvinylpyrrolidone coating. Each bead measures 300–800 μm in size and each g of material has a surface of 850 $m^2$ [75]. Beads are slightly larger than a grain of salt, blood-compatible, porous, and highly adsorbent. Pore diameter is sufficient to allow passage of molecules up to 50,000 Da. This implies that most relevant pro- and anti-inflammatory cytokines can be removed from blood and physiologic fluids. Substances entering the beads undergo hydrophobic interactions with the neutral lipophilic surface of the polymer making them firmly adhere to the beads' surface. Meanwhile, the large essential blood proteins can pass alongside the beads through the filter and back into the patient.

Treatment of septic animals with Cytosorb resulted in swift clearance of 50–80 % of circulating cytokines [76, 77], which exceeded by far the filtering potential of HCO or even highly adsorptive membranes [76, 77]. The sole clinical investigation randomized 43 patients to receive standard treatment associated or not with Cytosorb therapy (provided 6 h daily, for 7 days) [78]. Significant reduction of IL-1, MCP-1, IL-1ra, and IL-8 but not IL-10 was noticed. Twenty-eight-day mortality was significantly reduced ($p = 0.03$). A major disadvantage of CytoSorb, however, is its inability to adsorb endotoxin [77]. The CYT-860-DHP column has this capacity and can adsorb exotoxins as well [79, 80]. However, no clinical studies with this sorbent technique have been performed.

Awaiting more clinical trials, cytokine-adsorbing columns are actually applied as adjunctive therapy in conditions characterized by an ongoing hyperinflammatory

**Table 17.1** Characteristics of cytokine-adsorbing columns

|  | Cytosorb | CYT-860-DHP | Lixelle | CTR-001 | MPCF-X |
|---|---|---|---|---|---|
| Structure | Polystyrene divinyl copolymer beads | Polystyrene-based conjugated fibers | Porous cellulose beads | Porous cellulose beads | Cellulose beads |
| Surface | 850 m$^2$ | >500 m$^2$ | >500 m$^2$ | >500 m$^2$ | >500 m$^2$ |
| IL-6 reduction within the first 2 h | <50 % | 92 % | 82.9 % | 80 % | 98.9 % |
| Endotoxin adsorption | No | Yes | No data | No data | No data |

response (e.g. acute respiratory distress syndrome) although the evidences are weak [81–83]. This is somewhat the same as for new membranes that are to be considered as potential adjunctive therapies in sepsis with also weak evidences so far [84–87].

In Table 17.1 (modified from Taniguchi) [75], the characteristics of existing cytokine-adsorbing columns are summarized.

### 17.3.5.2 Sorbents Using an Apheresis System

The Prosorba column acts as a selective plasma exchanger [88]. Protein A, a major cell wall component of *Staphylococcus aureus*, binds human immunoglobulin (Ig) G with high affinity. In Prosorba columns, protein A is covalently bound to a silica matrix and used to purify the patient's plasma. Cells and plasma are separated with a continuous cell separator and 1,250 ml plasma passes through the column. Treated plasma is then reconstituted with cells and returned to the patient. This procedure was initially approved for treatment of idiopathic thrombocytopenic purpura. Later, Prosorba immune-adsorption was successfully used in rheumatoid arthritis [88] and was granted FDA approval for treatment of moderate to severe forms of this disease. Few reports discuss the use of apheresis in sepsis [89].

The mechanism underlying Prosorba-induced improvement in rheumatoid arthritis and sepsis is unknown. Obviously, direct removal of IgG plays no role because as little as 1.5 % of circulating Ig is removed, and levels of rheumatoid factor and circulating immune complexes are barely modified throughout the entire treatment cycle [90]. Additional factors, such as complement activation or production of anti-idiotype antibodies, likely do contribute to the observed clinical improvement [90]. Recently, Suda and coworkers developed a new type of sorbent that specifically targets HMGB-1 [91].

As for other sorbents and other related techniques, antimicrobial adsorption can be very high [92, 93] as described also for hyper-adsorptive membranes [94].

---

### Conclusions

CRRT in non-septic AKI can be is generally applied using a non-adsorptive biocompatible membrane of 1 m$^2$. However, some relatively cheap non-selective adsorptive membranes such as the AN69 ST type are already used on a large scale in this condition as well.

Regarding HVHF and after the two large randomized trials that are negative regarding mortality end points, HVHF is no longer recommended in clinical practice but may still be evaluated in appropriate trials.

The IVOIRE trial did suggest that an early start at AKI RIFLE injury score in septic shock with AKI may improve mortality as compared to a late start at AKI RIFLE failure score. Delay of therapy between ICU admission and CRRT start above 48 h may also impact negatively mortality according to IVOIRE. These data need to be further confirmed or not by randomized trials.

High cut-off membranes can remove cytokines and are under evaluation for treatment of rhabdomyolysis and sepsis. However, a cut-off of 60,000 Da enhances albumin loss. Instead, medium cut-off membranes (e.g. cut-off at 50,000 Da) should be preferred.

To increase removal of inflammatory mediators in septic AKI, the use of highly adsorptive filters that can be considered in CRRT such as the AN69 ST, septeX, PMMA, and Oxiris membranes but without strong clinical evidences.

The CytoSorb membrane binds cytokines and is seems a promising membrane for sepsis treatment, though it fails to capture endotoxin and IL-10. So far, there is more evidence for HCO and PMX filters. The AN 69 Oxiris membrane may be a valid alternative as it does capture both endotoxin and cytokines. AN69 ST also adsorbs the important upstream mediator HMGB-1. PMMA is a powerful scavenger of endotoxin and numerous other cytokines. Finally, high porosity septeX membranes may perform well especially when used in CVVH mode.

Clinical evidence for the benefit of adsorptive columns and selective plasma exchange is still scarce.

More studies are definitely needed to identify the ideal membrane or sorbent for adjuvant treatment of sepsis.

The highly adsorptive membranes AN69 ST and PMMA may capture significant amounts of crucial antibiotics such as colistin, amikacin, and vancomycin necessitating dose adaptation.

Heparin-coated membranes do not preclude the use of anticoagulation.

**Key Messages**
- HVHF is not recommended anymore in clinical practice, but appropriate studies are still wanted. A prescribed dose of 30–35 ml/kg/h is enough in order to deliver 25 ml/kg/h.
- In septic shock with AKI, it is suggested to start CRRT earlier, at RIFLE injury (after the results of the IVOIRE trial).
- New membranes and sorbents are promising but cannot be recommended at this stage in clinical practice, but well-designed trials are wanted.
- High-cut-off (HCO) membranes designed for sepsis and rhabdomyolysis are under investigation but cannot yet be recommended in daily routine clinical practice.

## References


1. Palewsky PM, Zhang JH, O'Connor TZ, et al., for the VA/NIH Acute Renal Failure Trial Network. Intensity of renal support in critically ill patients with acute kidney injury. N Engl J Med. 2008; 359:7–20.
2. Bellomo R, Cass A, Cole L, Finfer S, et al., for the RENAL replacement Therapy Study Investigators. Intensity of continuous renal-replacement therapy in critically ill patients. N Engl J Med. 2009;361:1627–38.
3. Morgera S, Haase M, Kuss T, et al. Pilot study on the effects of high cutoff hemofiltration on the need for norepinephrine in septic patients with acute renal failure. Crit Care Med. 2006;34:2099–104.
4. Yumoto M, Nishida O, Moriyama K, et al. In vitro evaluation of high mobility group box 1 protein removal with various membranes for continuous hemofiltration. Ther Apher Dial. 2011;15:385–93.
5. Thomas M, Moriyama K, Ledebo I. AN69: evolution of the world's first high permeability membrane. Contrib Nephrol. 2011;173:119–29.
6. Cruz DN, Antonelli M, Fumagalli R, et al. Early use of polymyxin B hemoperfusion in abdominal septic shock: the EUPHAS randomized controlled trial. JAMA. 2009;301:2445–52, (electronic supplemental material).
7. Yaroustovsky M, Abramyan M, Popok Z, et al. Preliminary report regarding the use of selective sorbents in complex cardiac surgery patients with extensive sepsis and prolonged intensive care stay. Blood Purif. 2009;28:227–33.
8. Honoré PM, Jamez J, Wauthier M, Lee PA, Dugernier T, Pirenne B, Hanique G, Matson JR. Prospective evaluation of short-term, high-volume isovolemic hemofiltration on the hemodynamic course and outcome in patients with intractable circulatory failure resulting from septic shock. Crit Care Med. 2000;28:3581–7.
9. Joannes-Boyau O, Rapaport S, Bazin R, Fleureau C, Janvier G. Impact of high volume hemofiltration on hemodynamic disturbance and outcome during septic shock. ASAIO J. 2004;50:102–9.
10. Boussekey N, Chiche A, Faure K, Devos P, Guery B, d'Escrivan T, Georges H, Leroy O. A pilot randomized study comparing high and low volume hemofiltration on vasopressor use in septic shock. Intensive Care Med. 2008;34:1646–53.
11. Herrera-Gutiérrez ME, Seller-Pérez G, Arias-Verdu D, Delgado-Amaya M. Hemodynamic improvement after continuous renal replacement therapies: not only immunomodulation. J Transl Intern Med. 2014;2:11–7.
12. Joannes-Boyau O, Honoré PM, Gauche B, et al. High volume versus standard-volume haemofiltration for septic shock patients with acute kidney injury(IVOIRE study):a multicentre randomized Controlled trial. Intensive Care Med. 2013;39:1535–46.
13. Zhang P, Yang Y, Lv R, Zhang Y, Xie W, Chen J. Effect of the intensity of continuous renal replacement therapy in patients with sepsis and acute kidney injury: a single-center randomized clinical trial. Nephrol Dial Transplant. 2012;27:967–73.
14. Honore PM, Jacobs R, Joannes-Boyau O, Boer W, De Regt J, De Waele E, Van Gorp V, Verfaillie L, Spapen HD. Moving from a cytotoxic to a cytokinic approach in the blood purification labyrinth– have we finally found the ariadne thread ? Mol Med. 2012. doi:10.2119/molmed.2012.00300.
15. Joannes-Boyau O, Honore PM, Boer W, Collin V. Are the synergistic effects of high volume haemofiltration and enhanced adsorption the missing key in sepsis modulation? Nephrol Dial Transplant. 2009;24:354–7.
16. Tetta C, Bellomo R, Inguaggiato P, Wratten ML, Ronco C. Endotoxin and cytokine removal in sepsis. Ther Apher. 2002;6:109–15.
17. Deans KJ, Haley M, Natanson C, Eichacker PQ, Minneci PC. Novel therapies for sepsis: a review. J Trauma. 2005;58:867–74.

18. Ronco C, Tetta C, Mariano F, Wratten ML, Bonello M, Bordoni V, Cardona X, Inguaggiato P, Pilotto L, d'Intini V, Bellomo R. Interpreting the mechanisms of continuous renal replacement therapy in sepsis: the peak concentration hypothesis. Artif Organs. 2003;27:792–801.
19. Honoré PM, Matson JR. Extracorporeal removal for sepsis: acting at the tissue level–the beginning of a new era for this treatment modality in septic shock. Crit Care Med. 2004;32:896–7.
20. Di Carlo JV, Alexander SR. Hemofiltration for cytokine-driven illnesses: the mediator delivery hypothesis. Int J Artif Organs. 2005;28:777–86.
21. Honore PM, Jacobs R, Boer W, Joannes-Boyau O, De Waele E, De Regt J, Van Gorpe V, Collin V, Spapen N. New insights regarding rationale, therapeutic target and dose of hemofiltration and hybrid therapies in septic AKI. Blood Purif. 2012;33:44–51.
22. Peng Z, Singbartl K, Simon P, Rimmele T, Bishop J, Clermont G, Kellum JA. Blood purification in sepsis: a new paradigm. Contrib Nephrol. 2010;165:322–8.
23. Rimmele T, Kellum JA. Clinical review: blood purification for sepsis. Crit Care. 2011;15:205.
24. Honoré PM, Joannes-Boyau O, Kotulak T. Report of the working party on high volume hemofiltration including definitions and classification. Proceedings of 2nd Czech Conference on Critical Care Nephrology, Pardubice; 2007. p. 11–4.
25. Rimmelé T, Kellum JA. High-volume hemofiltration in the intensive care unit: a blood purification therapy. Anesthesiology. 2012;116:1377–87.
26. Honoré PM, Joannes-Boyau O, Boer W, Rose T, Jennes S. Continuous renal replacement therapy (CRRT) & role of haemofiltration in critical care: time for revisiting in 2009? Minerva Anaesthesilogica. 2009;75:228–30.
27. Vinsonneau C, Camus C, Combes A, Costa de Beauregard MA, Klouche K, Boulain T, Pallot JL, Chiche JD, Taupin P, Landais P, Dhainaut JF, Hemodiafe Study Group. Continuous venovenous haemodiafiltration versus intermittent haemodialysis for acute renal failure in patients with multiple-organ dysfunction syndrome: a multicentre randomised trial. Lancet. 2006;368:379–85.
28. Palevsky PM, Zhang JH, O'Connor TZ, Chertow GM, Crowley ST, Choudhury D, Finkel K, Kellum JA, Paganini E, Schein RM, Smith MW, Swanson KM, Thompson BT, Vijayan A, Watnick S, Star RA, Peduzzi P. Intensity of renal support in critically ill patients with acute kidney injury. N Engl J Med. 2008;359:7–20.
29. Bellomo R, Cass A, Cole L, Finfer S, Gallagher M, Lo S, McArthur C, McGuinness S, Myburgh J, Norton R, Scheinkestel C, Su S. Intensity of continuous renal-replacement therapy in critically ill patients. N Engl J Med. 2009;361:1627–38.
30. Clark E, Molnar AO, Joannes-Boyau O, Honoré PM, Sikora L, Bagshaw SM. High-volume hemofiltration for septic acute kidney injury: a systematic review and meta-analysis. Crit Care. 2014;18:R7.
31. Ronco C, Honore PM. Renal support in critically ill patients with acute kidney injury. N Engl J Med. 2008;359:1959–62.
32. Ronco C, Cruz D, Oudemans-van-Straaten HM, Honoré PM, House A, Bin D, Gibney N. Dialysis dose in acute kidney injury: no time for therapeutic nihilism – a critical appraisal of the Acute Renal Failure Trial Network study. Crit Care. 2008;12:308.
33. Payen D, Mateo J, Cavaillon JM, Fraisse F, Floriot C, Vicaut E. Impact of continuous venovenoushemo filtration on organ failure during the early phase of severe sepsis: a randomized controlled trial. Crit Care Med. 2009;37:803–10.
34. Haase M, Kellum JA, Ronco C. Subclinical AKI–an emerging syndrome with important consequences. Nat Rev Nephrol. 2012;12:735–9.
35. Ronco C, Bellomo R, Homel P, Brendolan A, Dan M, Piccinni P, La Greca G. Effects of different doses in continuous veno-venous haemofiltration on outcomes of acute renal failure: a prospective randomised trial. Lancet. 2000;356:26–30.
36. Oudemans-van-straaten HM, Bosman RJ, van der Spoel JI, Zandstra DF. Outcome of critically ill patients treated with intermittent high-volume haemofiltration: a prospective cohort analysis. Intensive Care Med. 1999;25:814–21.

37. Bouman C, Oudemans-Van Straaten HM, Tijssen JG, Zandstra DF, Kesecioglu J. Effects of early high-volume continuous venovenous hemofiltration on survival and recovery of renal function in intensive care patients with acute renal failure: a prospective, randomized trial. Crit Care Med. 2002;30:2205–11.
38. Oudemans-van Straaten HM, Ostermann M. Bench-to-bedside review: citrate for continuous renal replacement therapy, from science to practice. Crit Care. 2012;16:249.
39. Baldwin I, Tan HK, Bridge N, Bellomo R. Possible strategies to prolong circuit life during hemofiltration: three controlled studies. Ren Fail. 2002;24:839–48.
40. Lindsay RM, Rourke JT, Reid BD, Linton AL, Gilchrist T, Courtney J, Edwards RO. The role of heparin on platelet retention by acrylonitrile co-polymer dialysis membranes. J Lab Clin Med. 1977;89:724–34.
41. Joannidis M, Oudemans-van Straaten HM. Clinical review: patency of the circuit in continuous renal replacement therapy. Crit Care. 2007;11:218.
42. Abe T, Kato K, Fujioka T, Akizawa T. The blood compatibilities of blood purification membranes and other materials developed in Japan. Int J Biomater. 2011;2011:375390. Epub Sep 28.
43. Sirolli V, Ballone E, Di Stante S, Amoroso L, Bonomini M. Cell activation and cellular-cellular interactions during hemodialysis: effect of dialyzer membrane. Int J ArtifOrgans. 2002;25:529–37.
44. Harig F, Feyrer R, Mahmoud FO, Blum U, von der Emde J. Reducing the post-pump syndrome by using heparin-coated circuits, steroids, or aprotinin. Thorac Cardiovasc Surg. 1999;47:111–8.
45. Désormeaux A, Moreau ME, Lepage Y, Chanard J, Adam A. The effect of electronegativity and angiotensin-converting enzyme inhibition on the kinin-forming capacity of polyacrylonitrile dialysis membranes. Biomaterials. 2008;29:1139–46.
46. Honore PM, Clark W. Novel therapeutical concepts for extracorporeal treatment of hyper-inflammation and sepsis: immunomodulation approach with a novel high Cut-OFF membrane: the SepteX membrane. Proceedings of 10th Congress of World Federation of CCU (WFSICCM), Florence; 2009. p. 17–21.
47. Honoré PM, Jacobs R, Boer W, et al. New insights regarding rationale, therapeutic target and dose of hemofiltration and hybrid therapies in septic acute kidney injury. Blood Purif. 2012;33:44–51.
48. Naka T, Haase M, Bellomo R. 'Super high-flux' or 'high cut-off' hemofiltration and hemodialysis. Contrib Nephrol. 2010;166:181–9.
49. Lee WC, Uchino S, Fealy N, et al. Super high flux hemodialysis at high dialysate flows: an ex vivo assessment. Int J Artif Organs. 2004;27:24–8.
50. Naka T, Jones D, Baldwin I, et al. Myoglobin clearance by super high-flux hemofiltration in a case of severe rhabdomyolysis: a case report. Crit Care. 2005;9:R90–5.
51. Honoré PM, Jacobs R, Joannes-Boyau O, Lochy S, Boer W, De Waele E, Van Gorp V, De Regt J, Collin V, Spapen HD. Continuous renal replacement therapy-related strategies to avoid colistin toxicity: a clinically orientated review. Blood Purif. 2014;37:291–5.
52. Premru V, Kovač J, Buturović-Ponikvar J, Ponikvar R. High cut-off membrane hemodiafiltration in myoglobinuric acute renal failure: a case series. Ther Apher Dial. 2011;15:287–91.
53. Stollwerck PL, Namdar T, Stang FH, Lange T, Mailänder P, Siemers F. Rhabdomyolysis and acute renal failure in severely burned patients. Burns. 2011;37:240–8.
54. Honore PM, Jacobs R, Joannes-Boyau O, et al. Septic AKI in ICU patients diagnosis, pathophysiology, and treatment type, dosing, and timing: a comprehensive review of recent and future developments. Ann Intensive Care. 2011;1:32.
55. Akizawa T, Koshikawa S, Nakazawa R, Yoshida T, Kaneko M, Nitadori Y. Elimination of beta 2-microglobulin by a new polyacrylonitrile membrane dialyser: mechanism and physiokinetics. Nephrol Dial Transplant. 1989;4:356–65.
56. Honoré PM, Joannes-Boyau O, Collin V, Boer W, Jennes S. Continuous hemofiltration in 2009: what is new for clinicians regarding pathophysiology, preferred technique and recommended dose? Blood Purif. 2009;28:135–43.

57. Rogiers P, Zhang H, Pauwels D, Vincent JL. Comparison of polyacrylonitrile (AN69) and polysulphone membrane during hemofiltration in canine endotoxic shock. Crit Care Med. 2003;31:1219–25.
58. Hu D, Sun S, Zhu B, et al. Effects of coupled plasma filtration adsorption on septic patients with multiple organ dysfunction syndrome. Ren Fail. 2012;34:834–9.
59. Honore PM, Joannes-Boyau O, Collin V, Boer W, Gressens B, Janvier G. Practical daily management of extra-renal continuous removal. Reanimation. 2008;17:472–8.
60. Hirayama Y, Oda S, Wakabayashi K, et al. Comparison of interleukin-6 removal properties among hemofilters consisting of varying membrane materials and surface areas: an in vitro study. Blood Purif. 2011;31:18–25.
61. Honoré PM, Joannes-Boyau O, Gressens B. CRRT technology and logistics: is there a role for a medical emergency team in CRRT? Contrib Nephrol. 2007;156:354–64.
62. Schetz M, Van Cromphaut S, Dubois J, Van den Berghe G. Does the surface-treated AN69 membrane prolong filter survival in CRRT without anticoagulation? Intensive Care Med. 2012;38:1818–25.
63. Nakada TA, Oda S, Matsuda K, Sadahiro T, Nakamura M, Abe R, Hirasawa H. Continuous hemodiafiltration with PMMA Hemofilter in the treatment of patients with septic shock. Mol Med. 2008;14:257–63.
64. Yamashita AC, Tomisawa N. Membrane materials for blood purification in critical care. Contrib Nephrol. 2010;166:112–8.
65. Davies B, Cohen J. Endotoxin removal devices for the treatment of sepsis and septic shock. Lancet Infect Dis. 2011;11:65–71.
66. Bosch T. Recent advances in therapeutic apheresis. J Artif Organs. 2003;6:1–8.
67. Rimmelé T, Assadi A, Cattenoz M, et al. High-volume haemofiltration with a new haemofiltration membrane having enhanced adsorption properties in septic pigs. Nephrol Dial Transplant. 2009;24:421–7.
68. Hirasawa H. Indications for blood purification in critical care. Contrib Nephrol. 2010;166: 21–30. Review.
69. Sakai Y. Polymethylmethacrylate membrane with a series of serendipity. Contrib Nephrol. 2011;173:137–47.
70. Nakamura M, Oda S, Sadahiro T, Hirayama Y, Watanabe E, Tateishi Y, Nakada TA, Hirasawa H. Treatment of severe sepsis and septic shock by CHDF using a PMMA membrane hemofilter as a cytokine modulator. Review Contrib Nephrol. 2010;166:73–82. http://www.ncbi.nlm.nih.gov/pubmed/20472994.
71. Cruz DN, Perazella MA, Bellomo R, et al. Effectiveness of polymyxin B-immobilized fiber column in sepsis: a systematic review. Crit Care. 2007;11:R47. Review.
72. Cantaluppi V, Assenzio B, Pasero D, et al. Polymyxin-B hemoperfusion inactivates circulating proapoptotic factors. J Am Soc Nephrol. 2008;19:1904–18.
73. Vincent JL, Polymyxin B. Hemoperfusion and mortality in abdominal septic shock. JAMA. 2009;302:1968–9.
74. Ruberto F, Pugliese F, D'Alio A, et al. Clinical effects of direct hemoperfusion using a polymyxin-B immobilized column in solid organ transplanted patients with signs of severe sepsis and septic shock. A pilot study. Int J Artif Organs. 2007;30:915–22.
75. Taniguchi T. Cytokine adsorbing columns. Contrib Nephrol. 2010;166:134–41.
76. Peng ZY, Carter MJ, Kellum JA. Effects of hemoadsorption on cytokine removal and short-term survival in septic rats. Crit Care Med. 2008;36:1573–7.
77. Kellum JA, Song M, Venkataraman R. Hemoadsorption removes tumor necrosis factor, interleukin-6, and interleukin-10, reduces nuclear factor-kappaB DNA binding, and improves short-term survival in lethal endotoxemia. Crit Care Med. 2004;32:801–5.
78. Quintel M. "CytoSorb™ whole blood cytokine adsorption – results of a controlled randomized trial". Presentation at the 32 ISICEM, Brussels; 20–23 Mar 2012.
79. Kobe Y, Oda S, Matsuda K, Nakamura M, Hirasawa H. Direct hemoperfusion with a cytokine-adsorbing device for the treatment of persistent or severe hypercytokinemia: a pilot study. Blood Purif. 2007;25:446–53.

80. Bosch T. Therapeutic apheresis–state of the art in the year 2005. Ther Apher Dial. 2005;9: 459–68. Review.
81. Mitaka C, Tomita M. Polymyxin B-immobilized fiber column hemoperfusion therapy for septic shock. Shock. 2011;36:332–8.
82. Tsuchida K, Yoshimura R, Nakatani T, Takemoto Y. Blood purification for critical illness: cytokines adsorption therapy. Ther Apher Dial. 2006;10:25–31.
83. Honore PM, Jacobs R, Joannes-Boyau O, De Regt J, De Waele E, van Gorp V, Boer W, Verfaillie L, Spapen HD. Newly designed CRRT membranes for sepsis and SIRS–a pragmatic approach for bedside intensivists summarizing the more recent advances: a systematic structured review. ASAIO J. 2013;59:99–106.
84. Honoré PM, Joannes-Boyau O, Gressens B. Blood and plasma treatments: high-volume hemofiltration–a global view. Contrib Nephrol. 2007;156:371–86. Review.
85. Jacobs R, Honore PM, Joannes-Boyau O, et al. Septic acute kidney injury: the culprit is inflammatory apoptosis rather than ischemic necrosis. Blood Purif. 2011;32:262–5.
86. Bellomo R, Palevsky PM, Honore PM, et al. Recent trials in critical care nephrology. Contrib Nephrol. 2010;165:299–309.
87. Matsumura Y, Oda S, Sadahiro T, et al. Treatment of septic shock with continuous HDF using 2 PMMA hemofilters for enhanced intensity. Int J Artif Organs. 2012;35:3–14.
88. Mugnier B, Poullin P, Lefevre P, Roudier J. Clinical improvement in a patient with severe rheumatoid arthritis and chronic hepatitis B after prosorba column immunoadsorption: a one-year followup. Arthritis Rheum. 2003;49:722–3.
89. Mattsby-Baltzer I, Bergstrom T, McCrea K, Ward R, Adolfsson L, Larm O. Affinity apheresis for treatment of bacteremia caused by Staphylococcus aureus and/or methicillin-resistant S. aureus (MRSA). J Microbiol Biotechnol. 2011;21:659–64.
90. Sato H, Yamagata Y, Kidoka T. Studies on quantitative levels of complement activation induced by immobilized and soluble forms of protein A: relevance to extracorporeal immunoadsorption. Trans Sci. 1991;12:299–305.
91. Suda K, Takeuchi H, Hagiwara T, et al. Spherical sulfated cellulose adsorbs high-mobility-group box chromosomal protein 1 in vitro and in vivo. ASAIO J. 2010;56:210–4.
92. Ruggero MA, Argento AC, Heavner MS, Topal JE. Molecular Adsorbent Recirculating System (MARS(®)) removal of piperacillin/tazobactam in a patient with acetaminophen-induced acute liver failure. Transpl Infect Dis. 2013;15:214–8. Review.
93. Page M, Cohen S, Ber CE, Allaouchiche B, Kellum JA, Rimmelé T. In vivo antibiotic removal during coupled plasma filtration adsorption: a retrospective study. ASAIO J. 2014;60:70–5.
94. Honore PM, Jacobs R, Joannes-Boyau O, Boer W, De Waele E, Gorp VV, Spapen HD. Continuous renal replacement therapy allows higher colistin dosing without increasing toxicity. J Transl Intern Med. 2013;1:6–8.

# Drug Removal by CRRT and Drug Dosing in Patients on CRRT

**18**


Miet Schetz, Olivier Joannes-Boyau, and Catherine Bouman


Give a man a fish and you feed him for a day. Teach a man to fish and you feed him for a lifetime – Maimonides

## 18.1 Introduction

Adequate drug therapy can be lifesaving in critically ill patients. Adequate not only means the correct drug choice but also the correct drug dose that maximizes efficacy while minimizing toxicity. This especially applies to antibiotics that should reach sufficient concentrations at the site of infection to prevent treatment failure and/or selection of resistant pathogens. Successful drug dosing should take into account the substantial and dynamic pharmacokinetic alterations that take place during critical illness. These alterations mainly include increases in volume of distribution ($V_d$) (capillary leak, fluid resuscitation, etc.) and changes in clearance (Cl) (altered organ function) and protein binding (PB) (hypoalbuminemia, acute phase reactants) [1, 2]. The application of continuous renal replacement


M. Schetz, MD, PhD (✉)
Clinical Division of Intensive Care Medicine, Department of Cellular and Molecular Medicine, University of Leuven, Leuven 3000, Belgium
e-mail: marie.schetz@uzleuven.be

O. Joannes-Boyau, MD
Service d'Anesthésie-Réanimation, Centre Hospitalier Universitaire (CHU) de Bordeaux, Bordeaux 33000, France
e-mail: olivier.joannes-boyau@chu-bordeaux.fr

C. Bouman, MD, PhD
Department of Intensive Care, Academic Medical Center, University of Amsterdam, PO Box 22660, Amsterdam 1100 DD, The Netherlands
e-mail: c.s.bouman@amc.uva.nl



© Springer International Publishing 2015
H.M. Oudemans-van Straaten et al. (eds.), *Acute Nephrology for the Critical Care Physician*, DOI 10.1007/978-3-319-17389-4_18

**Table 18.1** Factors affecting sieving coefficient and dialysate saturation

|                             | $S$    | $S(d)$ |
| --------------------------- | ------ | ------ |
| Molecular weight            | −      | +      |
| Protein binding             | ++++   | ++++   |
| Drug–membrane interactions  | +      | +      |
| Membrane thickness          | −      | +      |
| Membrane pore size          | −      | +      |
| Dialysate/blood flow        | −      | +      |

therapy (CRRT) adds another factor of uncertainty. A wide variability of drug concentrations has indeed been noted in patients receiving CRRT [3–5]. This chapter will summarize the factors affecting drug removal during CRRT and their implications for drug dosing regimens. These CRRT-induced changes should be interpreted in the context of the general pharmacokinetic alterations in critically ill patients.

## 18.2 Drug Removal with CRRT

The main factors affecting drug removal during CRRT are $V_d$, effluent flow rate ($Q_{effl}$) and PB, although modality, the drug's molecular weight (MW) and the choice of the membrane may also contribute [6–9].

### 18.2.1 Protein Binding

The drug fraction that is not bound to proteins is not only responsible for its efficacy and toxicity but it is also the only fraction that can cross the membrane of a renal replacement therapy. The ability of a solute to cross the membrane is expressed in the sieving coefficient ($S$) during hemofiltration and in dialysate saturation ($S(d)$) during hemodialysis. S and $S(d)$ equal the ratio of the drug's concentration in the effluent ($C_{effl}$) to its plasma concentration ($C_p$).

$$S(d) = C_{effl} / C_p$$

PB is the main determinant of $S$ and $S(d)$ that both approximate the free drug fraction (1−PB). The more the drug is bound by protein, the less it can be removed. Acidic drugs typically bind to albumin whereas basic drugs bind to acute phase reactant proteins such as alpha-1-acid glycoprotein. Critically ill patients have a high incidence of hypoalbuminemia and this will especially affect the unbound fraction of drugs with high PB such as ceftriaxone and flucloxacillin. Other factors affecting PB include temperature, pH and the presence of displacing substances such as other drugs, bilirubin or organic acids that are retained in uremia [10]. These changes in PB may at least partially explain the reported differences between a drug's free fraction (as reported in the literature) and measured sieving coefficients [11, 12] (Table 18.1).

## 18.2.2 Effluent Flow Rate

The second and most important factor affecting extracorporeal drug removal during CRRT is "dialysis dose" or $Q_{effl}$. Extracorporeal drug clearance ($Cl_{EC}$) equals the product of $S(d)$ and $Q_{effl}$ [6–9].

$$Cl_{EC} = S(d) \times Q_{effl}$$

Lower antibiotic concentrations have indeed been found in patients treated with high-volume hemofiltration [13–15]. The dose-effect also implies that (frequently occurring) differences between prescribed and delivered CRRT dose should be taken into account.

The prefilter infusion of the replacement solution in predilution hemofiltration or hemodiafiltration decreases plasma concentration in the filter and thus also extracorporeal drug removal. The above equation should therefore be adapted with a correction factor where $Q_b$ is the blood flow and $Q_{S_{pre}}$ is the prefilter replacement rate [6–9].

$$Cl_{EC} = S(d) \times Q_{effl} \times \left[ Q_b / \left( Q_{S_{pre}} + Q_b \right) \right]$$

## 18.2.3 Modality and Molecular Weight

Solute transport during hemofiltration is based on convection whereas hemodialysis uses diffusive transport. Convective solute removal is independent of MW up to the cut-off of the membrane (which is much higher than the MW of the majority of the drugs). Diffusion, on the other hand, is dependent on MW and this will potentially lead to a lower extracorporeal removal (compared to hemofiltration) of drugs with relatively high MW such as vancomycin (MW 1,480 Da) [16], teicoplanin (MW 1,880 Da), daptomycin (MW 1,620 Da), bivalirudin (MW 2,180 Da) or colistin (1,160 Da). This is especially the case when achieving equilibrium between blood and dialysate is hampered by the use of low-flux membranes [17], membranes with low surface area [18] and/or high dialysate flow rates [18–20]. Interaction of diffusion and convection in hemodiafiltration may also reduce the clearance of larger solutes compared to pure hemofiltration [21].

## 18.2.4 Membrane

Theoretically extracorporeal drug removal can also be affected by drug–membrane interactions. These interactions may be the result of drug charge and the so-called Gibbs–Donnan effect where negatively charged proteins along the membrane result in the retention of cationic drugs. Anionic drugs may experience the opposite effect explaining why drug concentrations in the effluent may be higher than the plasma concentration.

Another drug–membrane interaction is drug adsorption to the membrane that depends on drug and membrane characteristics. Drug adsorption has been described for levofloxacin, aminoglycosides and vancomycin with the polyacrylonitrile membrane [22–26]. The phenomenon rapidly reaches saturation and the clinical importance is not clear. It may influence aminoglycoside blood levels after the first dose, but, due to membrane saturation, the next dose will not be affected if the membrane has not been changed. Drug–membrane interactions provide another explanation for the reported differences between a drug's free fraction and $S(d)$ [11, 12].

## 18.2.5 Volume of Distribution

RRT only clears the plasma, which means that drugs with large $V_d$ are less efficiently cleared by extracorporeal therapy. This explains why intermittent RRT is often followed by a rebound of the plasma concentration due to re-equilibration between central and peripheral compartments. CRRT has access to the total $V_d$ due to continuous re-equilibration between the different compartments. For the same daily extracorporeal clearance, CRRT will therefore increase drug removal compared with intermittent hemodialysis. However, due to the limited plasma concentration of drugs with large $V_d$ the amount eliminated will anyway be small compared to the total amount present in the body. Here too, changes in $V_d$ induced by critical illness and its recovery should be taken into account.

## 18.3  Is Extracorporeal Drug Removal Clinically Important?

The clinical importance of $Cl_{EC}$ is determined by its contribution to total body clearance, which is the sum of all regional clearances including $Cl_{EC}$, residual renal clearance ($Cl_R$), hepatic drug metabolism and other non-renal clearances ($Cl_{NR}$). The contribution of a regional clearance to the total body clearance is called a fractional clearance (FrCl) [6–9].

$$Fr\,Cl = Regional\ Cl\,/\,total\,body\,Cl$$
$$FrCl_{EC} = Cl_{EC}\,/\left(Cl_{EC} + Cl_{R} + Cl_{NR}\right)$$

Any regional clearance is only clinically important if its contribution to total body clearance exceeds 25 %. Concomitant hepatic impairment, residual kidney function and the intensity of CRRT may all affect fractional extracorporeal clearance ($FrCl_{EC}$). In addition, the effect of AKI on drug metabolism should also be taken into account [27, 28].

## 18.4  Drug Dosing Regimens

In many cases drug dosing in critically ill patients will have to compromise between the risk of insufficient efficacy and the risk of toxicity. For instance, the dosing of antibiotics should take into account the severity of the infection, whether the patient's immune system is compromised, the minimal inhibitory concentration (MIC) of the most resistant (presumed) pathogen, the pharmacodynamics of the antibiotic, its potential toxicity and the changes in pharmacokinetics induced by critical illness.

The loading dose of a drug only depends on the volume of distribution and body weight (BW) and should thus be adapted for the changes in $V_d$ induced by critical illness, however, not for CRRT itself.

$$\text{Loading dose} = \text{Target level} \times V_d^{\,*}$$

Different approaches can be used for the selection of a maintenance dose. For antibiotics, the dosing schedule should take into account the pharmacodynamic profile (time-dependent or concentration-dependent bacterial killing). For time-dependent antibiotics, such as the beta-lactams, a continuous or extended infusion may be the optimal method to deliver the maintenance dose [29, 30].

## 18.4.1 Literature Data

Published dosing guidelines on drug dosing during CRRT are generally based on studies involving small and heterogeneous patient populations treated with heterogeneous (modality, intensity, membrane) CRRT [7, 31, 32]. Their applicability on individual patients is therefore questionable. In addition, many clinical trials in this field poorly report CRRT settings [33, 34] or report pharmacokinetics during CRRT thus reflecting the combined effect of critical illness and CRRT [35]. Understanding the basic principles of solute removal with CRRT (besides the pharmacokinetics and pharmacodynamics of critically ill patients) is therefore of utmost importance [6, 8, 9].

## 18.4.2 Drugs with Measurable Clinical Effect

Medications with real-time measurable clinical effect such as vasoactive drugs or sedatives can be titrated to their effect and therefore do not represent a problem.

## 18.4.3 Drugs with Available Monitoring

In most clinical settings therapeutic drug monitoring (TDM) is limited to aminoglycosides, glycopeptides and some anti-epileptics that have a narrow therapeutic index. CRRT can even be used to reduce toxicity of antibiotics that require high peak levels for efficacy such as the aminoglycosides. Reducing toxicity may require an intensified CRRT [36].

Beta-lactam and quinolone antibiotics have a wide safety margin. However, the frequently reported subtherapeutic levels in patients on CRRT [3, 5] that may result in treatment failure and selection of resistant pathogens argue for an expansion of TDM to these classes of antibiotics, not just for minimizing toxicity but mainly for ensuring efficacy [37–39].

Adaptation to the required drug level can use the following formula:

$$\text{Dose} = \left(\text{Target level} - \text{Actual level}\right) \times V_d^{\,*}$$

### 18.4.4  Drug with High Protein Binding

Protein binding is the main determinant of $S(d)$. This explains why the extracorporeal elimination of drugs with high PB can be expected to be limited. However, changes in PB due to critical illness must be taken into account and may explain why drugs with high PB in healthy volunteers such as ceftriaxone may be significantly removed with CRRT [40].

### 18.4.5  Drugs with Predominant Non-renal Clearance

The concept of fractional extracorporeal clearance explains why extracorporeal removal with CRRT will not be clinically important for drugs with predominant non-renal clearance such as voriconazole [41], amphotericin [42], echinocandins [43] or benzodiazepines [44]. Reduction in hepatic drug clearance induced by the patient's condition should be accounted for and may increase the clinical importance of extracorporeal clearance. In addition, (eventually active) metabolites may be significantly cleared [45].

### 18.4.6  Drugs with Predominant Renal Clearance

Drugs with predominant renal clearance generally require dosage adaptation for CRRT. Whether dosage adaptation should include a change in dosing interval or maintenance dose depends on the pharmacodynamics [8, 46–48].

The simplest way to perform this dosage adaptation is to determine extracorporeal creatinine clearance ($=Q_{\text{effl}}$ corrected for predilution) and to administer the dose that applies for a patient with comparable renal creatinine clearance [6, 9], eventually taking into account residual renal clearance. The major drawback of this method is the assumption that renal drug clearance is only by glomerular filtration. However, many drugs undergo tubular reabsorption or tubular secretion. Since the extracorporeal system only mimics glomerular filtration and not the tubular function, this may result in underdosing of drugs that undergo tubular reabsorption and overdosing in drugs that undergo tubular secretion, as illustrated in Fig. 18.1.

The best example of this problem is fluconazole that has an almost exclusive renal elimination. In the normal kidney, fluconazole is substantially reabsorbed resulting in a $Cl_R$ that is much lower than glomerular filtration. During CRRT, this reabsorption does not take place and the $Cl_{EC}$ may therefore be even higher than normal $Cl_R$ in healthy subjects. Supranormal doses of fluconazole will therefore be required in patients on CRRT especially with relatively high $Q_{\text{effl}}$ [49–52]. Another antibiotic that undergoes substantial tubular reabsorption is colistin [53].

Another method for dosage adaptation consists of reducing the dose in proportion to the reduction in total body clearance [54].

$$\text{Actual Cl} = Cl_{EC} + Cl_{NR} + Cl_R \left(\text{residual}\right)$$
$$\text{Dose} = \text{Normal dose} \times \text{Actual Cl} / \text{Normal Cl}$$

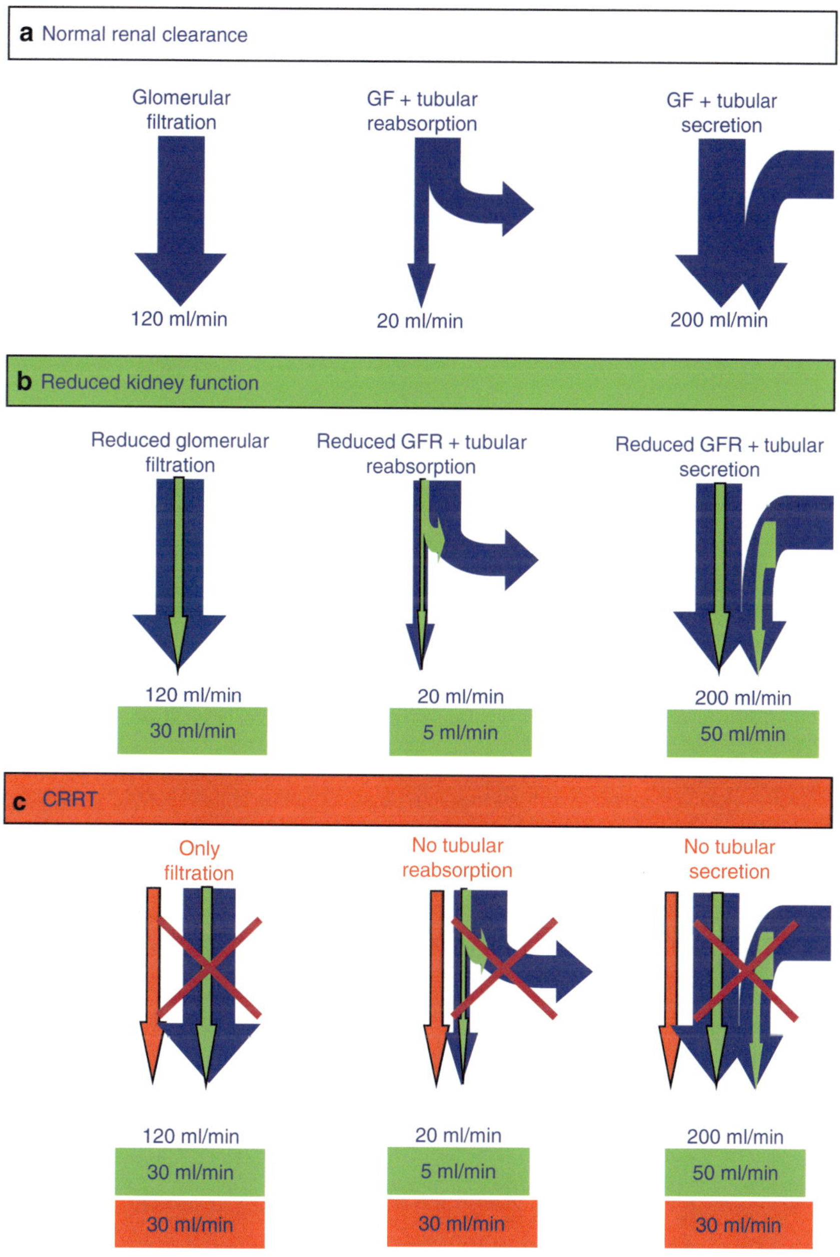


**Fig. 18.1** Extracorporeal removal of drugs with tubular secretion or reabsorption. (**a**) Figure representing renal clearance of a drug undergoing tubular reabsorption or tubular secretion in a patient with normal GFR. (**b**) With reduced kidney function (and assuming a similar decrease of glomerular and tubular function) clearance of drugs with tubular secretion and reabsorption will be reduced in proportion to the reduction in GFR. (**c**) CRRT with an extracorporeal clearance that is similar to the renal clearance under **b**. Due to the absence of tubular function, the clearance of a drug with tubular reabsorption will be less reduced and may be even higher than with normal kidney function. For drugs with tubular secretion, the reduction of drug clearance will be more pronounced compared with reduced kidney function

This approach is more complicated because it requires knowledge of the normal and the non-renal clearance (always taking into account the effect of critical illness).

A third approach starts from the anuric dose or dosing interval (as found in the literature) with adaptations based on the $FrCl_{EC}$ [20, 55].

$$Maintenance\,dose = Anuric\,dose\,/\left(1 - FrCl_{EC}\right)$$

$$Dosing\,intervel = Anuric\,dosing\,interval \times \left(1 - FrCl_{EC}\right)$$

However, anuric doses reported in the literature are often derived from patients with chronic kidney disease and may not apply to the situation of AKI.

---

### Conclusion

Understanding the basic principles and weighing the risks and benefits of over- and underdosing are key in drug management during CRRT. Clinically relevant extracorporeal removal can be expected for drugs with predominant renal clearance, especially if they have a poor PB. It is also important to realize that RRT is only one of the factors contributing to uncertainty with regard to a drug's fate in critically ill patients. The multitude of factors affecting drug disposal and the spectrum of variability within each of these factors explains why adequate prediction of drug levels in an individual ICU patient is almost impossible. Further expanding the possibilities for therapeutic drug monitoring is therefore indispensable in order to prevent over- and underdosing of potentially lifesaving/toxic drugs in critically ill patients.

---

**Key Messages**

1. Critical illness induces important alterations in pharmacokinetics. CRRT is therefore only one of the factors contributing to uncertainty with regard to a drug's fate in the body.
2. The most important factors affecting extracorporeal drug removal are effluent flow rate, protein binding and volume of distribution.
3. As a general rule, drugs with important renal elimination also require dosage adaptation for CRRT.
4. The simplest method for drug dosage adaptation during CRRT is based on total creatinine clearance (sum of residual renal clearance + effluent flow rate), but its limitations for drugs undergoing tubular secretion or reabsorption should be acknowledged.
5. Adaptation of maintenance doses of antibiotics should take into account their pharmacodynamic profile (time- or concentration-dependent bacterial killing).
6. Expanding the possibilities of therapeutic drug monitoring is the only way forward to improve accuracy of drug dosing in critically ill patients with CRRT.

## References


1. Smith BS, Levasseur-Franklin KE, Forni A, Fong J. Introduction to drug pharmacokinetics in the critically ill patient. Chest. 2012;141:1327–36.
2. Udy AA, Roberts JA, Lipman J. Clinical implications of antibiotic pharmacokinetic principles in the critically ill. Intensive Care Med. 2013;39:2070–82.
3. Seyler L, Cotton F, Taccone FS, De Backer D, Macours P, Vincent JL, et al. Recommended β-lactam regimens are inadequate in septic patients treated with continuous renal replacement therapy. Crit Care. 2011;15:R137.
4. Bauer SR, Salem C, Connor Jr MJ, Groszek J, Taylor ME, Wei P, et al. Pharmacokinetics and pharmacodynamics of piperacillin-tazobactam in 42 patients treated with concomitant CRRT. Clin J Am Soc Nephrol. 2012;7:452–7.
5. Roberts DM, Roberts JA, Roberts MS, Liu X, Nair P, Cole L, et al. Variability of antibiotic concentrations in critically ill patients receiving continuous renal replacement therapy: a multicentre pharmacokinetic study. Crit Care Med. 2012;40:1523–8.
6. Schetz M. Drug dosing in continuous renal replacement therapy: general rules. Curr Opin Crit Care. 2007;13:645–51.
7. Pea F, Viale P, Pavan F, Furlanut M. Pharmacokinetic considerations for antimicrobial therapy in patients receiving renal replacement therapy. Clin Pharmacokinet. 2007;46:997–1038.
8. Choi G, Gomersall CD, Tian Q, Joynt GM, Freebairn R, Lipman J. Principles of antibacterial dosing in continuous renal replacement therapy. Crit Care Med. 2009;37:2268–82.
9. Awdishu L, Bouchard J. How to optimize drug delivery in renal replacement therapy. Semin Dial. 2011;24:176–82.
10. Roberts JA, Pea F, Lipman J. The clinical relevance of plasma protein binding changes. Clin Pharmacokinet. 2013;52:1–8.
11. Golper TA. Update on drug sieving coefficients and dosing adjustments during continuous renal replacement therapies. Contrib Nephrol. 2001;132:349–53.
12. Bouman CS, van Kan HJ, Koopmans RP, Korevaar JC, Schultz MJ, Vroom MB. Discrepancies between observed and predicted continuous venovenous hemofiltration removal of antimicrobial agents in critically ill patients and the effects on dosing. Intensive Care Med. 2006;32:2013–9.
13. Bilgrami I, Roberts JA, Wallis SC, Thomas J, Davis J, Fowler S, et al. Meropenem dosing in critically ill patients with sepsis receiving high-volume continuous venovenous hemofiltration. Antimicrob Agents Chemother. 2010;54:2974–8.
14. Frazee EN, Kuper PJ, Schramm GE, Larson SL, Kashani KB, Osmon DR, et al. Effect of continuous venovenous hemofiltration dose on the achievement of adequate vancomycin trough concentrations. Antimicrob Agents Chemother. 2012;56:6181–5.
15. Joannes-Boyau O, Honoré PM, Perez P, Bagshaw SM, Grand H, Canivet JL, et al. High-volume versus standard volume haemofiltration for septic shock patients with acute kidney injury (IVOIRE study): a multicentre randomized controlled trial. Intensive Care Med. 2013;39:535–46.
16. Jeffrey RF, Khan AA, Prabhu P, Todd N, Goutcher E, Will EJ, et al. A comparison of molecular clearance rates during continuous hemofiltration and hemodialysis with a novel volumetric continuous renal replacement system. Artif Organs. 1994;18:425–8.
17. Vilay AM, Shah KH, Churchwell MD, Patel JH, DePestel DD, Mueller BA. Modeled dalbavancin transmembrane clearance during intermittent and continuous renal replacement therapies. Blood Purif. 2010;30:37–43.
18. Schroeder TH, Krueger WA, Hansen M, Hoffmann E, Dieterich HJ, Unertl K. Elimination of meropenem by continuous hemo(dia)filtration: an in vitro one-compartment model. Int J Artif Organs. 1999;22:307–12.
19. Joy MS, Matzke GR, Frye RF, Palevsky PM. Determinants of vancomycin clearance by continuous venovenous hemofiltration and continuous venovenous hemodialysis. Am J Kidney Dis. 1998;31:1019–27.

20. Reetze-Bonorden P, Bohler J, Keller E. Drug dosage in patients during continuous renal replacement therapy. Pharmacokinetic and therapeutic considerations. Clin Pharmacokinet. 1993;24:362–79.
21. Brunet S, Leblanc M, Geadah D, Parent D, Courteau S, Cardinal J. Diffusive and convective solute clearances during continuous renal replacement therapy at various dialysate and ultrafiltration flow rates. Am J Kidney Dis. 1999;34:486–92.
22. Choi G, Gomersall CD, Lipman J, Wong A, Joynt GM, Leung P, et al. The effect of adsorption, filter material and point of dilution on antibiotic elimination by haemofiltration: an in vitro study of levofloxacin. Int J Antimicrob Agents. 2004;24:468–72.
23. Tian Q, Gomersall CD, Wong A, Leung P, Choi G, Joynt GM, et al. Effect of drug concentration on adsorption of levofloxacin by polyacrylonitrile haemofilters. J Antimicrob Agents. 2006;28:147–50.
24. Tian Q, Gomersall CD, Leung PP, Choi GY, Joynt GM, Tan PE, et al. The adsorption of vancomycin by polyacrylonitrile, polyamide, and polysulfone hemofilters. Artif Organs. 2008;32:81–4.
25. Tian Q, Gomersall CD, Ip M, Tan PE, Joynt GM, Choi GY. Adsorption of amikacin, a significant mechanism of elimination by hemofiltration. Antimicrob Agents Chemother. 2008;52:1009–13.
26. Lam KN, Tian Q, Ip M, Gomersall CD. In vitro adsorption of gentamicin and netilmicin by polyacrylonitrile and polyamide hemofiltration filters. Antimicrob Agents Chemother. 2010;54:963–5.
27. Vilay AM, Churchwell MD, Mueller BA. Clinical review: drug metabolism and nonrenal clearance in acute kidney injury. Crit Care. 2008;12:235.
28. Philips BJ, Lane K, Dixon J, Macphee I. The effects of acute renal failure on drug metabolism. Expert Opin Drug Metab Toxicol. 2014;10:11–23.
29. Macvane SH, Kuti JL, Nicolau DP. Prolonging β-lactam infusion: a review of the rationale and evidence, and guidance for implementation. Int J Antimicrob Agents. 2013. pii: S0924-8579(13)00378-6. doi:10.1016/j.ijantimicag.2013.10.021. [Epub ahead of print].
30. Falagas ME, Tansarli GS, Ikawa K, Vardakas KZ. Clinical outcomes with extended or continuous versus short-term intravenous infusion of carbapenems and piperacillin/tazobactam: a systematic review and meta-analysis. Clin Infect Dis. 2013;56:272–82.
31. Trotman RL, Williamson JC, Shoemaker DM, Salzer WL. Antibiotic dosing in critically ill adult patients receiving continuous renal replacement therapy. Clin Infect Dis. 2005;41:1159–66.
32. Choi G, Gomersall CD, Tian Q, Joynt GM, Li AM, Lipman J. Principles of antibacterial dosing in continuous renal replacement therapy. Blood Purif. 2010;30:195–212.
33. Li AM, Gomersall CD, Choi G, Tian Q, Joynt GM, Lipman J. A systematic review of antibiotic dosing regimens for septic patients receiving continuous renal replacement therapy: do current studies supply sufficient data? J Antimicrob Chemother. 2009;64:929–37.
34. Vaara S, Pettila V, Kaukonen KM. Quality of pharmacokinetic studies in critically ill patients receiving continuous renal replacement therapy. Acta Anaesthesiol Scand. 2012;56:147–57.
35. Udy AA, Covajes C, Taccone FS, Jacobs F, Vincent JL, Lipman J, et al. Can population pharmacokinetic modelling guide vancomycin dosing during continuous renal replacement therapy in critically ill patients? Int J Antimicrob Agents. 2013;41:564–8.
36. Layeux B, Taccone FS, Fagnoul D, Vincent JL, Jacobs F. Amikacin monotherapy for sepsis caused by pan-resistant Pseudomonas aeruginosa. Antimicrob Agents Chemother. 2010;54:4939–41.
37. Sime FB, Roberts MS, Peake SL, Lipman J, Roberts JA. Does Beta-lactam pharmacokinetic variability in critically ill patients justify therapeutic drug monitoring? A systematic review. Ann Intensive Care. 2012;2:35.
38. Pea F. Plasma pharmacokinetics of antimicrobial agents in critically ill patients. Curr Clin Pharmacol. 2013;8:5–12.
39. Hayashi Y, Lipman J, Udy AA, Ng M, McWhinney B, Ungerer J, et al. β-Lactam therapeutic drug monitoring in the critically ill: optimising drug exposure in patients with fluctuating renal function and hypoalbuminaemia. Int J Antimicrob Agents. 2013;41:162–6

40. Matzke GR, Frye RF, Joy MS, Palevsky PM. Determinants of ceftriaxone clearance by continuous venovenous hemofiltration and hemodialysis. Pharmacotherapy. 2000;20:635–43.
41. Radej J, Krouzecky A, Stehlik P, Sykora R, Chvojka J, Karvunidis T, et al. Pharmacokinetic evaluation of voriconazole treatment in critically ill patients undergoing continuous venovenous hemofiltration. Ther Drug Monit. 2011;33:393–7.
42. Bellmann R, Egger P, Djanani A, Wiedermann CJ. Pharmacokinetics of amphotericin B lipid complex in critically ill patients on continuous veno-venous haemofiltration. Int J Antimicrob Agents. 2004;23:80–3.
43. Weiler S, Seger C, Pfisterer H, Stienecke E, Stippler F, Welte R, et al. Pharmacokinetics of caspofungin in critically ill patients on continuous renal replacement therapy. Antimicrob Agents Chemother. 2013;57:4053–7.
44. Swart EL, de Jongh J, Zuideveld KP, Danhof M, Thijs LG, Strack van Schijndel RJ. Population pharmacokinetics of lorazepam and midazolam and their metabolites in intensive care patients on continuous venovenous hemofiltration. Am J Kidney Dis. 2005;45:360–71.
45. Bolon M, Bastien O, Flamens C, Paulus S, Boulieu R. Midazolam disposition in patients undergoing continuous venovenous hemodialysis. J Clin Pharmacol. 2001;41:959–62.
46. Roberts JA, Joynt GM, Choi GY, Gomersall CD, Lipman J. How to optimise antimicrobial prescriptions in the Intensive Care Unit: principles of individualised dosing using pharmacokinetics and pharmacodynamics. Int J Antimicrob Agents. 2012;39:187–92.
47. McKenzie C. Antibiotic dosing in critical illness. J Antimicrob Chemother. 2011;66 Suppl 2:ii25–31.
48. Petrosillo N, Drapeau CM, Agrafiotis M, Falagas ME. Some current issues in the pharmacokinetics/pharmacodynamics of antimicrobials in intensive care. Minerva Anestesiol. 2010;76:509–24.
49. Nicolau DP, Crowe H, Nightingale CH, Quintiliani R. Effect of continuous arteriovenous hemodiafiltration on the pharmacokinetics of fluconazole. Pharmacotherapy. 1994;14:502–5.
50. Yagasaki K, Gando S, Matsuda N, Kameue T, Ishitani T, Hirano T, et al. Pharmacokinetics and the most suitable dosing regimen of fluconazole in critically ill patients receiving continuous hemodiafiltration. Intensive Care Med. 2003;29:1844–8.
51. Bergner R, Hoffmann M, Riedel KD, Mikus G, Henrich DM, Haefeli WE, et al. Fluconazole dosing in continuous veno-venous haemofiltration (CVVHF): need for a high daily dose of 800 mg. Nephrol Dial Transplant. 2006;21:1019–23.
52. Patel K, Roberts JA, Lipman J, Tett SE, Deldot ME, Kirkpatrick CM. Population pharmacokinetics of fluconazole in critically ill patients receiving continuous venovenous hemodiafiltration – using Monte Carlo Simulations to predict doses for specified pharmacodynamic targets. Antimicrob Agents Chemother. 2011;55:5868–73.
53. Garonzik SM, Li J, Thamlikitkul V, Paterson DL, Shoham S, Jacob J, et al. Population pharmacokinetics of colistin methanesulfonate and formed colistin in critically ill patients from a multicenter study provide dosing suggestions for various categories of patients. Antimicrob Agents Chemother. 2011;55:3284–94.
54. Kroh UF. Drug administration in critically ill patients with acute renal failure. New Horiz. 1995;3:748–59.
55. Schetz M, Ferdinande P, Van den Berghe G, Verwaest C, Lauwers P. Pharmacokinetics of continuous renal replacement therapy. Intensive Care Med. 1995;21:612–20.

# Renal Replacement Therapy for Intoxications

**19**

Anne-Cornélie J.M. de Pont

## 19.1 Introduction

Intoxications are common in emergency medicine: in the United States, more than two million poison exposures are reported each year and more than 100,000 of these patients are admitted to critical care units because of a serious intoxication. Most of these intoxications involve analgesics, sedatives and cardiovascular drugs [1]. Although in the past, decontamination techniques such as gastric lavage and administration of activated charcoal have been advocated, their clinical benefit has not been confirmed in controlled studies and their use has substantially declined during recent years [1, 2]. Nevertheless, enhanced elimination of the toxic agent remains one of the cornerstones of the management of the intoxicated patient. In this chapter, we will give an overview of the indications and techniques for the elimination of toxic agents.

## 19.2 Indications

The use of renal replacement therapy to remove a toxin is justified if there is an indication of severe toxicity (Table 19.1) and if the total body elimination of the toxin can be increased by 30 % or more using this technique [3]. Whether removal of toxins by means of renal replacement therapy is possible depends on characteristics of the toxin itself and of the elimination technique used (Table 19.2) [4, 5].

A.C.J.M. de Pont
Department of Intensive Care, Academic Medical Center, University of Amsterdam,
Amsterdam, The Netherlands
e-mail: a.c.depont@amc.uva.nl

© Springer International Publishing 2015
H.M. Oudemans-van Straaten et al. (eds.), *Acute Nephrology for the Critical
Care Physician*, DOI 10.1007/978-3-319-17389-4_19

**Table 19.1**  Indications of severe toxicity

| |
|---|
| Ingested quantity associated with severe toxicity |
| Ingestion of a toxin with serious delayed effects |
| Natural removal mechanisms impaired |
| Clinical condition deteriorating |
| Clinical evidence of severe toxicity: hypotension, coma, metabolic acidosis, respiratory depression, dysrhythmias, cardiac decompensation |

**Table 19.2**  Necessary properties for extracorporeal removal by three different techniques

| | Hemodialysis | Hemofiltration | Hemoperfusion |
|---|---|---|---|
| Solubility | water | water | water or lipid |
| Molecular weight | <500 Da | <40,000 Da | <40,000 Da |
| Protein binding | Low (<80 %) | Low | Low or high |
| Volume of distribution | <1 L/kg | <1 L/kg | <1 L/kg |
| Endogenous clearance | <4 mL/min/kg | <4 mL/min/kg | <4 mL/min/kg |
| Distribution time | Short | Longer | Short |

## 19.3  Techniques

Hemodialysis, hemofiltration, and hemoperfusion can all be used to remove toxins from the blood. However, hemodialysis is most suitable to remove water-soluble toxins with a low molecular weight (Table 19.2). Taken into account these restrictions, hemodialysis is by far the most efficient technique in terms of clearance.

## 19.4  Techniques Based on Diffusion

### 19.4.1  Hemodialysis

During hemodialysis, small molecules are cleared from the blood by diffusion across a semipermeable membrane down a concentration gradient from blood into dialysate. The clearance of a substance depends on its molecular weight, the membrane surface area and type, as well as on blood and dialysate flow rates [6, 7]. Newer high-flux membranes can also remove high-molecular weight substances. Increasing blood and dialysate flow rates can increase the concentration gradient between blood and dialysate, thus increasing the rate of diffusion and elimination. Intermittent hemodialysis typically uses a blood flow rate of 200–500 mL/min and a dialysate flow rate of 500–1,000 mL/min [7, 8]. When a high-flux, high-efficiency membrane is used, a urea clearance exceeding 200 mL/min can be reached [9]. Hemodialysis is therefore the most efficient technique in terms of clearance. The major drawback is the risk of rebound toxicity due to redistribution of the toxin after stopping the treatment. In addition, hemodynamically unstable patients generally do not tolerate the high blood flows used in intermittent hemodialysis.

## 19.4.2 Sustained Low Efficiency Dialysis

Sustained low efficiency dialysis (SLED) or prolonged intermittent renal replacement therapy (PIRRT) is a diffusive technique comparable to hemodialysis. In contrast, SLED is used continuously with lower rates of blood and dialysate flow than intermittent hemodialysis, typically 200 and 100 mL/min, respectively [10]. With these settings, a urea clearance of 70–80 mL/min can be reached [11]. Therefore, SLED is less efficient in removing toxic substances than hemodialysis. However, since flow rates are lower and treatment duration is longer, it is better tolerated by hemodynamically unstable patients and the risk of rebound toxicity is diminished.

## 19.4.3 Continuous Venovenous Hemodialysis (CVVHD)

Continuous venovenous hemodialysis (CVVHD) is another technique based on diffusion. However, blood flow and dialysis flow used are much lower than during SLED, typically 100–200 mL/min and 10–30 mL/min, respectively [5]. Current international guidelines recommend delivering an effluent volume of 20–25 mL/kg/h (www.KDIGO.com). Therefore, urea clearance is low (20–30 mL/min), which makes the technique unsuitable for the treatment of intoxications.

## 19.5 Techniques Based on Convection

## 19.5.1 Hemofiltration

During hemofiltration, plasma ultrafiltrate is produced under influence of a pressure gradient across the hemofiltration membrane. Molecules up to 40 kDa can thus be cleared from the blood convectively. The plasma ultrafiltrate is replaced by a buffered replacement fluid, infused either before (predilution) or after the filter (postdilution). In postdilutional hemofiltration, clearance equals the ultrafiltration rate, typically ranging from 10 to 30 mL/min, with 20–25 mL/kg/h being the current recommendation for renal replacement therapy. When using high-volume hemofiltration, a clearance up to 85 mL/min can be reached, which makes the efficiency of this technique equal to SLED [5]. However, for small water-soluble molecules, extracorporeal removal by hemodialysis is much more efficient.

## 19.5.2 Continuous Venovenous Hemodiafiltration (CVVHDF)

In continuous venovenous hemodiafiltration (CVVHDF), a dialysis component is added to conventional hemofiltration, by means of which the clearance can be increased [5]. However, the efficiency of this technique is insufficient for the treatment of intoxications.

### 19.5.3 Hemoperfusion

During hemoperfusion, the blood passes through a cartridge containing a sorbent material. In order to be able to be removed by hemoperfusion, the toxic substance must have binding affinity to the sorbent in the cartridge and a low volume of distribution (Table 19.2). Despite their efficacy, the use of hemoperfusion cartridges has declined over the last 20 years due to limitations of their indications and shelf life [7, 12, 13].

## 19.6 Intoxications for Which Extracorporeal Removal May be Indicated

Due to the characteristics required for extracorporeal removal, the number of substances suitable for this technique is limited. Drugs for which extracorporeal removal is indicated are summarized in Table 19.3 and will be discussed in alphabetical order. When an intoxication with one of these agents is suspected, consultation of a nephrologist and pharmacologist is warranted [7, 14].

### 19.6.1 Barbiturates

The physicochemical and pharmacokinetic properties of barbiturates determine their suitability for extracorporeal elimination [15]. Their protein binding ranges from 5 % for barbital to 70 % for secobarbital, and their endogenous clearance ranges from 3 mL/min for barbital to 53 mL/min for secobarbital. Although for all barbiturates extracorporeal clearance is higher than endogenous clearance, barbital, phenobarbital, and secobarbital are most suitable for this technique because of their low endogenous clearance [15]. The choice for extracorporeal treatment in case of barbiturate overdose depends on the severity of the toxicity rather than on the serum level and should be considered in cases of severe hypotension, respiratory depression, or deep and prolonged coma. Until recently, hemoperfusion was the treatment of choice. However, with the use of high-flux, high-efficiency membranes, similar or even better elimination can be obtained with hemodialysis [16, 17].

**Table 19.3** Substances for which extracorporeal removal may be indicated

| Substance | Preferred method |
| --- | --- |
| Barbiturates | Hemoperfusion/hemodialysis |
| Lithium | Hemodialysis |
| Metformin | Hemodialysis |
| Salicylates | Hemodialysis |
| Theophylline | Hemoperfusion/hemodialysis |
| Toxic alcohols | Hemodialysis |
| Valproic acid | Hemodialysis |

## 19.6.2 Lithium

Lithium is widely used in the treatment of bipolar affective disorders. It has a molecular weight of 74 Da, a distribution volume of 0.6–0.9 L/kg body weight, and it is not protein bound, which makes it an ideal substance to be removed by renal replacement therapy. With hemodialysis, an extraction ratio of 90 % and a clearance ranging from 63 to 114 mL/min can be achieved [18]. Hemodialysis is even more effective in removing lithium than the kidney itself, since 70–80 % of lithium filtered by the kidney is reabsorbed in the proximal tubule. Hemodialysis should be started in case of confusion, stupor, coma, or seizures. Although the serum lithium level is effectively lowered by hemodialysis, a rebound rise in serum levels occurs 6–8 h after cessation of the treatment, since lithium redistributes to the circulation from the interstitial space [19]. Therefore, hemodialysis should be continued until the serum lithium level remains below 1 mEq/L.

## 19.6.3 Metformin

The biguanide metformin is the most widely used oral antidiabetic agent in the world. Yet it carries the risk of metformin associated lactic acidosis (MALA), which usually occurs in cases of overdose or renal failure. Although rare, MALA carries a mortality risk of 50 % [20]. Metformin has a molecular weight of 166 Da, is not protein bound, and is excreted by the kidney by means of glomerular filtration and tubular secretion. Its renal clearance therefore exceeds the creatinine clearance and ranges from 552 to 642 mL/min, reaching a plasma elimination half-life of 1.5–4.7 h [21]. Metformin intoxication itself can induce acute renal failure, which aggravates toxicity. By means of hemodialysis, metformin can be removed with clearances up to 170 mL/min [22]. Extracorporeal treatment should be performed in cases of refractory lactic acidosis or impaired renal function [23–25].

## 19.6.4 Salicylates

At therapeutic levels, salicylates have over 90 % protein binding, which decreases to 50–75 % at toxic levels, due to saturation. Salicylates are metabolized in the liver and excreted by the kidney. The elimination half-life is dose dependent, ranging from 2 h at a low dose to 30 h at a high dose. Treatment with hemodialysis should be started when the serum level exceeds 700 mg/L or when the clinical situation deteriorates (altered mental status, respiratory failure, pulmonary edema, severe acid-base disturbances, renal failure) [26]. Hemodialysis is recommended as the extracorporeal treatment of choice, since it more rapidly corrects metabolic acidosis and electrolyte disturbances [27].

### 19.6.5 Theophylline

Theophylline is more than 50 % protein bound and under normal conditions metabolized by the p450 enzyme in the liver. At therapeutic levels its elimination obeys first order kinetics, while limitation of the enzyme capacity results in zero order kinetics at higher concentrations [28]. Since theophylline binds readily to charcoal, hemoperfusion is the treatment of choice. In acute toxicity, it should be started at serum levels greater than 90 μg/mL and in chronic intoxications at levels greater than 40 μg/mL in the presence of signs of severe toxicity. When hemoperfusion is not available, hemodialysis is also effective.

### 19.6.6 Toxic Alcohols

The toxic alcohols include ethylene glycol, methanol, and isopropanol. Ethylene glycol is a compound used in antifreeze and windshield washer solutions. It is converted by alcohol dehydrogenase to glycolate, which causes renal failure and pulmonary and cerebral edema. Therefore, the mainstay of the treatment of ethylene glycol poisoning is the inhibition of alcohol dehydrogenase with ethanol or fomepizole [29, 30]. Hemodialysis should be started when signs and symptoms of severe toxicity are present (deteriorating vital signs, severe metabolic acidosis, acute kidney injury, pulmonary or cerebral edema) or when the serum level exceeds 0.5 g/L [30]. Hemodialysis effectively eliminates glycolate with an elimination half-life of $155 \pm 474$ min, compared with a spontaneous elimination half-life of $625 \pm 474$ min [30, 31].

Under physiological circumstances, methanol is metabolized by alcohol dehydrogenase to formaldehyde, and by aldehyde hydrogenase to formic acid, which is responsible for the acidosis and toxic manifestations. Therefore, the primary step in the treatment of methanol intoxication is inhibition of alcohol dehydrogenase with ethanol or fomepizole [29, 30]. The usual criteria for hemodialysis include severe acidosis, visual impairment, renal failure, electrolyte disturbances or a plasma methanol concentration greater than 0.5 g/L [32]. Hemodialysis does not substantially enhance the endogenous clearance of formate. The endogenous half-life of formic acid is $205 \pm 25$ min, whereas the hemodialysis half-life is $185 \pm 63$ min [33].

Isopropanol is a colorless liquid with a bitter taste, used in the manufacturing of acetone and glycerin. The minimal lethal dose for adults is approximately 100 mL. Unlike ethylene glycol and methanol, most of the toxic effects of isopropanol are due to the parent compound itself. Isopropanol is metabolized to acetone by alcohol dehydrogenase. The clinical signs of intoxication occur within 1 h of ingestion and include gastrointestinal symptoms, confusion, stupor, and coma. Severe intoxications may present with hypotension due to cardiac depression and vasodilatation [34]. Hypotension is the strongest predictor of mortality. Inhibition of alcohol dehydrogenase is not indicated, since acetone is less toxic than isopropanol. Hemodialysis is indicated for patients with an isopropanol level greater than 4 g/L and significant central nervous system depression, renal failure, or hypotension [34].

## 19.6.7 Valproic Acid

Valproic acid is a 144 Da branched chain carboxylic acid primarily metabolized in the liver. At therapeutic levels it is 90 % protein bound, but protein binding decreases at toxic serum levels due to saturation. Valproic acid has a small volume of distribution (0.1–0.5 L/kg) and a plasma half-life of 6–16 h [35]. Clinical manifestations of toxicity vary from mild confusion and lethargy to coma and death. In addition to neurological symptoms, valproate can cause hypothermia, hypotension, tachycardia, gastrointestinal disturbances, and hepatotoxicity as well as hypernatremia, hyperosmolarity, hypocalcemia, and metabolic acidosis. Valproic acid can be eliminated by hemodialysis with an elimination half-life of 2–4 h [35–38]. Extracorporeal treatment is justified in cases of refractory hemodynamic instability or metabolic acidosis [39].

---

**Conclusion**

In case of severe toxicity, renal replacement therapy is justified if the technique is able to increase the total body elimination of the toxin by 30 % or more. The possibility for a toxin to be removed from the blood by means of renal replacement therapy depends on its molecular weight, protein binding, volume of distribution, and solubility in water. Hemodialysis is the most efficient technique in terms of the clearance of water-soluble toxins with a low molecular weight. Rebound toxicity requires longer treatment times.

**Key Notes**
- In case of severe toxicity, renal replacement therapy is justified if the technique is able to increase the total body elimination of the toxin by 30 % or more.
- The possibility for a toxin to be removed from the blood by means of renal replacement therapy depends on its molecular weight, protein binding, volume of distribution, and solubility in water.
- Hemodialysis is the most efficient technique in terms of the clearance of water-soluble toxins with a low molecular weight.
- Drawbacks for the use of hemodialysis in intoxicated patients are rebound toxicity due to redistribution and hemodynamic instability.
- The risk of rebound toxicity and hemodynamic instability can be diminished by using sustained low efficiency hemodialysis (SLED).
- Drugs suitable for removal by renal replacement therapy are barbiturates, lithium, metformin, salicylates, theophylline, toxic alcohols, and valproic acid.

# References


1. Bronstein AC, Spyker DA, Cantilena LR. 2011 Annual report of the American Association of Poison Control Centers' National Poison Data System (NPDS): 29th Annual Report. Clin Toxicol. 2012;50:911–1164.
2. Soar J, Perkins GD, Abbas G, et al. European Resuscitation Council guidelines for resuscitation 2010 section 8: cardiac arrest in special circumstances: electrolyte abnormalities, poisoning, drowning, accidental hypothermia, hyperthermia, asthma, anaphylaxis, cardiac surgery, trauma, pregnancy, electrocution. Resuscitation. 2010;18:1400–33.
3. Orlowski JM, Hou S, Leikin JB. Extracorporeal removal of drugs and toxins. In: Ford M, Delaney KA, Ling L, et al., editors. Clinical toxicology. 1st ed. St. Louis: WB Saunders Company; 2001. p. 43–50.
4. de Pont AC. Extracorporeal treatment of intoxications. Curr Opin Crit Care. 2007;13:668–73.
5. Ronco C. Recent evolution of renal replacement therapy in the critically ill patient. Crit Care. 2006;10:123.
6. Matzke GR, Aronoff GR, Atkinson Jr AJ, et al. Drug dosing consideration in patients with acute and chronic kidney disease – a clinical update from Kidney Disease: Improving Global Outcomes (KDIGO). Kidney Int. 2011;80:1122–37.
7. Fertel BS, Nelson LS, Goldfarb DS. Extracorporeal removal techniques for the poisoned patient: a review for the intensivist. J Intensive Care Med. 2010;25:139–48.
8. Suresh M, Farrington K. Principles of extracorporeal therapy: haemodialysis, haemofiltration and haemodiafiltration. In: Jörres A, Ronco C, Kellum J, editors. Management of acute kidney problems. 1st ed. Berlin/Heidelberg: Springer; 2010. p. 481–9.
9. Munshi R, Ahmad S. Comparison of urea clearance in low efficiency low-flux vs. high-efficiency high-flux dialyzer membrane with reduced blood and dialysate flow: an in vitro analysis. Hemodial Int. 2014;18:172–4.
10. Vinsonneau C, Benyamina M. Intermittent hemodialysis. In: Jörres A, Ronco C, Kellum J, editors. Management of acute kidney problems. 1st ed. Berlin/Heidelberg: Springer; 2010. p. 515–23.
11. Bogard KN, Peterson NT, Plumb TJ, et al. Antibiotic dosing during sustained low efficiency dialysis: special considerations in adult critically ill patients. Crit Care Med. 2011;39:560–70.
12. Barshes NR, Gay N, Williams B, et al. Support for the acutely failing liver: a comprehensive review of historic and contemporary strategies. J Am Coll Surg. 2005;201:458–76.
13. Shalkham AS, Kirrane BM, Hoffman RS, et al. The availability and use of charcoal hemoperfusion in the treatment of poisoned patients. Am J Kidney Dis. 2006;48:239–41.
14. Erickson TB, Thompson TM, Lu JJ. The approach to the patient with an unknown overdose. Emerg Med Clin North Am. 2007;25:249–81.
15. Roberts DM, Buckley NA. Enhanced elimination in acute barbiturate poisoning – a systematic review. Clin Toxicol (Phila). 2011;49:2–12.
16. Palmer BF. Effectiveness of hemodialysis in the extracorporeal therapy of phenobarbital overdose. Am J Kidney Dis. 2000;36:640–3.
17. Jacobs F, Brivet FG. Conventional haemodialysis significantly lowers toxic levels of phenobarbital. Nephrol Dial Transplant. 2004;19:1663–4.
18. Eyer F, Pfab R, Felgenhauer N, et al. Lithium poisoning: pharmacokinetics and clearance during different therapeutic measures. J Clin Pharmacol. 2006;26:325–30.
19. Borras-Blasco J, Sirvent AD, Navarro-Ruiz A, et al. Unrecognized delayed toxic lithium peak concentration in acute poisoning with sustained release lithium product. South Med J. 2007;100:321–3.
20. Galea M, Jelacin N, Bramham K, et al. Severe lactic acidosis and rhabdomyolysis following metformin and ramipril overdose. Br J Anaesth. 2007;98:213–5.
21. Davidson MB, Peters AL. An overview of metformin in the treatment of type 2 diabetes mellitus. Am J Med. 1997;102:99–110.

22. Lalau JD, Andrejak M, Morinière P, et al. Hemodialysis in the treatment of lactic acidosis in diabetics treated by metformin: a study of metformin elimination. Int J Clin Pharmacol Ther Toxicol. 1989;27:1285–8.
23. Spiller HA, Sawyer TS. Toxicology of oral antidiabetic medications. Am J Health Syst Pharm. 2006;63:929–38.
24. Alivanis P, Giannikouris I, Paliuras C, et al. Metformin associated lactic acidosis treated with continuous renal replacement therapy. Clin Ther. 2006;28:396–400.
25. Guo PY, Storsley LJ, Finkle SN. Severe lactic acidosis treated with prolonged hemodialysis: recovery after massive overdoses of metformin. Semin Dial. 2006;19:80–3.
26. O'Malley GF. Emergency department management of the salicylate poisoned patient. Emerg Med Clin North Am. 2007;25:333–46.
27. Dargan PI, Wallace CI, Jones AL. An evidence based flowchart to guide the management of acute salicylate (aspirin) overdose. Emerg Med J. 2002;19:206–9.
28. Henderson JH, McKenzie CA, Hilton PJ, et al. Continuous venovenous haemofiltration for the treatment of theophylline toxicity. Thorax. 2001;56:242–3.
29. Mycyk MB, DesLauriers C, Metz J, et al. Compliance with poison center fomepizole recommendations is suboptimal in cases of toxic alcohol poisoning. Am J Ther. 2006;13:485–9.
30. Mégarbane B, Borron SW, Baud FJ. Current recommendations for treatment of severe toxic alcohol poisonings. Intensive Care Med. 2005;31:189–95.
31. Moreau CL, Kerns II W, Tomaszewski CA, et al. Glycolate kinetics and hemodialysis clearance in ethylene glycol poisoning. J Toxicol Clin Toxicol. 1998;36:659–66.
32. Barceloux DG, Bond GR, Krenzelok EP, et al. American Academy of Clinical Toxicology practice guidelines on the treatment of methanol poisoning. J Toxicol Clin Toxicol. 2002;40:415–46.
33. Kerns II W, Tomaszewski C, McMartin K, et al. Formate kinetics in methanol poisoning. J Toxicol Clin Toxicol. 2002;40:137–43.
34. Abramson S, Singh AK. Treatment of the alcohol intoxications: ethylene glycol, methanol and isopropanol. Curr Opin Nephrol Hypertens. 2000;9:695–701.
35. Al Aly Z, Yalamanchili P, Gonzalez E. Extracorporeal management of valproic acid toxicity: a case report and review of the literature. Semin Dial. 2005;18:62–6.
36. Meek MF, Broekroelofs J, Yska JP, et al. Valproic acid intoxication: sense and nonsense of haemodialysis. Neth J Med. 2004;62:333–6.
37. Singh SM, McCormick BB, Mustata S, et al. Extracorporeal management of valproic acid overdose: a large regional experience. J Nephrol. 2004;17:43–9.
38. Goodman JW, Goldfarb DS. The role of continuous venovenous replacement therapy in the treatment of poisoning. Semin Dial. 2006;19:402–7.
39. Sztajnkrycer MD. Valproic acid toxicity: overview and management. J Toxicol Clin Toxicol. 2002;40:789–801.

# Pediatric CRRT

Zaccaria Ricci and Stuart L. Goldstein

## 20.1 Epidemiology of pCRRT and the ppCRRT Registry

Information available on pediatric patients requiring continuous renal replacement therapy (CRRT) is scant and partially deriving from the adult critically ill patients: in many cases pediatric CRRT (pCRRT) is prescribed according to local expertise and without the utilization of any specific recommendation. The prospective pCRRT (ppCRRT) registry was created in order to improve and increase observational information on pCRRT practice of several US centers and it is currently the only source, worlwide, which gathered the experience derived from hundreds of treated children [1]. The ppCRRT registry was founded in 2001 and comprises 13 pediatric centers in the USA. So far, the ppCRRT enrolled 344 patients with age ranging from 1 day to 25 years and weights ranged from 1.3 to 160 kg; 11 different primary diagnoses were described in the registry the most represented of which are sepsis, stem cell transplantation, cardiac disease, liver disease, and malignancies [1]. The overall survival of these patients was 58 % and it appeared to be significantly reduced in patients with multiple organ dysfunction syndrome and fluid overload, weighing less than 10 kg or receiving stem cell transplantation [1]. Provided this unique set of information (and other related to technical aspects such as position and size of dialysis catheters, the association with filter lifespan or anticoagulation) the ppCRRT registry left several questions unanswered: optimal timing of pCRRT has still to be

Z. Ricci, MD (✉)
Pediatric Cardiac Intensive Care Unit, Department of Pediatric Cardiology and Cardiac Surgery, Bambino Gesù Children's Hospital, IRCCS, Piazza S. Onofrio 4, Rome, 00165, Italy
e-mail: z.ricci@libero.it

S.L. Goldstein, MD
Division of Nephrology, Center for Acute Care Nephrology,
Cincinnati Children's Hospital Medical Center,
3333 Burnet Avenue, MLC 7022, Cincinnati, OH 45206, USA
e-mail: stuart.goldstein@cchmc.org

© Springer International Publishing 2015
H.M. Oudemans-van Straaten et al. (eds.), *Acute Nephrology for the Critical Care Physician*, DOI 10.1007/978-3-319-17389-4_20

clarified (although it is now clear that it should be considered before fluid is accumulated in children), optimal dosing of CRRT prescription is currently unknown (even if, after adult experience and the possibility to easily achieve highest doses in such small patients, this may not be an issue significantly affecting outcomes) and, above all, long-term outcomes of acute kidney injury (AKI) children undergoing CRRT are still to be explored (it is possible that patients surviving a CRRT treatment suffer a reduced renal reserve with a significant risk of becoming chronic renal failure patients).

## 20.2 Timing to Start and Stop pCRRT

Although the analysis of timing of pCRRT may appear difficult due to the lack of prospective evidence, the lack of absolute indications for dialysis inception and the lack of a common definition of "timing", as a common sense rule "timely" CRRT start has been advocated by several authors [2]. It seems particularly important that the pCRRT start occurs before the fluid overload threshold of 10–20 % has been reached in an AKI pediatric patient [3]. A recent small retrospective observation of pCRRT patients undergoing extracorporeal membrane oxygenation (ECMO) showed that not only mortality is affected by the level of fluid overload achieved at the time of CRRT start, but also that it seems hard to "force" fluid removal in order to improve patient outcomes [4]. In light of this, a post hoc analysis of the RENAL trial showed that apart from what level of fluid overload is reached at CRRT start (in adult patients), mortality was affected by the level of fluid balance reached in the first 48 h: critically ill adult patients tended to survive more if a negative level of fluid balance was rapidly achieved [5]. In a large retrospective 10-year cohort analysis, a thorough analysis of timing of pCRRT initiation was recently attempted [6]. The authors defined timing as the time from intensive care unit (ICU) admission to CRRT initiation. They found that late initiators (>5 days) had higher mortality than early initiators (≤5 days) with a hazard ratio of 1.56 (95 % confidence interval: 1.02–2.37) with an increase of 5 % in mortality for every day of delay in CRRT initiation after adjusting for significant confounders. On multivariable regression, independent predictors of mortality were also fluid overload, indication for CRRT initiation (simultaneous presence of renal dysfunction and fluid overload), severity of illness at ICU admission, and active oncologic diagnosis. Interestingly, according to pediatric-modified risk, injury, failure, loss, and end stage (pRIFLE) classification, the authors seemed to realize that many severe cases at ICU admission were more likely to be treated earlier (hence, most severe pRIFLE classes were more common in the survivor group); on the other side, if a patient slightly but significantly progressed to higher AKI stages during the course of ICU admission, the treatment was delayed and a correlation between pRIFLE progression and time to CRRT start was found. It is possible that this subgroup of patients may receive the most benefit from an earlier CRRT start. Pediatric CRRT has to be started before 5 days from ICU admission if a patient has AKI in order to be effective in terms of mortality [6].

## 20.3    The Modern Practice of CRRT in Infants

Currently, the two dialysis modalities most frequently used in infants are peritoneal dialysis (PD) and CRRT. PD is currently the RRT treatment of choice in neonates, unless specific contraindications are present (i.e. peritonitis, abdominal masses, or bleeding) [7]. PD uses peritoneum as a semipermeable membrane to achieve solute diffusion and plasma water ultrafiltration: dialysate is infused through an abdominal catheter and after a period of so-called "dwell time", waste solution is drained from the abdomen. Typically, in pediatric cardiac surgery neonates, in order to avoid excessive intra-abdominal pressure rise during dialysis solution infusion and to prevent hemodynamic instability, a "low flow" prescription of 10 ml/kg dialysate is recommended [8]. Dwell times may vary from 10 to 30 min according to the need for higher to lower solute clearances. Water ultrafiltration may be regulated by dialysate tonicity (provided by glucose concentration, 1.36–2.5 %). PD is a simple and safe technique, which does not require dedicated technology or a steep learning curve and may be administered by ICU nurses without specific nephrologic exper tise. Nonetheless, it must be acknowledged that PD is limited by a relative lack of efficiency especially in water removal which may be particularly relevant in severely overloaded patients. Furthermore, the most important side effects of PD in neonates may be interstitial fluid accumulation in case of suboptimal dialysate drainage, hyperglycemia, and higher risk of peritoneal infection. PD is finally contra-indicated in patients with recent abdominal surgery or abdominal bleeding [7]. However, PD in the post-operative phase may be applied proactively and in a very early phase of oliguria or fluid retention. PD has been recently showed to be associated with improved survival in a large cohort of post-cardiac surgery neonates if started in the first 24 post-operative hours when compared with patients who received PD after the second post-operative day [9].

Extracorporeal dialysis in children can be managed with a variety of modalities, including intermittent hemodialysis, and CRRT, delivered as hemofiltration, hemodialysis or hemodiafiltration [10]. The choice of dialysis modality to be used is influenced by several factors, including the goals of dialysis, the unique advantages and disadvantages of each modality, and institutional resources. Intermittent dialysis may not be well tolerated in infants because of its rapid rate of solute clearance and in particular in hemodynamically unstable pediatric critically ill patients. These children are generally treated by CRRT that seems to better provide both fluid and solute re-equilibration and pro-inflammatory mediators removal. Circuits with reduced priming volume together with monitors providing an extremely accurate fluid balance are still not commercially available [10]. Post-heart surgery patients, in particular, are a peculiar and interesting model of acute water accumulation and inflammation: they receive ultrafiltration soon after cardiopulmonary bypass weaning in order to remove water and inflammatory mediators before the harmful effects of inflammation and fluid overload become clinically relevant [10]. Several studies showed a statistical difference in the percentage of fluid overload of children with severe renal dysfunction requiring RRT. At the time of dialysis initiation, survivors tend to have less fluid overload than non-survivors, especially in the setting of

MODS [11]. For this reason, in children now priority indication is given to the correction of water overload. In fact, differently from the adult patients where dialysis dose may play a key role, an adequate water content in small children is the main independent predictor of outcome.

With regard to the CRRT modality, Parakininkas, compared in vitro the solute clearance in three modes of CRRT at the low blood flow rates typically used in pediatric patients and concluded that post-dilution CVVH and CVVHD gave nearly equivalent clearances [12]. At the low blood flow rates used in pediatric patients, which raise concerns about high filtration fractions during post-dilution CVVH causing excessive hemoconcentration and filter clotting, CVVHD appeared to be the optimal modality for maximizing clearance of small solutes during CRRT. Nevertheless, if we consider the advantages of hemofiltration with respect to hemodialysis on the clearance of medium and higher molecular weight solutes together with the increased risk of filter clotting, predilution hemofiltration might be the preferred modality in small patients. There is no randomized trial guiding the prescription of CRRT in children: a small solute clearance of 2 L/h*1.73 m$^2$ may be recommended in children and it is typically utilized in the USA [13].

## 20.4 Technical Aspects of pCRRT and Future Directions

In recent years, in spite of significant advances in critical care technology, a truly pediatric CRRT system has never been developed. From one side, current CRRT machines have been equipped with pediatric circuits and lines demonstrating an attempt to comply with the specific requirements of the very small patient. On another side, most machines if not all, are used off label when patients below 10 kg are treated. The small number of cases, together with the limited interest of industry to develop a fully integrated device specifically designed for the pediatric population. Current CRRT machines present significant limitations for the pediatric population and in some cases, severe complications have occurred. In current practice, clinical application of dialysis equipment to pediatric patients is substantially adapted to smaller patients with great concerns about outcomes and side effects of such extracorporeal therapy. In these conditions, whereas adult critically ill patients receive renal support with modern devices and very strict safety features, smaller patients cannot rely on a very accurate delivery of therapy especially as far as fluid balance is concerned. On the other hand, it is extremely difficult to treat a small infant with a dialysis monitor providing accurate blood flow rates in the range of 10–50 ml/min and hourly ultrafiltration error below 5 ml/h. The accuracy of current systems is much lower than requested and fatal errors may occur in the very small patient. Since manufacturers of dialysis or CRRT machines do not perform specific tests for treatments in patients weighing less than 10–15 kg and safety features in these patients are not specifically created, legal concerns may arise when operators decide to prescribe these therapies. The Cardio-Renal, Pediatric Dialysis Emergency Machine (CARPEDIEM) project was designed in Vicenza in order to create the basis for the conception of a renal replacement therapy equipment specifically dedicated to newborns and small infants with a weight range of 2.0–9.9 kg and with an approximate body surface area from 0.15 to 0.5 m². In these patients, the total blood volume ranges from less than 200 ml to about 1 l meaning that total body water content varies from 1 to 5 l: in such conditions, circuits priming volumes should be reduced to a minimum level and roller pumps should be able to run at slow speed, maintaining a good level of accuracy together with the possibility of warranting lines integrity (small roller pumps running small tubes are expected to cause a quick decline in their performance) [14].

## 20.5 CRRT in ECMO Patients

A peculiar and complex category of critically ill patient is the one requiring both RRT and ECMO. This clinical picture is frequently seen in the pediatric setting. AKI occurs to the vast majority of ECMO children, who suffered from severe cardiac dysfunction (cardio-renal syndrome) or required aggressive mechanical ventilation (lung-renal syndrome). The CRRT circuit may be placed in parallel (blood flows in the same direction of the ECMO circuit) or in series (countercurrent to the ECMO circuit). Santiago and coauthors described how to connect the CRRT device into the ECMO circuit [15]: the inlet (arterial) line of the CRRT circuit was connected after the ECMO blood pump by a three-way tap that was also used for the infusion of heparin, and the outlet (venous) line was connected to the circuit at another tap before the oxygenator. Differently from what suggested by the authors, the inlet of the CRRT machine may be connected after the ECMO pump and the filter outlet then returned to the ECMO circuit before the pump (into the reservoir, if present): the CRRT circuit, running countercurrent to extracorporeal assistance, allows the RRT blood to be aspired from the arterial ECMO section (where blood returns to the patient) and then to be infused into the venous ECMO section (where the patient is drained) [16]. This second set-up might reduce blood flow resistance and turbulence after the centrifugal pump and improve reservoir drainage when a roller pump is present. The blood recirculation induced by these circuit set-ups is negligible, considering that the CRRT to ECMO blood flow ratio is never superior to 0.1. Dr. Shaheen and colleagues [17] presented their experience with two different subgroups of children: one group that required hemofiltration alone and the other group that required both hemofiltration and ECMO. Not surprisingly, the authors identified a higher mortality rate in those patients requiring both CVVH and ECMO compared with those patients requiring hemofiltration alone. The authors promoted the concept that certain therapies should be reserved to experienced teams. Performing CVVH in a heterogeneous population with large age and weight ranges poses significant clinical and technical challenges. The low frequency of CVVH use in ECMO, as well as the use of other extracorporeal therapies, also raises problems with maintaining nursing skills. Objective clinical and biochemical markers for commencing CVVH alone or in combination with ECMO remain to be defined. Several studies, however, already showed safety and feasibility of this connection in the pediatric setting [18] and, even if some worries on such difficult interaction have been raised (i.e. fluid balance accuracy [19]), today the application of CRRT to all ECMO is indeed recommended by some authors [20, 21]: in a matched control study, 15 ECMO newborns, with continuous hemofiltration added to the ECMO circuit were matched with 46 historical controls. Time on extracorporeal assistance and on mechanical ventilation was significantly reduced in the CRRT population: such strategy might improve fluid balance management and capillary leak syndrome. Furthermore, according to these authors, fewer blood transfusions are needed and overall costs per extracorporeal membrane oxygenation run are lower.

## Conclusion

AKI is a severe clinical condition that is further complicated in critically ill children by some peculiar problems of these patients. Early diagnosis, prevention, conservative measures, and renal replacement therapies are all part of a common approach that must be undertaken in these high risk patients. The outcomes may vary significantly depending on the underlying disease, the severity of illness, and the time of intervention. A multidisciplinary approach should be encouraged to reach the best possible care of these patients and to utilize the highest levels of competence in each single branch of the intensive care medicine. So far, however, outcomes of critically ill children requiring CRRT are poor and strongly need a strategy for improvement. In this scenario, new technological advances such as miniaturized circuits and membranes, accurate CRRT machines and effective prescription schedules promise to help the clinician in improving quality of treatment.

### Key Messages
- pCRRT may be delivered with peritoneal dialysis (typically in neonates) or with extracorporeal RRT: in such case, generally CVVHD or pre-dilution CVVH are prescribed.
- Fluid overload prevention and aggressive treatment have a key role in pCRRT patients mortality improvement.
- Current pCRRT technology requires dedicated development and technical evolution in order to improve ease of application, to broaden indications to treatment and to anticipate CRRT start.

## References


1. Sutherland SM, Goldstein SL, Alexander SR. The Prospective Pediatric Continuous Renal Replacement Therapy (ppCRRT) Registry: a critical appraisal. Pediatr Nephrol. 2014;29(11):2069–76.
2. Ricci Z, Ronco C. Timing, dose and mode of dialysis in acute kidney injury. Curr Opin Crit Care. 2011;17:556–61.
3. Sutherland SM, Zappitelli M, Alexander SR, Chua AN, Brophy PD, Bunchman TE, Hackbarth R, Somers MJ, Baum M, Symons JM, Flores FX, Benfield M, Askenazi D, Chand D, Fortenberry JD, Mahan JD, McBryde K, Blowey D, Goldstein SL. Fluid overload and mortality in children receiving continuous renal replacement therapy: the prospective pediatric continuous renal replacement therapy registry. Am J Kidney Dis. 2010;55:316–25.

4. Selewski DT, Cornell TT, Blatt NB, Han YY, Mottes T, Kommareddi M, Gaies MG, Annich GM, Kershaw DB, Shanley TP, Heung M. Fluid overload and fluid removal in pediatric patients on extracorporeal membrane oxygenation requiring continuous renal replacement therapy. Crit Care Med. 2012;40:2694–9.
5. The RENAL Replacement Therapy Study Investigators. An observational study fluid balance and patient outcomes in the randomized evaluation of normal vs. augmented level of replacement therapy trial. Crit Care Med. 2012;40:1753–60.
6. Modem V, Thompson M, Gollhofer D, Dhar AV, Quigley R. Timing of continuous renal replacement therapy and mortality in critically ill children. Crit Care Med. 2014;42(4):943–53.
7. Morelli S, Ricci Z, Di Chiara L, Stazi GV, Polito A, Vitale V, Giorni C, Iacoella C, Picardo S. Renal replacement therapy in neonates with congenital heart disease. Contrib Nephrol. 2007;156:428–33.
8. Ricci Z, Morelli S, Ronco C, Polito A, Stazi GV, Giorni C, Di Chiara L, Picardo S. Inotropic support and peritoneal dialysis adequacy in neonates after cardiac surgery. Interact Cardiovasc Thorac Surg. 2008;7:116–20.
9. Bojan M, Gioanni S, Vouhé PR, Journois D, Pouard P. Early initiation of peritoneal dialysis in neonates and infants with acute kidney injury following cardiac surgery is associated with a significant decrease in mortality. Kidney Int. 2012;82:474–81.
10. Picca S, Ricci Z, Picardo S. Acute kidney injury in an infant after cardiopulmonary bypass. Semin Nephrol. 2008;28(5):470–6.
11. Goldstein SL, Somers MJ, Baum MA, Symons JM, Brophy PD, Blowey D, Bunchman TE, Baker C, Mottes T, McAfee N, Barnett J, Morrison G, Rogers K, Fortenberry D. Pediatric patients with multi-organ dysfunction syndrome receiving continuous renal replacement therapy. Kidney Int. 2005;67:653–8.
12. Parakininkas D, Greenbaum LA. Comparison of solute clearance in three modes of continuous renal replacement therapy. Pediatr Crit Care Med. 2004;5:269–74.
13. Askenazi DJ, Goldstein SL, Koralkar R, Fortenberry J, Baum M, Hackbarth R, Blowey D, Bunchman TE, Brophy PD, Symons J, Chua A, Flores F, Somers MJ. Continuous renal replacement therapy for children ≤10 kg: a report from the prospective pediatric continuous renal replacement therapy registry. J Pediatr. 2013;162(3):587–592.e3.
14. Ronco C, Garzotto F, Ricci Z. CA.R.PE.DI.E.M. (Cardio-Renal Pediatric Dialysis Emergency Machine): evolution of continuous renal replacement therapies in infants. A personal journey. Pediatr Nephrol. 2012;27:1203–11.
15. Santiago MJ, Sánchez A, López-Herce J, Pérez R, del Castillo J, Urbano J, Carrillo A. The use of continuous renal replacement therapy in series with extracorporeal membrane oxygenation. Kidney Int. 2009;76:1289–92.
16. Ricci Z, Ronco C, Picardo S. CRRT in series with extracorporeal membrane oxygenation in pediatric patients. Kidney Int. 2010;77:469–70.
17. Shaheen IS, Harvey B, Watson AR, Pandya HC, Mayer A, Thomas D. Continuous venovenous hemofiltration with or without extracorporeal membrane oxygenation in children. Pediatr Crit Care Med. 2007;8:362–5.
18. Symons JM, McMahon MW, Karamlou T, Parrish AR, McMullan DM. Continuous renal replacement therapy with an automated monitor is superior to a free-flow system during extracorporeal life support. Pediatr Crit Care Med. 2013;14(9):e404–8.
19. Ricci Z, Morelli S, Vitale V, Di Chiara L, Cruz D, Picardo S. Management of fluid balance in continuous renal replacement therapy: technical evaluation in the pediatric setting. Int J Artif Organs. 2007;30:896–901.
20. Hoover NG, Heard M, Reid C, Wagoner S, Rogers K, Foland J, Paden ML, Fortenberry JD. Enhanced fluid management with continuous venovenous hemofiltration in pediatric respiratory failure patients receiving extracorporeal membrane oxygenation support. Intensive Care Med. 2008;34:2241–7.
21. Blijdorp K, Cransberg K, Wildschut ED, Gischler SJ, Jan Houmes R, Wolff ED, Tibboel D. Haemofiltration in newborns treated with extracorporeal membrane oxygenation: a case-comparison study. Crit Care. 2009;13:R48.

# 21

Ian Baldwin

## 21.1 Introduction

Continuous renal replacement therapy (CRRT) use in the ICU for over 25 years has yielded new nursing knowledge and a body of literature is building. This chapter provides a contemporary approach for training and education, useful to maintain competence in CRRT listing useful lecture topics and describes how when linked to simulation a powerful education process can occur. The most common question to experienced users – 'which machine should I use' – along with other technical questions for the CRRT machine and circuit are answered. Another concern is the lack of local information for CRRT users; policy and protocol documents are discussed as they are a foundation resource in the ICU using CRRT ensuring some safety and quality. As a key quality indicator, monitoring the filter 'life' is discussed to suggest this data point can represent success or failure for the many facets of CRRT use in the ICU. Finally, undertaking research and questioning use of CRRT not only provides feedback and useful clinical data but stimulates interest for this aspect of critical illness nursing. This approach develops a culture and nursing skills base where other blood purification techniques may be possible and performed safely when needed.

## 21.2 Training, Education and Prep for CRRT

As continuous therapies were introduced to the ICU during the 1980s and early 1990s, much education and training was required [1–4]. This was because many ICU's were undertaking a switch from intermittent to continuous treatment for acute renal failure support. Accompanying this change was moving responsibility

I. Baldwin, RN, PhD, ACCCN
Department of Intensive Care, Austin Health, Heidelberg, VIC 3084, Australia
e-mail: Ian.baldwin@austin.org.au

© Springer International Publishing 2015

263

H.M. Oudemans-van Straaten et al. (eds.), *Acute Nephrology for the Critical Care Physician*, DOI 10.1007/978-3-319-17389-4_21

for patient care from the dialysis to ICU nurse or a collaborative approach sharing the work and expertise [5–7]. In many centres, the training and education was for large groups or entire ICU staffing cohorts, and accompanied by new purpose-built CRRT machines or the use of adapted or modified blood pumps and intravenous pumps configured to provide CRRT but with limited automation and safety [8, 9]. The literature at this time reflected information describing and defining CRRT, the basic technology used, differences in modes (diffusive or convective) and provided circuit diagrams to explain this, and outlined additional nursing care and tasks in the ICU [1–3, 10–12]. In current day, more than 25 years later with CRRT well imbedded in the ICU and a nursing independence evident [13–16]. The education focus has been for smaller groups associated with ICU orientation for new staff and specialist training for nursing now taught a more established CRRT curriculum, and new learning for advanced treatments. In this case or when a smaller ICU begins CRRT with no background in artificial renal failure support, a 1-day or series of small presentations is appropriate [17, 18] and can include the topics listed in Fig. 21.1 provided in three sequential sessions with time variability depending on the audience demographic. The didactic delivery of these topics becomes a powerful approach when supplemented with simulation activities linked to live patient care and bedside clinical support [19, 20]. A recent report [21] suggests when simulation is added to didactic CRRT education programmes, an improvement in CRRT functional time (filter 'life') is observed – a direct benefit to users, less cost and better for patients [21].

CRRT machine vendors, product suppliers or conference websites can now provide many education recourses for CRRT in the ICU [22] and many of these free web-based offerings are suitable [23]. The key to successful CRRT education and training is nurses with a clinical background managing CRRT in the ICU and teaching qualifications to conduct the teaching. This may require a nurse being allocated to this role within an award structure such as clinical nurse specialist (CNS) or where educators are in place for the wider ICU education [1, 19]. In addition to the teachers, identifying a small number of nurses as CRRT 'champions' for this initial training and the ongoing support when CRRT is in progress is a common and successful approach [1, 17–19].

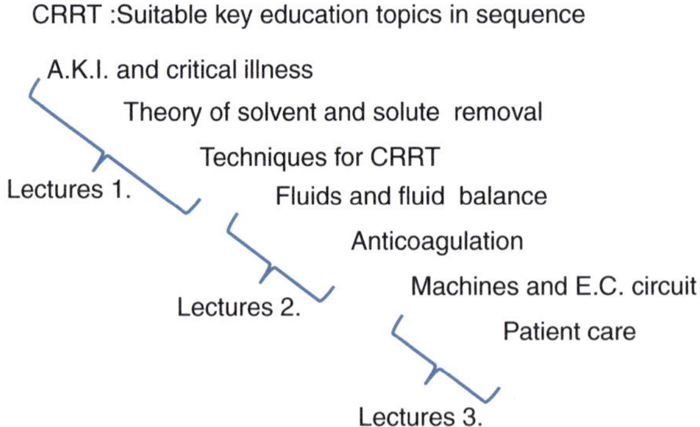


**Fig. 21.1** Suitable schedule and sequence for CRRT education; grouped into three classes

## 21.3    Machines and Technology for CRRT: Selection and Other

The most common question asked of experienced nurses in the ICU where CRRT is performed frequently is their opinion for machine choice and other treatment preferences. Depending on global location, regional availability, past or existing hospital contracts, leading physician input, and available budget, the choice will vary widely. Many suppliers are now offering flexible contracts where the high purchase cost is removed for acquisition of machines, but built into an anticipated consumables use contract over a number of years into the future.

While interface and appearance will differ, machines for CRRT mostly differ in the manner in which they control fluids measurement to achieve fluid balance [24, 25]. They all offer a version of pre-assembled disposable circuitry, colour monitor screen user interface with touch or control knob navigation and roller pumps to provide blood and fluids flow [8, 26, 27]. An internal computer manages the system reliant on pressure readings, sensors and detectors from the circuit to facilitate correct software function from the priming phase and during use. This functionality is to detect errors preventing major failure likely to cause death such as air embolism [28] or fluid imbalance [24, 25]. This is a complex requirement and generally done well by manufacturers. Figure 21.2 provides a generic circuit diagram for any automated CRRT machine and circuit indicating key sensors and

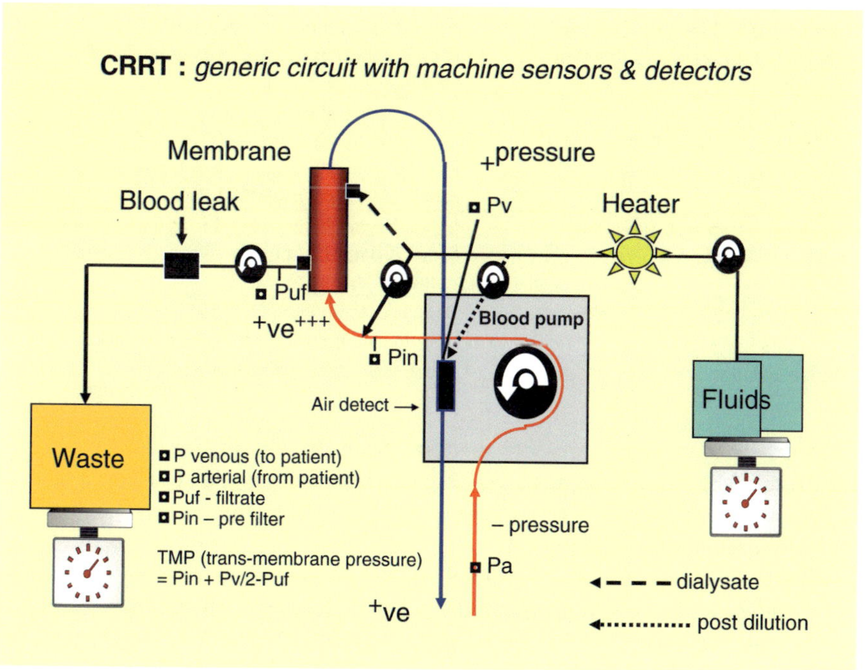


**Fig. 21.2** Circuit diagram for CRRT indicating sensors for pressure and detectors for air and blood. See Table 21.1 for normal ranges

**Table 21.1** Nursing check list for CRRT when in use – during shift

| Shift check and simple troubleshooting list: CRRT as CVVH using scales-automated CRRT machine | |
| --- | --- |
| Check | Rationale |
| Machine position relative to patient with blood lines not too tight – stretched | Patient movement could cause excess drag on access catheter and securing tape |
| Brakes ON | Machine must have brakes on to prevent inadvertent movement and risk of above |
| Fluids: correct for k+ and both bags hanging from same point – height, both line clamps open | Fluids should empty at similar rate, minimise mixing, scales and balance alarms more likely if the bags hanging at different heights |
| Venous – bubble chamber full and inspect for clot | Adjust this up slowly, using preferred method. Keep full to trap gas/ air and allow for the level to fall during use with gas entry associated with bicarbonate fluids ($CO_2$) when heated |
| Settings and alarms (*common settings*) | |
| Blood flow – speed | 200 ml/min standard |
| UF flow | 2000 ml/h standard CVVH |
| Manual pre-dilution % | 50:50 for CVVH |
| 'Weight loss' – fluid loss rate ml/h | Check orders – fluid loss target |
| Next intervention (h:min) | Time until fluids bag change or bottle empty |
| Temperature setting | Default at 37 °C, maybe ↑↓ to patient need |
| Venous +10 ----+150 (influenced by blood flow rate and chamber clotting, access function – blue lumen) | This pressure always positive, measured on the return limb of circuit. ~50–100 mmHg High pressure due to access kink or chamber clotting |
| Arterial −150 ---- −10 (influenced by blood flow rate and access function – red lumen) | This pressure always negative, measured on the outflow limb of circuit. ~−50 to −100 mmHg Excessive negative due to access kink or poor access placement – internal, clot |
| Trans-membrane pressure (TMP) $= (P_{in} + P_v)/2 - P_{uf}$ | Indicative of clotting/clogging in the membrane. Set at 200 mmHg initially. When 250+, usually terminate treatment |
| Blood leak line – detector in place | Detects colour change – blood leak very rare but reflects membrane failure – cease treatment |
| Anticoagulation and prescription orders | Check drug dose and orders correct |

detectors with common pressure readings from the circuit linked into machine software. Table 21.1 indicates a suitable troubleshooting and shift check for any automated scale-based CRRT machine associated with this circuit diagram and the pressures – sensors indicated.

Fluid measurement is done by direct volume measurement technology along the fluid pathways or by simple electronic scales assessing a change in substitution (decreasing weight) and waste (increasing) weights [24, 25]. A difference between these two measures is the fluid 'balance'; usually a loss, or more fluid in the waste compared to the fluid replacement.

Accuracy of the fluids management and how this links into the user interface setting for a desired treatment with accurate fluid removal is the challenge for manufacturers to provide safety with suitable alarms systems for the user to be aware of error. This aspect of CRRT machines creates the most concern for safe use, particularly in paediatrics with regulatory and published reports of morbidity and mortality due to fluid setting error or failure to respond to fluids alarms in adults, children and small babies [24]. When reviewing a number of different machines for purchase, a simple practical specifications table is useful. This allows the selection team to include the local preferences, required options and needs for comparison and review in order to support their final decision. A selection team needs to be inclusive of nurses, doctors, pharmacy, biomedical or technical support, fund or budget managers and nurse teachers. Practical bedside use is an important consideration throughout; therefore, machine footprint or monitor screen adjustment may need to be highly ranked in a selection table given the usual cluttered ICU bedside space or user interface with a focus on how easy the machine is to teach another nurse.

Another important consideration for machine choice is the disposable circuit necessary and how this is supplied and when fitted connects the machine to the patient, and importantly the composition and size of the membrane used, and costing for all. The circuit tubing configuration and quality of this vital component are often overlooked due to a focus on the software offerings and other options in a machine.

## 21.4 Protocols and Policy for CRRT

A protocol for CRRT in the ICU means a document with instructions for use designed and prepared by clinicians in a specific ICU. Although key aspects of a CRRT protocol may be applicable to any ICU, the idiosyncrasies and local context needs to be added and incorporated into this important resource for safe use of CRRT in your ICU. Using the protocol from another ICU is a mistake and should not be done, but is a useful guide or example to develop your own [17]. The protocol will have a practical focus with most content devoted to 'how to do' CRRT with the patients in your care, the machine used and the CRRT method chosen [1, 5, 17, 19].

Key headings for the protocol are set out in Fig. 21.3. This document is usually read as a digital file via bedside computer and allows use of colour diagrams, may include hyperlinks to different sections of the document from key words or as an index function at the front of the protocol. This allows readers to find what they need quickly. In addition, hyperlinks to other hospital policies and protocols relevant to CRRT within a local network, intranet or Internet (http:WWW) make for fast and helpful referencing. Reviewing and updating the CRRT protocol is a time-consuming task and needs to be done in-line with latest evidence, how this may alter practice, changes to consumables used and any new techniques developed such as plasma exchange (PE) or other blood purification methods; this is the role of a small interest group and the nurse and doctor champions or key experts in CRRT. Some sections of the protocol may be printed for single use or

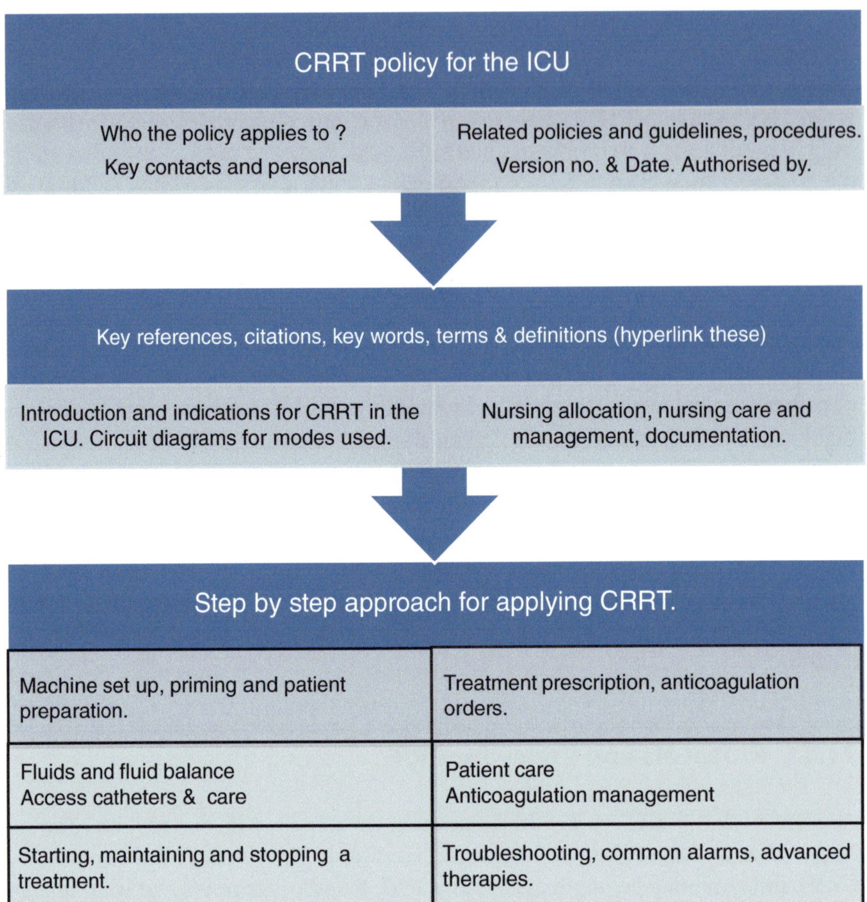


**Fig. 21.3** Policy and protocol concept map indicating key elements for CRRT in the ICU

laminated within plastic for use at a bedside by the nurse managing the CRRT repeatedly across several patients. Anticoagulation technique is a good example of this, where there may need to be drug infusion adjustments according to regular blood testing. Citrate anticoagulation is a good example where the ionised calcium level requires maintenance and is checked frequently for adjustment to calcium infusion supplementation [29, 30]. Reportable parameters for when acid–base and total calcium levels require intervention will also be included as they are not easy to remember and terminology and acronyms used may create confusion and error. There are some publications devoted to content of a CRRT protocol and provide a step-by-step approach beginning with criterion for starting CRRT, how to prepare the patient and the machine – circuit, connecting and beginning a treatment, manage and troubleshoot treatment in progress, commonly include a focus to anticoagulation approaches, and finally when and how to cease CRRT [15].

The protocol is not a machine instruction for use document and is different to the technical manual supplied with a machine; however, there may be some technical information in a manual useful to include in the protocol such as machine's battery life, significance of unusual error codes and maintenance or calibration requirements.

The protocol can be a useful educational tool, and should be used this way. Inclusion of research evidence with citations, weblinks, diagrams and tables will help keep the document limited in size and staff should be encouraged to have copies of the protocol. This will also help the reviewing team keep the protocol current and correct as these people will provide feedback if they encouraged to read, use and have their own copy.

## 21.5  Teaching CRRT and Maintaining Quality

Maintaining expertise using CRRT in the ICU will be influenced by the frequency of use or number of cases treated annually and the size of the user pool. Some programmes utilize regular competency checks and assessments [20, 21] and where use is frequent this is not done allowing the constant exposure of nurses to CRRT use provide the competency process. Different levels of skills sets can be determined for nurse to patient allocation; therefore, controlling learning and providing some safety for the patient being managed by a nurse with the appropriate CRRT skills set [1, 19]. In either case, when expert users or CNS nurses with CRRT expertise work adjacent to or close to new learners, they should be encouraged to review treatments, teach and advise. Teaching can be achieved by reviewing treatments, their progress and anticipated problems with live use of CRRT at the bedside, at the time; the teaching 'moment' such as this will be remembered by the learner, gives them reassurance and ensures safety as small errors may be detected before they create changes to patient stability. Electrolyte control such as potassium levels or anticoagulation dosing, for example. In addition to this framework and teaching culture among nurses in the ICU, pre-connection or preparation checklists, during use shift checklists (see Table 21.1), quick reference alarms and troubleshooting sheets available through bedside clinical information and e-protocol systems are very helpful to maintain skills and ensure standards are maintained. Regular group mini-simulations, review of incident or adverse events associated with CRRT, machine repair reports from technicians, tutorials, case presentations within an in-house education structure at nurse handover periods all ensure safety and quality is promoted [31].

A quick and useful outcome measure for quality when using CRRT is to document each hour the progressive 'life' of the circuit or haemofilter [32]. This data point may be collected automatically on a screen monitor with most CRRT machines. However, if also recorded on ICU bedside charts with pen on paper or electronically as part of the routine vital signs observations for the patient, this provides an instant audit for current and previous treatments. This variable is commonly cited as the outcome measure for many studies assessing different anticoagulation techniques, but may also be considered a measure of access catheter function and blood flow reliability, machine technical function and staff user competence. Furthermore, time between a circuit stopping and restarting or 'downtime' may be a measure of nurse expertise and the wider aspects of patient management in the ICU or the system of care generally. Long delays when using a continuous therapy will be associated with a loss of solute and fluid balance control [33, 34]. As circuit life is reported widely in the literature and often without a clear definition, multicentre controlled trial data inform us that a median life of 21 h is common [35, 36]. Many clinical studies report much higher values as the mean or average is reported at 50–70 h [37, 38] and without any clear definition. However, if any given circuit is functioning continuously for greater than 21 h, it could be concluded that standards and quality are being met, the patient solute and fluid balance is being achieved and they are safe. Shorter and low circuit life such as 4–6 h reflect significant problems and a focussed review before the next treatment begins as high cost will be associated, and will eventually be a consideration in the success of a CRRT programme if this is common and is not corrected. Figure 21.4 provides a concept graph to reflect that successful CRRT is when circuit life or continuous function is greater than 20⁺ hours. This is when most goals of CRRT are being met, usually due to all facets of the policy or protocol are being adhered to. Frequent clotting with circuit life at 6 h suggests there is a breakdown in the policy ideals somewhere. For example, failing access catheter, incorrect or insufficient anticoagulation, user errors or poor competence, machine technical errors, or patient agitation and delirium and frequent alarms stopping blood flow. Any of these can cause the extracorporeal circuit for CRRT to fail.

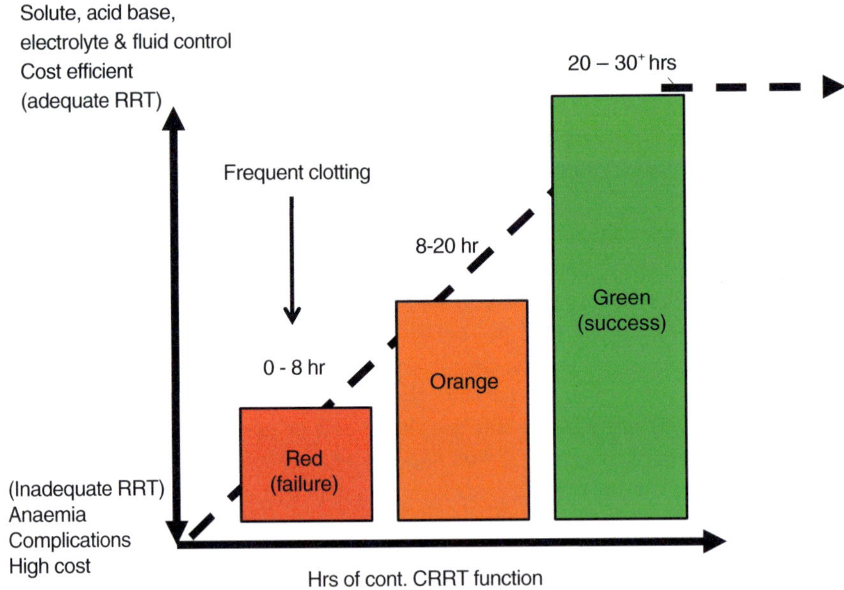



**Fig. 21.4** Filter life concept map to illustrate that filter life >20⁺ hours reflects effective CRRT and is an aim for successful CRRT program in ICU

## 21.6 Research

Research and quality activities are a useful component to a successful CRRT programme. Asking questions and testing hypotheses for the many aspects of CRRT use will only improve standards of care and provide an appropriate focus to patient care. These activities engage clinicians in thinking closely about technique and outcomes, safety and standards. A simple audit of filter life as previously discussed is an easy audit to complete monthly or for a number of patients to determine the median filter life in your ICU. Achieving fluid balance, acid–base control, electrolyte control, 'off-time', can all be audited. This type of quality activity is usually without any consent process; however, other questions where comparison and an experiment is done will require ethics permission and informed consent. As the literature is sparse, many aspects of CRRT application exist without data and evidence despite over 25 years of clinical application. Best practice is not well revealed and a key interest group in the ICU may easily formulate useful research questions for a single centre study.

## 21.7 Advanced Therapies

In some settings, basic nursing skills for CRRT use can be utilised for advanced and related therapies in the ICU such as plasma exchange (PE) [39–41], combined plasma filtration and adsorption (CPFA) [42] and the membrane adsorbing recirculating system (MARS) [43]. These treatments are possible in the general ICU, but will require the skills and confidence of experienced CRRT users, ICU physicians with an interest in blood purification techniques and close liaison with the relevant biomedical supplier. Whilst CPFA and MARS are available, expensive and with limited data reflecting best care [42, 44], PE is more likely to be prescribed in the ICU where some clear indications with data suggesting benefit are available in apheresis guidelines [45]. The technique simply requires a plasma exchange (separator) membrane inserted into the CRRT circuit set as convective clearance haemofiltration. This is plasma removal and plasma substitution, with no fluid loss set; an exchange. As the treatment is usually completed after 4–6 h or when 2.5–3.5 l of plasma is exchanged in an adult, this form of blood purification can be achieved in one nursing shift managed by an experienced ICU nurse with CRRT expertise. Some of these patients may then be further treated with CRRT in between PE treatments by less experienced staff.

### Conclusion

CRRT has now been available and performed by nurses in the ICU across multiple countries for over 25 years. Much has been learnt and a body of literature is building. However, much research is required to provide evidence for best practice in the ICU. This chapter has provided some brief insights into the issues of training and education useful to maintain competence in CRRT highlighting the useful lecture topics and how simulation with a practical focus led by CRRT *champions* is essential. The most common question to experienced users – 'which machine should I use' – along with some technical considerations for CRRT machines is outlined. The policy and protocol documents, best provided via e-systems are a foundation resource in the ICU using CRRT and provide much safety and quality if staff use them and can access these quickly. Quality indicators are numerous, but recording and monitoring filter 'life' when using CRRT is a quick and useful activity as this data can reflect success or failure in the multilayered context of CRRT use in the ICU. Finally, undertaking research and other activities to investigate and question your use of CRRT will provide interest and focus to this aspect of critical illness nursing and lead nurses towards advanced skills for other blood purification techniques.

## References


1. Baldwin IC, Elderkin TD. CVVH in intensive care. Nursing perspectives. New Horiz. 1995;3(4):738–47.
2. Baldwin IC, Bridge NP, Elderkin TD. Nursing issues, practices, and perspectives for the management of continuous renal replacement therapy in the intensive care unit. In: Bellomo R, Ronco C, editors. Critical care nephrology. Dordrecht: Kluwer Publishing Co. 1998. p. 1309–27.
3. Guiliano K, Pysznik E. Renal replacement therapy in critical care: implementation of a unit-based continuous venovenous hemodialysis program. Crit Care Nurse. 1998;18(1):40–51.
4. Martin R, Jurschak J. Nursing management of continuous renal replacement therapy. Semin Dial. 1996;9(2):192–9.
5. Mehta R, Martin R. Initiating and implementing a continuous renal replacement therapy program. Semin Dial. 1996;9(2):80–7.
6. Clevenger K. Setting up a continuous venovenous hemofiltration educational program. Crit Care Nurs Clin North Am. 1998;10(2):235–44.
7. Baldwin I, Elderkin T. Continuous hemofiltration: nursing perspectives in critical care. New Horiz. 1995;3(4):738–47.
8. Bellomo R, Baldwin I, Ronco C, Golper T. Atlas of hemofiltration. London: W.B. Saunders; 2001. Chapters 6 and 13.
9. Ronco C, Brendolan A, Belomo R. Current technology for continuous renal replacement therapies. In: Ronco C, Bello R, editors. Critical care nephrology. Dordrecht: Kluwer Academic Publishers; 1998. p. 1269–308.
10. Burchardi H. History development of continuous renal replacement techniques. Kidney Int. 1998;53 Suppl 66:S120–4.
11. Bellomo R, Ronco C. Continuous renal replacement therapy in the intensive care unit. Intensive Care Med. 1999;25:781–9.
12. Bellomo R, Ronco C. Continuous versus intermittent renal replacement therapy in the intensive care unit. Kidney Int. 1998;53(Supp. 66):S125–8.
13. Dirkes S, Hodge K. Continuous renal replacement therapy in the adult intensive care unit. History and current trends. Critical Care Nurs. 2007;27(2):61–80.
14. Baldwin I, Leslie G. Chapter 18. Support of renal function. In: Elliot D, Aitken L, Chaboyer W, Elliot D, Aitken L, Chaboyer W, editors. ACCCN's critical care nursing. 2nd ed. Sydney: Elsevier Pub, Mosby Co; 2012.
15. Baldwin I, Fealy N. Clinical nursing for the application of renal replacement therapies in the intensive care unit. Semin Dial. 2009;22(2):189–93.

16. Langford S, Slivar S, Tucker SM, Bourbonnais FF. Exploring CRRT practices in ICU: a survey of Canadian hospitals. Dynamics. 2008;19(1):18–23.
17. Baldwin I, Fealy N. Nursing for renal replacement therapies in the intensive care unit: historical, educational, and protocol review. Blood Purif. 2009;27:174–81.
18. Baldwin I. Training management and credentialing for CRRT in critical care. Am J Kidney Dis. 1997;30(5 S4):S112–6.
19. Graham P, Lischer E. Nursing issues in renal replacement therapy: organization, manpower assessment, competency evaluation and quality improvement processes. Semin Dial. 2011;24(2):183–7.
20. Hagaman C, Ballard-Hernandez J, Cabaluna V. Developing nursing competency in Continuous Renal Replacement Therapy (CRRT). Abstract in Critical Care Nurse. 2008;28(2):e5.
21. Mottes T, Owens T, Niedner M, Juno Julie S, Thomas P, Heung M. Improving delivery of continuous renal replacement therapy: impact of a simulation-based educational intervention. Pediatr Crit Care Med. 2013;14(8):747–54.
22. http://www.baxter.com/healthcare_professionals/therapies/renal/.html Retrieved 19 Feb 2014.
23. http://www.advancedrenaleducation.com and http://www.CRRTonline.com. Retrieved 19 Feb 2014.
24. Ronco C. Fluid balance in CRRT: a call to attention! Int J Artif Organs. 2005;28(8):763–4.
25. Bagshaw S, Baldwin I, Fealy N, Bellomo R. Fluid balance error in continuous renal replacement therapy: a technical note. Int J Artif Organs. 2007;30(5):435–40.
26. Ronco C. Chapter 29. Machines for continuous renal replacement therapy. In: Kellum J, Bellomo R, Ronco C, editors. Continuous renal replacement therapy. New York: Oxford Press; 2010.
27. Boyle M, Baldwin I. Understanding the continuous renal replacement therapy circuit for acute renal failure support; a quality issue in the intensive care unit. AACN Adv Crit Care. 2010;21(4):365–75.
28. Ku L, Weinberg L, Seevanayagam S, Baldwin I, Opdam H, Doolan L. Massive air embolism from continuous electromechanical dissociation in a cardiac surgical patient. Crit Care Resusc. 2012;14(2):154–8.
29. Davies H, Morgan D, Leslie G. A regional citrate anticoagulation protocol for pre-dilution CVVHDf: the "modified Alabama protocol". Aust Crit Care. 2009;21(3):154–65.
30. Tolwani A, Wille K. Anticoagulation for continuous renal replacement therapy. Semin Dial. 2009;22(2):141–5.
31. Baldwin I, Whiteman K. Educational resources. Chapter 31. In: Kellum J, Bellomo R, Ronco C, editors. Continuous renal replacement therapy. New York: Oxford Press; 2010.
32. Bellomo R, Baldwin I. Anticoagulation. Chapter 17. In: Kellum J, Bellomo R, Ronco C, editors. Continuous renal replacement therapy. New York: Oxford Press; 2010.
33. Fealy N, Baldwin I, Bellomo R. The effect of circuit "down time" on uraemic control during continuous veno-venous haemofiltration. Crit Care Resusc. 2002;4:266–70.
34. Bouchard J, et al. Fluid accumulation, survival and recovery of kidney function in critically ill patients with acute kidney injury. Kidney Int. 2009;76:422–7.
35. Palevsky PM, Zhang JH, O'Connor TZ, et al. Intensity of renal support in critically ill patients with acute kidney injury. N Engl J Med. 2008;359:7–20.
36. The RENAL replacement Therapy Study Investigators. Intensity of continuous renal replacement therapy in critically ill patients. N Engl J Med. 2009;361:1627–38.
37. Monchi M, Berghmans D, Ledoux D, Canivet JL, Dubois B, Damas P. Citrate vs. heparin for anticoagulation in continuous venovenous hemofiltration: a prospective randomized study. Intensive Care Med. 2004;30:260–5.
38. Kutsogiannis DJ, Gibney NRT, Stollery D, Gao J. Regional citrate versus systemic heparin anticoagulation for continuous renal replacement in critically ill patients. Kidney Int. 2005;67:2361–7.
39. Reeves J. Plasmapheresis in critical illness. In: Ronco C, Bellomo R, Kellum J, editors. Critical care nephrology. 2nd ed. Philadelphia: Saunders Elsevier; 2009. p. 1519–24.

40. Ward DM. Conventional apheresis therapies: a review. J Clin Apheresis. 2011;26(5):230–8. doi:10.1002/jca.20302.
41. Paton E, Baldwin I. Plasma exchange in the intensive care unit; a 10 year retrospective audit. Australian Crit Care. 2013. http://dx.doi.org/10.1016/j.aucc.2013.10.001.
42. Livigni S, Bertolini G, Rossi C, Ferrari F, Giardino M, Pozzato M, Remuzzi G, GiViTI: Gruppo Italiano per la Valutazione degli Interventi in Terapia Intensiva (Italian Group for the Evaluation of Interventions in Intensive Care Medicine) is an independent collaboration network of Italian Intensive Care units. Efficacy of coupled plasma filtration adsorption (CPFA) in patients with septic shock: a multicenter randomised controlled clinical trial. BMJ Open. 2014;4(1):e003536. doi:10.1136/bmjopen-2013-003536.
43. Wittebole X, Hantson P. Use of the molecular adsorbent recirculating system (MARS) for the management of acute poisoning with or without liver failure. Clin Toxicol. 2011;49:782–93.
44. Honore PM, Jacobs R, Joannes-Boyau O, De Regt J, De Waele E, van Gorp V, Boer W, Verfaillie L, Spapen HD. Newly designed CRRT membranes for sepsis and SIRS—a pragmatic approach for bedside intensivists summarizing the more recent advances: a systematic structured review. ASAIO J. 2013;59(2):99–106.
45. Szczepiorkowski ZM, Winters JL, Bandarenko N, Kim HC, Linenberger ML, Marques MB, et al. Guidelines on the use of therapeutic apheresis in clinical practice—evidence-based approach from the apheresis applications committee of the American Society for Apheresis. J Clin Apheresis. 2010;25(3):83–177. doi:10.1002/jca.20240.

# Index



© Springer International Publishing 2015
H.M. Oudemans-van Straaten et al. (eds.), *Acute Nephrology for the Critical Care Physician*, DOI 10.1007/978-3-319-17389-4

Made in the USA
Monee, IL
07 July 2026

56546131R00178